Integrating Lifestyle Medicine for Prediabetes, Type 2 Diabetes, and Cardiometabolic Disease

Lifestyle change is universally recommended for patients with type 2 diabetes and cardiometabolic disease, yet the majority of clinical practice, educational programs, and clinical trials within these chronic disease spaces focus on medication use and procedures, with insufficient emphasis on lifestyle medicine. The concept of lifestyle medicine can serve as a countermeasure, acting through aspects of personal choice, natural and built environments, cultural traditions, and socioeconomic influences that affect the metabolic health of an individual. *Integrating Lifestyle Medicine for Prediabetes, Type 2 Diabetes, and Cardiometabolic Disease* provides clinical evidence for and a mechanistic understanding of the six pillars of lifestyle medicine. It guides the reader to identify opportunities for early intervention rather than focus on the diagnosis and treatment of the established disease. Interventions at earlier points have the potential to mitigate progression, prevent complications, reduce costs, and improve a patient's overall health at all points in their lifetime.

Key Features

- Provides a mechanistic, epidemiological, and clinical understanding of all pillars of lifestyle medicine
- Presents information on mechanisms for lifestyle medicine in cardiometabolic disease
- Features a unique model that includes recognition of predisease and even pre-predisease with rationale for intervention
- Promotes evidence-based recommendations for all stages of cardiometabolic disease

This volume in the *Lifestyle Medicine* series is an essential resource for clinicians and students, providing them with information to help prevent complications, reduce costs, and improve a patient's overall health at all points in their lifetime.

Lifestyle Medicine

Series Editor:

James M. Rippe, Professor of Medicine, University of Massachusetts Medical School

Led by James M. Rippe, MD, the founder of the Rippe Lifestyle Institute, this series is directed to a broad range of researchers and professionals, consisting of topical books with clinical applications in nutrition and health, physical activity, obesity management, and applicable subjects in lifestyle medicine.

Increasing Physical Activity: A Practical Guide
James M. Rippe

Manual of Lifestyle Medicine
James M. Rippe

Obesity Prevention and Treatment: A Practical Guide
James M. Rippe and John P. Foreyt

Improving Women's Health Across the Lifespan
Michelle Tollefson, Nancy Eriksen, and Neha Pathak

Lifestyle Principles and Nursing Practice
Gia Merlo and Kathy Berra

Integrating Lifestyle Medicine in Cardiovascular Health and Disease Prevention
James M. Rippe

Integrating Lifestyle Medicine for Prediabetes, Type 2 Diabetes, and Cardiometabolic Disease
Michael A. Via and Jeffrey I. Mechanick

For more information, please visit: www.routledge.com/Lifestyle-Medicine/book-series/CRCLM

Integrating Lifestyle Medicine for Prediabetes, Type 2 Diabetes, and Cardiometabolic Disease

Edited by
Michael A. Via, MD
Jeffrey I. Mechanick, MD

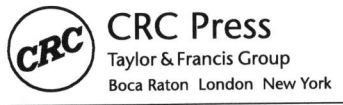

CRC Press
Taylor & Francis Group
Boca Raton London New York

CRC Press is an imprint of the
Taylor & Francis Group, an **informa** business

First edition published 2023
by CRC Press
6000 Broken Sound Parkway NW, Suite 300, Boca Raton, FL 33487-2742

and by CRC Press
4 Park Square, Milton Park, Abingdon, Oxon, OX14 4RN

CRC Press is an imprint of Taylor & Francis Group, LLC

© 2023 Taylor & Francis Group, LLC

Library of Congress Cataloging-in-Publication Data
Names: Via, Michael A., editor. | Mechanick, Jeffrey I., editor.
Title: Integrating Lifestyle medicine for prediabetes, type 2 diabetes and cardiometabolic disease / edited by Michael A. Via and Jeffrey Mechanick.
Other titles: Lifestyle medicine series (CRC Press)
Description: First edition. | Boca Raton, FL : CRC Press, 2023. |
Series: Lifestyle medicine | Includes bibliographical references and index. |
Summary: "This book outlines underlying mechanisms of disease and evidence for intervention for patients with all stages of the metabolic syndrome, insulin resistance, and cardiovascular disease. Evidence for actionable lifestyle components is examined including dietary patterns, physical activities, sleep hygiene, stress reduction, avoidance of endocrine disrupting compounds, and socioeconomic/cultural factors. The book incorporates studies in human behaviors, choices, and necessities that determine one's lifestyle and affect the risk for cardiovascular metabolic disease. The information imparts the ability to recognize patients with pre-clinical conditions and provide the tools to direct change"— Provided by publisher.
Identifiers: LCCN 2022050730 (print) | LCCN 2022050731 (ebook) |
ISBN 9781032072654 (paperback) | ISBN 9781032073828 (hardback) | ISBN 9781003206637 (ebook)
Subjects: MESH: Metabolic Syndrome—prevention & control |
Prediabetic State—prevention & control |
Diabetes Mellitus, Type 2—prevention & control | Risk Reduction Behavior
Classification: LCC RC662.18 (print) | LCC RC662.18 (ebook) | NLM WK 880 |
DDC 616.4/624–dc23/eng/20230201
LC record available at https://lccn.loc.gov/2022050730
LC ebook record available at https://lccn.loc.gov/2022050731

ISBN: 9781032073828 (hbk)
ISBN: 9781032072654 (pbk)
ISBN: 9781003206637 (ebk)

DOI: 10.1201/9781003206637

Typeset in Times
by codeMantra

Contents

Foreword

Integrating Lifestyle Medicine for Prediabetes, Type 2 Diabetes, and Cardiometabolic Disease, edited by Drs. Michael A. Via and Jeffrey I. Mechanick, is an important book that makes a significant impact on the understanding of the pathophysiology of metabolic diseases and their interrelationships.

In addition, this book makes a critical linkage between the role of lifestyle medicine modalities and the prevention and treatment of these diseases. I am delighted to include this book as a volume in the *Lifestyle Medicine Series* which I edit.

When the first edition of my *Lifestyle Medicine* textbook was published in 1999, which named this field in the academic literature (1), my vision was to underscore the ubiquitous and critical role of lifestyle habits and practices, both in preventing and in ameliorating chronic diseases. Even in 1999, there was already robust literature linking lifestyle habits and practices to reducing the risk of chronic diseases. However, this literature was spread over many disciplines and often not emphasized enough in mainstream medical treatment. This was my driving impetus to attempt to provide this literature in one place for physicians and other healthcare workers. Subsequent initiatives and the continued emergence of powerful data have confirmed the validity of this initial vision.

Our understanding of the profound role that lifestyle habits and practices play in combating chronic disease has become stronger every year. This critical understanding has also served as the basis for the major initiative from the World Health Organization on combating noncommunicable diseases (NCDs) (2) and the American Heart Association's emphasis on cardiometabolic disease and lifestyle medicine (3–5). It also served as the founding principle behind the establishment of the American College of Lifestyle Medicine (ACLM), which has become the fastest-growing organization within medicine (6).

Now, this wonderful book, edited by two distinguished physician researchers, takes us to the next step in the journey of embedding lifestyle medicine as a cornerstone of medical therapy. This volume provides compelling evidence for how habits and actions contribute to all stages of numerous metabolic diseases while underscoring the fundamental opportunity for lifestyle medicine to profoundly impact all stages of their prevention and treatment. This understanding carries profound importance since, as the WHO reports, NCDs now result in more than 70% of all mortality worldwide.

Central to the tenets of this book is the foundational role of insulin resistance as the precipitating cause of multiple adverse metabolic consequences uniting obesity, diabetes, and cardiometabolic diseases. Drs. Via and Mechanick present the stunning statistic that more than 75% of individuals in the USA already have insulin resistance although many of them are unaware of this given the difficulty in and the expense of obtaining insulin measurements.

Central to the breakthrough concepts presented by Drs. Via and Mechanick are three interrelated concepts: dysglycemia-based chronic disease (DBCD), adiposity-based chronic disease (ABCD), and cardiometabolic-based chronic disease (CMBCD).

While each of these frameworks relates to specific metabolic sequelae, their unifying principle is the common underlying pathophysiologic response to insulin resistance.

The importance of these frameworks resides in three related core concepts. First, all three of these frameworks rest on compelling pathophysiologic underpinnings.

Second, the broad context of these three frameworks allows much earlier intervention well before symptoms arise to help people avoid serious metabolic diseases. This is consistent with the American Heart Association's articulated goal of expanding cardiovascular practice into the area of "primordial" prevention (3). Third, these three frameworks place a laser focus on the key role of lifestyle measures.

Drs. Via and Mechanick have selected an outstanding group of expert contributors and have generated a book with a wide range of salient topics including traditional lifestyle medicine modalities such as physical activity, various aspects of nutrition, stress management, and sleep. They have further expanded the scope of their discussions with the insightful elucidation of evolutionary biology, endocrine-disrupting chemicals, and the important role of disseminating both lifestyle medicine practices and principles to a variety of different cultures. The book concludes with a valuable chapter synthesizing specific recommendations for how to use lifestyle medicine modalities to reduce metabolic risk.

I have been an admirer of the work of Drs. Via and Mechanick for many years, ever since they contributed brilliant chapters on their innovative concepts of DBCD and ABCD in the 3rd (7,8) and 4th (9–11) editions of my *Lifestyle Medicine* textbook. They have now expanded these concepts in the current book. The framework that they have developed for the interrelated underlying causes of metabolic diseases and the key role of lifestyle medicine modalities in ameliorating these diseases represents cutting-edge thinking.

The type of research-based evidence presented in this book represents the future of lifestyle medicine and, indeed, the future of both medicine and health care.

I am honored to publish this important book as the latest volume in the *Lifestyle Medicine Series*.

James M. Rippe, MD
Series Editor, Lifestyle Medicine Series
Professor of Medicine, UMass Chan Medical School

REFERENCES

1. Rippe JM. Lifestyle Medicine, Blackwell Science, Inc. (London), 1999.
2. The World Health Organization. Noncommunicable Diseases. Geneva, Switzerland. https://www.who.int/health-topics/noncommunicable-diseases#tab=tab_1 (Accessed July 26, 2022).
3. Lloyd-Jones DM, Hong Y, Labarthe D, Mozaffarian D, Appel LJ, Van Horn L, et al. Defining and setting national goals for cardiovascular health promotion and disease reduction: the American Heart Association's strategic Impact Goal through 2020 and beyond. Circulation. 2010;121(4):586–613.

4. American Heart Association. Council on Lifestyle and Cardiometabolic Health. Dallas, TX. https://professional.heart.org/en/partners/scientific-councils/lifestyle (Accessed July 26, 2022).

5. Eckel R, Jakicic J, Ard J, et al. 2013 AHA/ACC Guideline on Lifestyle Management to Reduce Cardiovascular Risk: A Report of the American College of Cardiology/American Heart Association Task Force on Practice Guidelines. Circulation. 2014;129 (25_suppl_2):S76–S99.

6. American College of Lifestyle Medicine. https://lifestylemedicine.org/ (Accessed July 26, 2022).

7. Via MA, Mechanick JI. The Impact of Lifestyle Medicine on Dysglycemia-Based Chronic Disease. In Rippe JM (ed): Lifestyle Medicine 3rd ed, CRC Press (Boca Raton), 2019.

8. Via MA, Mechanick JI. Adiposity-based Chronic Disease in a New Diagnostic Term. In Rippe JM (ed): Lifestyle Medicine 3rd ed, CRC Press (Boca Raton), 2019.

9. Via MA, Mechanic JI. Overview: Dysglycemia-Based Chronic Disease – Exposing Lifestyle Medicine Targets. In Rippe JM (ed): Lifestyle Medicine, 4th ed, CRC Press (Boca Raton), In Press.

10. Via MA, Mechanic JI. Adiposity-Based Chronic Disease. In Rippe JM (ed): Lifestyle Medicine, 4th ed, CRC Press (Boca Raton), In Press.

11. Malick W, Mechanick JI. Context: Impact of Dysglycemia and Lifestyle Medicine on Cardiometabolic-Based Chronic Disease In Rippe JM (ed) Lifestyle Medicine, 4th ed, CRC Press (Boca Raton). In Press.

Preface

Here's the rub: In the majority of research, educational, and clinical programs in diabetes and cardiovascular disease, lifestyle change is deemed paramount, but in reality, the majority of clinical trials, educational programs, and clinical practice in these chronic disease spaces focus on medication use and procedures, with a minimal emphasis on lifestyle medicine. Why? The answer can be dispassionate, scientific, and pragmatic, or it can be emotional, quick, and superficial, but ultimately it is not surprising and simply reinforces the need for transformative thinking, action, and innovation. Indeed, the burgeoning specialty of "Lifestyle Medicine" is categorically relevant.

In contemporary societies, degrading metabolic health is clearly recognized as a pervasive, ongoing trend. Not surprisingly, references to this are easily recognizable in popular culture: newspaper headlines, online postings and content, movies, books, and advertisements. Entire magazines are often dedicated to improving lifestyle and health through sometimes dubious claims, with cultural icons such as movie stars and well-known athletes commonly providing specific advice that typically lacks scientific evidence and may even be harmful. Above this fray and the advice commonly given by anyone's mother, "eat your vegetables," "go outside and play," and "get to bed early" rank among the most efficacious. While not as edgy and somewhat incomplete, these rules and the implicit warnings that accompany any thoughts of misbehavior promote metabolic health, and many would benefit from strong reminders about healthy living. Notwithstanding these admonitions, the field of lifestyle medicine includes many other aspects of life such as natural and built environments, cultural traditions, and socioeconomic influences. One goal of this book is to provide clinical evidence for and a mechanistic understanding of the pillars of lifestyle medicine.

Another goal is to promulgate a certain rethinking in medicine. The approach currently espoused by training programs in health care focuses on the diagnosis and treatment of established disease, largely in the setting of abnormal tests or significant symptomatology, missing opportunities for early intervention. In the case of cardiometabolic conditions, such as obesity, type 2 diabetes, hypertension, and atherosclerotic cardiovascular disease, the pathophysiology that leads to acute and chronic disease states begins decades before clinical presentation. Moreover, pharmacological or surgical therapies that introduce costs and risks may not be suitable in these early predisease or pre-predisease states. For example, in the case of type 2 diabetes, prevalence rates have skyrocketed over the past 60 years; moreover, the prevalence of the predisease known as prediabetes has nearly tripled, and the pre-predisease known as insulin resistance is even more common, approximately twice as prevalent as prediabetes. Nearly three-quarters of the population is affected by this pre-predisease and is at risk of complications. Both microvascular and macrovascular complications observed in patients with type 2 diabetes are known to affect patients with prediabetes as well. The concept of ongoing pathophysiology that predates clinical diagnosis in cardiometabolic conditions calls for action. Interventions at earlier points have the potential to mitigate the progression and impede the development of complications that may develop later. Early interventions with lifestyle medicine can also improve a patient's overall health at all points in their lifetime, in addition to reducing costs. If a widespread implementation can be achieved, lifestyle medicine stands to impact the public health threat of noncommunicable diseases.

A premise to this is perseverance at later stages: Once the disease develops and, further, after significant complications arise, the role of lifestyle becomes complementary to medical and surgical treatments. Meaningful benefits are still demonstrable through interventions such as increased physical activity, tobacco cessation, and dietary change. The observation of residual cardiovascular risk exhibited by advanced patients on optimal medical therapies further suggests the need for lifestyle medicine in the care of patients.

In *Integrating Lifestyle Medicine for Prediabetes, Diabetes, and Cardiometabolic Disease*, we reverse-engineer the answer we believe is most relevant to the problems just outlined: to ideally have a strategy with long-term deliverables based on core recommendations and pragmatically have a tactical plan for implementation comprised of action steps, so readers can more easily actualize their intent and aspirations. Therefore, the primary content of the book is organized and fleshed out to lead to these core recommendations and action steps. Readers are encouraged to approach chapters in the order in which they are presented, but naturally to feel free to peruse and even get a sneak preview of the "answer" in the last chapter if more context is needed.

Editing books and writing chapters are fun. We have a vision, shared by many, and the energy to bring this project to fruition. But many others made this possible and added to the enormous enjoyment of witnessing our thoughts and ideas mature and crystalize here. We thank Beth Grady for the expert administrative support, Randy Brehm at CRC Press for her ongoing advice and guidance, and Dr. James Rippe for his constant encouragement and laudatory emails that kept us going. Naturally, we thank our families for their patience, our colleagues for their wisdom, and our patients for their expressions of truth.

Michael A. Via, M.D.
Associate Professor of Medicine
Fellowship Program CoDirector
Division of Endocrinology, Diabetes, and Bone Disease
Icahn School of Medicine at Mount Sinai

Jeffrey I. Mechanick, M.D.
Professor of Medicine
Medical Director, Kravis Center for
Cardiovascular Health at Mount Sinai Heart
Director, Metabolic Support
Division of Endocrinology,
Diabetes and Bone Disease
Icahn School of Medicine at Mount Sinai

Editors

Dr. Michael Via is a Clinical Endocrinologist and an Associate Professor of Medicine at the Icahn School of Medicine at Mount Sinai. He is the co-director for the Icahn School of Medicine at Mount Sinai endocrinology fellowship training program. Dr. Via has authored over 50 articles and chapters on topics in nutritional, biochemical, and metabolic science. He serves as a chair of the Nutrition Committee at his institution as well as the director of the metabolic support service. He also serves as the editor for the lipids, obesity, and nutrition section of the American College of Endocrinology Self-Assessment Program.

Dr. Via completed undergraduate study in biochemistry at Cornell University, with an honors thesis on omega-3 fatty acid metabolism. He received his M.D. from New York University School of Medicine, and he completed residency training in internal medicine at Brown University as well as fellowship in endocrinology and metabolism at Mount Sinai in NY. He carries Board Certifications in both Endocrinology and Nutritional Sciences.

Dr. Jeffrey Mechanick is a Professor of Medicine and Medical Director of The Marie-Josée and Henry R. Kravis Center for Cardiovascular Health at Mount Sinai Heart, and Director of Metabolic Support in the Division of Endocrinology, Diabetes and Bone Disease, Icahn School of Medicine at Mount Sinai. He received his M.D. from the Icahn School of Medicine at Mount Sinai, completed an Internal Medicine residency at Baylor College of Medicine, and completed Endocrine Fellowship at The Mount Sinai Hospital. Dr. Mechanick has authored over 400 publications in Endocrinology, Metabolism, and Nutrition Support with 289 PubMed citations, 75 chapters, and 10 books currently. He served as the Past President of the American College of Endocrinology during 2016–2017, Past President of the American Association of Clinical Endocrinology during 2013–2014, and Past President of the American Board of Physician Nutrition Specialists during 2005–2006. Dr. Mechanick was appointed a member of the President's Council on Fitness, Sports and Nutrition (PCFSN) Science Board during 2010–2013. He was the Editor-in-Chief during 2013–2015 and is currently Editor-in-Chief Emeritus of the PCFSN quarterly publication *Elevate Health*. Dr. Mechanick is Past Chair of the Physician Engagement Committee of the American Association for Parenteral and Enteral Nutrition. He continues to chair the International Transcultural Diabetes Nutrition Algorithm Working Group, and METRICS – a global cardiometabolic research consortium. Dr. Mechanick also currently serves as Chair of the Board of Visitors for the College of Computer, Mathematics, and Natural Sciences at the University of Maryland at College Park and was the 2011 recipient of the University of Maryland Industry Impact Award and the 2011 University of Maryland Biology Alumnus Award. Dr. Mechanick's research interests are in the fields of nutrition and metabolic support, preventive cardiology, and lifestyle medicine.

Contributors

Hajira Amir
Division of Endocrinology, Diabetes, and Bone Disease, Mount Sinai Beth Israel
Icahn School of Medicine at Mount Sinai
New York City, New York

Dushyanthy Arasaratnam
Division of Endocrinology, Diabetes, and Bone Disease, Mount Sinai Beth Israel
Icahn School of Medicine at Mount Sinai
New York City, New York

Geetika Arora
Department of Medicine, Mount Sinai Beth Israel
Icahn School of Medicine at Mount Sinai
New York City, New York

Neal D. Barnard
Department of Medicine
George Washington University School of Medicine and Health Sciences Physicians Committee for Responsible Medicine
Washington, DC

Stephanie Behringer-Massera
Division of Endocrinology, Diabetes, and Bone Disease
Icahn School of Medicine at Mount Sinai
New York City, New York

Amanda Bonano-Carambot
Department of Medicine, Mount Sinai Beth Israel
Icahn School of Medicine at Mount Sinai
New York City, New York

Ana Devesa
Centro Nacional de Investigaciones Cardiovasculares (CNIC)
Madrid, Spain
The Zena and Michael A. Wiener Cardiovascular Institute, Icahn School of Medicine at Mount Sinai
New York City, New York
BioMedical Engineering and Imaging Institute
Icahn School of Medicine at Mount Sinai
New York City, New York

Rodrigo Fernandez-Jimenez
Centro Nacional de Investigaciones Cardiovasculares (CNIC)
Madrid, Spain
Hospital Universitario Clínico San Carlos
Madrid, Spain
Centro de Investigación Biomédica En Red en enfermedades CardioVasculares (CIBERCV)
Madrid, Spain

Valentin Fuster
Centro Nacional de Investigaciones Cardiovasculares (CNIC)
Madrid, Spain
The Zena and Michael A. Wiener Cardiovascular Institute, Icahn School of Medicine at Mount Sinai
New York City, New York

Juan P. González-Rivas
International Clinical Research Center
    (ICRC)
St Anne's University Hospital (FNUSA)
    Brno
Brno, Czech Republic
Departments of Global Health and
    Population and Epidemiology
Harvard University TH Chan School of
    Public Health
Boston, Massachusetts
Foundation for Clinic, Public Health,
    and Epidemiological Research of
    Venezuela (FISPEVEN INC)
Barquisimeto, Venezuela

Keerthana Haridas
Department of Medicine, Mount Sinai
    Morningside – West
Icahn School of Medicine at Mount
    Sinai
New York City, New York

María M. Infante-García
International Clinical Research Center
    (ICRC)
St Anne's University Hospital (FNUSA)
    Brno
Brno, Czech Republic
Foundation for Clinic, Public Health,
    and Epidemiological Research of
    Venezuela (FISPEVEN INC)
Barquisimeto, Venezuela

Hana Kahleova
Physicians Committee for Responsible
    Medicine
Washington, DC

Gary D. Lopaschuk
Department of Pediatrics,
    Cardiovascular Research Centre
University of Alberta
Edmonton, Alberta

Kaveeta Marwaha
Division of Endocrinology, Diabetes,
    and Bone Disease
Icahn School of Medicine at Mount
    Sinai
New York City, New York

Jeffrey I. Mechanick
Department of Cardiology
Kravis Center for Cardiovascular Health
    at Mount Sinai Heart
Division of Endocrinology, Diabetes
    and Bone Disease
Icahn School of Medicine at Mount
    Sinai
New York City, New York

Ramfis Nieto-Martínez
Departments of Global Health and
    Population and Epidemiology
Harvard University TH Chan School of
    Public Health
Boston, Massachusetts
Foundation for Clinic, Public Health,
    and Epidemiological Research of
    Venezuela (FISPEVEN INC)
Barquisimeto, Venezuela
LifeDoc Health
Memphis, Tennessee

Andrea Delgado Nieves
Department of Medicine, Mount Sinai
    Beth Israel
Icahn School of Medicine at Mount
    Sinai
New York City, New York

Gloria Santos-Beneit
The Zena and Michael A. Wiener
    Cardiovascular Institute
Icahn School of Medicine at Mount
    Sinai
New York City, New York
Foundation for Science, Health and
    Education (SHE)
Barcelona, Spain

Reshmi Srinath
Division of Endocrinology, Diabetes
    and Bone Disease
Icahn School of Medicine at Mount
    Sinai Hospital
New York City, New York

Qiuyu Sun
Department of Pediatrics,
    Cardiovascular Research Centre
University of Alberta
Edmonton, Alberta

Alexandra Turco
The Zena and Michael A. Wiener
    Cardiovascular Institute
Icahn School of Medicine at Mount
    Sinai
New York City, New York

Michael A. Via
Division of Endocrinology, Diabetes,
    and Bone Disease, Mount Sinai Beth
    Israel Medical Center
Icahn School of Medicine at Mount
    Sinai
New York City, New York

Alexa Yuen
Division of Endocrinology, Diabetes
    and Bone Disease
Icahn School of Medicine at Mount
    Sinai Hospital
New York City, New York

1 Epidemiology, Drivers, and Public Health Challenges of Prediabetes, Type 2 Diabetes, and Cardiometabolic-Based Chronic Disease

Michael A. Via
Icahn School of Medicine at Mount Sinai

Jeffrey I. Mechanick
Kravis Center for Cardiovascular Health at Mount Sinai Heart
Icahn School of Medicine at Mount Sinai

CONTENTS

DOI: 10.1201/9781003206637-1

1

1.1   INTRODUCTION

Noncommunicable disease has been identified as a premier health challenge of the 21st century.[1] Public health and individual implications of chronic metabolic health conditions arise within the pathophysiological setting of insulin resistance. This central pathway of dysregulated metabolism commonly progresses to manifest as prediabetes and type 2 diabetes (T2D), both of which have increased potential to develop complications such as atherosclerosis or microvascular disease.[2] A relatively recent (since the 1960s) and continual rise in the prevalence of all of these conditions that represent predisease, disease, and secondary disease outcomes can lead to both great personal and societal costs.[2] Direct effects include the impact on physical and psychological health of the individual patient, reduced quality of life, increased burden on family members or caregivers, and increased economic costs through consumption of health resources and diminished productivity.[3]

The model of dysglycemia-based chronic disease (DBCD) centers around insulin resistance and its sequelae and serves to stratify the level of risk to an individual patient with implications on course of treatment and prevention.[2] This staged classification system defines chronic metabolic disease that is commonplace and driven by dysglycemia, with insulin resistance as an initial and progressive process that leads to prediabetes, T2D, vascular complications, and, most importantly, cardiometabolic-based chronic disease – a central theme of this book. The potential for progression of DBCD and for the development of complications at any stage is suggestive of a strong role for lifestyle medicine as a modality to address this condition.

Outside of DBCD, a series of modifiable risk factors that contribute to atherosclerotic cardiovascular disease must also be considered in a comprehensive approach to lifestyle medicine. These include tobacco cessation, reduction in excess alcohol consumption, as well as other lifestyle approaches to hypertension, dyslipidemia, and excessive adiposity that each are associated with insulin resistance and DBCD.

1.2   THE DYSGLYCEMIA-BASED CHRONIC DISEASE MODEL

In the earliest stage of DBCD, insulin resistance (stage 1) exerts numerous metabolic regulatory effects. As this condition progresses, patients may develop prediabetes

(DBCD stage 2), T2D (DBCD stage 3), or T2D with complications (microvascular and macrovascular/atherosclerotic disease; DBCD stage 4). This progression is not necessarily linear; for example, an individual patient can skip over stages, or they may experience regression to earlier stages, with or without subsequent re-progression. The adverse outcomes of cardiovascular and microvascular disease, defined as DBCD stage 4, can occur among higher-risk (e.g., when other metabolic syndrome [MetS] traits are present) patients with both prediabetes and insulin resistance.[4] Thus, the course an individual patient with DBCD may experience can vary. However, this framework highlights the concept that DBCD and cardiometabolic disease have early beginnings, amenable to early prevention, and, over a prolonged time course, can traverse a lifetime.[2]

Along this trajectory, patients with DBCD commonly develop conditions associated with insulin resistance, including overweight or obesity, hepatosteatosis, hypertriglyceridemia, hypertension, MetS, polycystic ovary syndrome (PCOS), obstructive sleep apnea (OSA), hypertriglyceridemia, and gestational diabetes mellitus (GDM). As with the stages of DBCD, the current prevalence rates of each of these related conditions are high.

1.3   DEFINITION OF DBCD STAGES

1.3.1   DBCD STAGE 1: INSULIN RESISTANCE

Insulin resistance may be present for years or even decades before progression brings clinical attention. Blood glucose levels are normal during this time, and since levels of insulin are not routinely measured, insulin resistance almost always goes undiagnosed.[5] The presence of insulin resistance may be suggested by abdominal adiposity, a family history of T2D, weight gain, presence of acanthosis nigricans on examination, or a history of any condition associated with DBCD, such as PCOS, GDM, MetS, hypertension, and OSA. Hopefully, at some future time, commercially available insulin levels or other markers can be validated as sensitive and specific indicators of an insulin-resistant state.[6]

1.3.2   DBCD STAGE 2: PREDIABETES

Patients with insulin resistance eventually develop defects in pancreatic β-cell function where insulin secretion cannot meet requirements for euglycemia and therefore mildly elevated plasma glucose levels result. This connection between insulin resistance and β-cell function has been explained in terms of various mechanisms, including lipotoxicity, macrophage activation, abnormal metabolism-secretion coupling, and apoptosis.[7] At present, there is no consensus standard definition for prediabetes,[4] but it is reasonable to classify a patient with this condition as having glucose levels above normal and less than cutoff thresholds for T2D. More specifically, this includes a hemoglobin A1c (A1C) between 5.7% and 6.4% (inclusive),[5] impaired fasting glucose 100–125 mg/dL (inclusive), or impaired glucose tolerance with a 2-hour post-challenge (i.e., after 75 g oral glucose) glucose 140–199 mg/dL (inclusive).[4]

A 20% increased risk for cardiovascular events and a nearly 10-fold increased risk for heart failure are noted among patients with prediabetes.[4,8] The presence of microvascular complications commonly seen in patients with T2D is also observed in patients with prediabetes. In one study of 1,391 patients with prediabetes, 4.2% had retinopathy, 5.3% had severe neuropathy, and 5.7% had renal insufficiency.[9] This potential for both macrovascular and microvascular complications in patients with prediabetes highlights the urgency for intervention and may cause one to question its "predisease" designation (as opposed to an "early disease" designation).[5]

1.3.3 DBCD Stage 3: Type 2 Diabetes

As pancreatic β-cell function deteriorates further in the chronic insulin-resistant state, greater amounts of hyperglycemia result. A clear clinical definition for T2D includes any patient with either a fasting blood glucose ≥126 mg/dL, two random blood glucose levels ≥200 mg/dL, a 2-hour post-challenge blood glucose ≥200 mg/dL, or A1C ≥6.5%.[10] The increased level of risk for cardiovascular and microvascular complications warrants medical and/or surgical interventions at this stage. Additionally, lifestyle choices are central in the treatment of T2D to diminish drivers of complications[11] and to promote durability of a therapeutic regimen.[11,12]

1.3.4 DBCD Stage 4: Type 2 Diabetes with Complications

Patients with T2D are at risk for certain vascular complications, generally considered in terms of macrovascular/atherosclerotic (primarily due to the insulin-resistant state and involving various arterial beds: coronary, carotid/cerebrovascular, peripheral, aortic, etc.) and microvascular (primarily due to the hyperglycemic state and involving various organs: myocardium, brain, retinal, renal, perineural, etc.). Patients at this stage are at high risk for heart failure, atrial fibrillation, and cardiovascular/cerebrovascular events.[13] In addition, peripheral ischemia can lead to lower extremity ulcerations and risk for amputation; advanced renal disease can lead to hemodialysis. Despite the ominous natural history of this advanced DBCD stage and need for oftentimes acute intervention, lifestyle improvement can still retard underlying drivers that impel disease progression, thereby improving quality of life and reducing risks for additional complications.[14,15]

1.4 DBCD PREVALENCE

The four-stage DBCD model describes dysregulated metabolic conditions that are highly prevalent (Table 1.1). Cross-sectional studies using the Homeostasis Model Assessment of Insulin Resistance (HOMA-IR) demonstrate an approximate 75% prevalence of insulin resistance in populations studied.[16,17] This finding is significantly higher than the prevalence of MetS, which is approximately 35% using the National Cholesterol Education Program definition.[18] The extremely high prevalence of insulin resistance in current populations suggests a clinical approach that includes a high index of suspicion for case finding and lifestyle intervention.

TABLE 1.1

Prevalence of DBCD by Stage[4,16,17,19,20,26]

	Prevalence		
	USA	Czech Republic	Worldwide
DBCD stage 1: Insulin resistance	74.5%	54%	50%–60%
DBCD stage 2: Prediabetes	28%–35%	10.3%	30%–45%
DBCD stage 3: Type 2 diabetes	10.5%	3.7%	7.2%
DBCD stage 4: Type 2 diabetes with vascular complications	6.0%	1.2%	1%–2%

TABLE 1.2

Prevalence of Conditions Associated with Insulin Resistance[21–25]

	Prevalence	
	USA	Worldwide
Obesity	42.4%	8.7%
Hypertension	45.4%	17.1%
The metabolic syndrome	35.0%	20%–40%
Hypertriglyceridemia	25.9%	29.6%
Hepatosteatosis	24.1%	24.5%
Obstructive sleep apnea – moderate to severe (men)	25.0%	4.0%
Obstructive sleep apnea – moderate to severe (women)	9.0%	2.0%
Polycystic ovary syndrome (among women of reproductive age; Rotterdam criteria)	6%–21%	6%–21%
Gestational diabetes (among pregnant women)	7.0%	10.3%

Using A1c of 6 to <6.5% as a definition, the US prevalence for prediabetes is reported as 28%–35%.[4] The US prevalence of T2D is reported as 10.5%, and the prevalence of T2D with complications is 6%.[19] Worldwide in 2021, over 537 million people have T2D (7.2% prevalence), a number that is expected to rise to 735 million by 2045.[20]

Other conditions associated with insulin resistance are also common (Table 1.2). Approximately 42% of the US population has obesity (body mass index [BMI] ≥30 kg/m^2). Hypertension is present in 45% of US adults, and hepatosteatosis is present in 24%.[21] Hypertriglyceridemia is present in 25%–30% of the population and as high as 40% among patients with T2D.[22] MetS, OSA, PCOS, and GDM are also highly prevalent in the USA and worldwide.[23,24]

In a recent cohort study conducted in the Czech Republic, many of the conditions associated with insulin resistance increase in prevalence substantially at each progressive stage of DBCD.[26] For example, prevalence of hypertension is increased by a factor of 2.3, 4.3, 5.0, and 10.9 in DBCD stages 1, 2, 3, and 4, respectively, compared to patients without DBCD.[26] Similarly, obesity (BMI $\geq$30 kg/m²) is increased by a factor of 225, 348, 1,109, and 878 in DBCD stages 1, 2, 3, and 4, respectively.[26] Epidemiological details for these DBCD drivers and components are given below.

1.5   ATHEROSCLEROTIC RISK FACTORS

Outside of insulin resistance, modifiable risk factors including tobacco use, excess alcohol consumption, hyperlipidemia, hypertension, and adiposity-based chronic disease (ABCD) represent reasonable targets for lifestyle medicine. The American Heart Association recognizes Life's Simple 7 cardiometabolic risk factors that represent actionable targets in lifestyle medicine (Table 1.3).[27] While there is considerable overlap between many of these risk categories and insulin resistance, especially in the cases of ABCD or hypertension, strategies to mitigate the effects of these modifiable risk factors must be included in a comprehensive lifestyle approach to patients with prediabetes, T2D, and cardiometabolic-based chronic disease (CMBCD). The overarching CMBCD framework is interpreted as a chronic pathophysiologic state (disease) affecting the cardiovascular system with key mechanistic metabolic drivers that include abnormal adiposity, dysglycemia, hypertension, and dyslipidemia.[28,29]

TABLE 1.3

US Adults (Age $\geq$45) Meeting Ideal Levels for Each of the American Heart Association Defined Life's Simple 7 Cardiometabolic Risk Factors (Achieved Without Medications)[27]

	Adults ($\geq$45) Meeting Ideal Targets
Blood pressure <120/<80 mm Hg	20%
Fasting glucose <100 mg/dL	64%
Total cholesterol < 200 mg/Dl	38%
BMI <25 kg/m²	25%
Physical activity Four times per week	30%
Diet ªREGARDS survey	0%
Smoking Never or quit >12 months	84%

ª   Ideal diet in the REGARDS survey is defined as four or more of the following: fruits and vegetables $\geq$4.5 cups/day; fish 3.5 ounces $\geq$2 servings/week; sodium <1,500 mg/ day; sugar-containing beverages $\leq$450 kcal/week; whole grains $\geq$3 servings per day.

1.5.1 Tobacco Use

Tobacco use is a well-established risk for atherosclerotic disease and continues to burden global health initiatives. Nearly 8 million deaths and 200 million disability life years are attributed to tobacco use in 2019, with approximately one-third of these secondary to atherosclerotic disease.[30] Mechanistically, exposure to tobacco smoking leads to generation of reactive oxygenation species (ROS) and consumption of tissue antioxidants.[31] Reduced nitric oxide production and increased adhesion protein expression contribute further to dysfunction of the vascular endothelium.[31] Subsequent inflammation leads to atherosclerotic plaque generation and instability, driving cardiovascular disease. Platelet activation within an induced prothrombotic state can lead to acute vascular occlusion.[31]

In 2019, approximately 1.14 billion people were identified as current smokers (15% prevalence), which represents a decrease by 27% in men and by 38% in women since 1990.[30] An international treaty, sponsored by the World Health Organization and signed by 182 countries, has taken effect in 2005 and mandates taxation for reduced tobacco affordability, package warnings, restricted advertising, and establishment of designated smoke-free areas.[32] The success in tobacco use reduction thus far may be partially attributed to these policies. In patients who continue to smoke, cessation is universally recommended.[10,28]

1.5.2 Excessive Alcohol Consumption

Excessive alcohol intake is associated with increased cardiovascular risk, and current guidelines recommend curtailing its consumption. Excess alcohol is responsible for 4.2% of global burden of disease, assessed by disability-adjusted life years.[33] The US prevalence of heavy alcohol consumption, defined as three or more drinks per day for men, and two or more drinks per day for women, is approximately 8%.[34] Binge drinking, defined as consumption of five or more alcoholic beverages at one sitting, is also considered as heavy alcohol consumption.[34] The worldwide prevalence of abstinence from alcohol within the past year is approximately 57%, while the prevalence of moderate consumption (<24 g/day) is 24% and heavy consumption prevalence is 19%.[35]

With regard to alcohol, the controversy that continues is whether full abstinence confers the highest health benefit, or is moderation acceptable or even beneficial. Moderate wine is an integral component in many versions of the Mediterranean diet. A study of 224 subjects with T2D randomized to 150 mL of either red wine, white wine, or mineral water daily demonstrated cardiovascular benefits with wine consumption after 2 years of follow-up.[36] In the white wine group, fasting glucose decreased by 17 mg/dL and HOMA-IR score decreased by 1.2. In the red wine group, the HOMA-IR score decreased by glucose by 0.77 and the number of diagnostic criteria for MetS decreased by 0.3 on average, high-density lipoprotein levels increased by 2 mg/dL, and triglycerides decreased by 12 mg/dL.[36] Unfortunately, the scientific literature has many similar small studies that rely on surrogate cardiovascular endpoints due to underpowered study size. Nevertheless, several larger studies have been recently published. One study that included 48,423 patients with previous myocardial infarction followed for 8.7 years demonstrated a "J-curve" association between alcohol consumption and all-cause mortality (relative risk [RR] 0.79), cardiovascular mortality (RR 0.73), and cardiovascular events (RR 0.5).[37] The lowest risk for each was between 6 and 8 g alcohol consumption daily (approximately 0.8–1 alcoholic beverage per day).[37] A recent meta-analysis of 83 studies that included 599,912 patients demonstrated findings consistent with modest cardiovascular benefit, with the lowest cardiovascular risk among patients who consumed 0–14 g alcohol per day.[38] On the other hand, a survey of 371,463 patients demonstrated that light alcohol consumption showed a minimal (RR 1.1) increase in cardiovascular events after adjusting for other healthy lifestyle factors that are commonly associated with light alcohol consumption.[39] Other health risks associated with alcohol must also be considered, including potential dependence and cognitive impairment, especially when operating vehicles or machinery. These findings, the potential risks, and global disease burden of noncommunicable disease suggest overall risk derived from any level of alcohol consumption may outweigh the measured benefits.[33]

1.5.3 HYPERLIPIDEMIA

Cholesterol, which contributes to atherosclerotic plaque development and activates inflammatory pathways, especially when oxidized, is another well-established cardiovascular risk factor. The most recent published analysis from the 2005 to 2008 National Health and Nutrition Survey demonstrates approximately 71 million adults (33.5%) with elevated low-density lipoprotein-cholesterol (LDL-c) levels, defined as above National Cholesterol Education Program (NCEP) guidelines determined by individual cardiovascular risk (100 mg/dL; 130 mg/dL; or 160 mg/dL for high, moderate, and low risks, respectively).[40] More recent data from the 2019 Korean National Health Survey show a similar prevalence of 21% of adults with hyperlipidemia within the South Korean population.[41] Meeting the targeted LDL-c goals set by the NCEP is estimated to prevent 20,000 myocardial infarctions and 10,000 deaths from cardiovascular disease annually in the USA.[42] Lifestyle interventions to reduce LDL-c levels are part of a comprehensive approach. In many cases, interventions such as adaptation of a Mediterranean or plant-based diet that are beneficial within other cardiometabolic fronts (e.g., T2D prevention) also show benefit in LDL-c reduction.[43,44]

1.5.4 HYPERTENSION

Hypertension also represents a well-established cardiovascular risk, though the pathophysiology remains incompletely understood. Insulin resistance, which is central to DBCD, is also associated with development of hypertension and vice versa.[45] The presence of insulin resistance confers a 2- to 3-fold increase in risk of hypertension.[46] Data published in 1992 suggest that approximately 50% of patients with essential hypertension have insulin resistance.[45] This figure may have increased in the interim, as the overall prevalence of insulin resistance has risen to 75% within the general population.[16] The presence of hypertension also predicts the development of

T2D, with a 49% incident risk for T2D among patients with systolic blood pressure >160 mm Hg and a 30% incident risk for T2D for patients with systolic blood pressure between 130 and 159 mm Hg.[47]

The role of insulin signaling to activate endothelial nitric oxide synthase, which promotes vasodilation through nitric oxide production, has been implicated as a common pathophysiology between hypertension and DBCD.[48] More general processes of vascular endothelial dysfunction and systemic inflammation that are present in patients with DBCD further drive hypertension.[48] Additionally, both the renin–angiotensin system and sympathetic pathways are activated in patients with insulin resistance, which also promotes the development of hypertension.[48] From an interventional standpoint, lifestyle changes that show benefit in markers of insulin resistance can also reduce blood pressure.[2,28]

One lifestyle factor specific to hypertension is sodium intake. (Although high sodium consumption is associated with increased processed food consumption and consequent insulin resistance, sodium itself confers a specific risk for hypertension.) Excessive sodium intake is directly associated with development of hypertension,[49] and as an extension to cardiovascular risk, data from 2017 suggest excessive dietary sodium is responsible for 11 million deaths worldwide annually and 255 million disability-adjusted life years.[50] A reduction in sodium intake by 2,200 mg per day yields decreased blood pressure by 5.4/2.8 mm Hg (systolic/diastolic) among patients with hypertension.[49] Limiting total daily sodium intake to approximately 2,000 mg or less is associated with the lowest level of cardiovascular risk.[51]

1.5.5 ADIPOSITY-BASED CHRONIC DISEASE

Adiposity-based chronic disease (ABCD) is a new model for understanding and managing abnormal adiposity (amount, distribution, and function).[52] Similar to the DBCD and CMBCD driver-based chronic disease models, ABCD progresses from "risk" to "predisease" (e.g., overweight) to "disease" (e.g., obesity) to "complications." Patients with ABCD can have increased central and visceral adipose depots, with disrupted adipokine signaling, as well as activated, systemic inflammatory pathways. Consequently, insulin resistance and advanced DBCD stages, dyslipidemia, hypertension, and cardiovascular disease can develop.[52]

The relative narrow term *obesity* (ABCD stage 3), which is based simply on BMI above 30 kg/m^2, is not adequate to estimate risk in certain populations, such as Asians.[53] In fact, the distribution pattern of adiposity has significant predictive value for cardiometabolic risk, especially in Asians.[52] Additionally, controversy continues over the concept of metabolically healthy obesity (MHO) and the obesity paradox, which is predicated on BMI-centric definitions of abnormal adiposity.[54,55] Some authors argue that the subset of patients with BMI ≥30 kg/m^2 who exhibit only modest increases in insulin resistance may not be sufficiently affected for this to be considered as a disease state.[56] Still, this hypothesized group of patients with MHO demonstrates some insulin resistance and the supposed lower cardiovascular risk may only be transient.[54,57] In sum, these limitations of the use of BMI to define cardiometabolic risk are avoided in the ABCD model.[52]

1.6   DRIVERS OF INSULIN RESISTANCE AND CARDIOMETABOLIC-BASED CHRONIC DISEASE

1.6.1   PRIMARY DRIVERS

An array of primary drivers contributes to the prevalence of insulin resistance and CMBCD. Genetic susceptibility plays a small role, followed by epigenetic phenomena that influence gene expression over several generations.[58] Pathophysiological changes in metabolic control within the individual patient, coupled with environmental factors, fashion individual behavior choices and lifestyle that create abnormal adiposity, insulin resistance, and other early stages of ABCD, DBCD, and CMBCD.[2] Outside of genetics, all of these factors can be influenced by lifestyle change.

1.6.2   GENETICS AND EPIGENETICS

The "thrifty gene hypothesis" proposes that ancestral conditions are selected for highly efficient metabolic machinery to promote survival in times of scarcity.[59] In modern times, changes in dietary abundance, physical activity, and other lifestyle factors within this vestigial "thrifty" genetic background may be responsible for the development of ABCD and DBCD. While genome-wide association studies have demonstrated approximately 400 genetic variants that increase risk for insulin resistance, obesity, T2D, and cardiovascular disease, cohort studies suggest genetic factors explain only 2.7% of the variance for development of these conditions.[58,60] This modest genetic contribution supports the observation that the rise in prevalence for each stage of DBCD was relatively recent. The prevalence of T2D has risen 10-fold in the last 60 years, and the prevalence of obesity has nearly tripled since 1985.[19] These changes are much faster than what any maladaptive variations in population genetics could explain.[58]

Epigenetic processes mediate the effect of certain environmental factors on the regulation of gene expression; this occurs via DNA methylation, histone modification, and noncoding RNA-associated gene silencing.[61] These chemical modifications to the genetic machinery may be passed along generations enabling a species to adapt over to environmental changes over several generations. In the case of DBCD, a number of epigenetic phenomena have been described that adversely affect cardiometabolic risk. For example, histone acetylation can impair pancreatic β-cell function.[61] In another study of visceral adipose tissue, 538 genes have been identified that demonstrate enhanced DNA methylation in patients with obesity and insulin resistance.[62] Many of these modified genes are known to be involved in metabolic regulation, including PPARγ and ZNF34 among others.[62] Further study using techniques to identify genome-wide methylation suggests that 18% of the variance in weight gain in patients with overweight and obesity may be explained by differences in DNA methylation.[63] Changes in lifestyle can affect the epigenetics of an individual patient and future generations, such as by reducing DNA methylation and histone acetylation processes.[58]

1.6.3 ENVIRONMENTAL AND BEHAVIORAL FACTORS

Environmental factors can significantly lead to metabolic dysregulation through epigenetic effects on gene expression, direct effects on pathophysiology, and complex effects on human behavior.[2,64] This nexus of primary drivers – genetics, environment, and behavior – ultimately determines one's particular lifestyle. Behaviors that are characteristic of modern lifestyles have developed following industrialization and information age technologies. These modern trends generally promote unhealthy choices related to foods/dietary patterns, sedentariness, poor sleep hygiene, disruptive lighting and screen usage, as well as alcohol consumption. In addition to these general behaviors, social determinants of health, including daily work schedule and conditions, food and housing security, crime, and culture, among other elements of structural disruption/crisis affect DBCD and CMBCD risk.[2]

1.6.4 SECONDARY/METABOLIC DRIVERS

Once primary drivers and a specific lifestyle are established, steering physiology toward health or illness, various metabolic processes modulate and impel this trajectory. The prototypical example would be an unhealthy lifestyle leading to abnormal adiposity, then insulin resistance, then DBCD and other MetS traits, and then cardiovascular disease.[65] Specifically, insulin resistance leads to changes in adiposity amount, distribution, and function.[66] Inefficient uptake of free fatty acids (FFA) by visceral adipose leads to higher circulating FFA levels. Consequently, tissues such as skeletal muscle, cardiac muscle, liver, kidney, vascular endothelium, and pancreas increase FFA uptake (creating ectopic fat), worsening insulin resistance, inflammation, and the emergence of MetS traits.[28]

Adipokines are signaling molecules produced by adipose tissue in patterns that reflect different inflammatory states in DBCD.[66] For instance, circulating levels of adiponectin, the most abundant adipokine, are diminished with central and visceral adipose distribution.[67] This leads to insulin resistance in hepatocytes and skeletal muscle, reduced efficiency of pancreatic β-cells, as well as further adipocyte dysfunction through reduced PPARγ activity.[68,69] Production of leptin, another prominent adipokine, is increased in association with adipose accumulation. However, hypothalamic resistance to leptin can develop and lead to decreased food satiety, increased caloric intake, development of obesity, and increased atherosclerotic risk.[70] Systemic inflammation is also driven by changes in adipose function and within the vascular endothelium. As insulin resistance and obesity develop, levels of cytokines, including tumor necrosis factor-α, interleukin (IL)-1β, IL-6, and IL-10 levels, increase.[71] Macrophages are activated through adipose and vascular endothelial surface signaling.[71] In this condition, systemic inflammation is also associated with increased production of ROS,[71] increased misfolded proteins in the setting of endoplasmic reticulum stress,[72] and reduced clearance with increased formation of advanced glycosylated end-products.[73] Within the vascular endothelium, insulin resistance leads to reduced lipoprotein lipase activity, resulting in reduced triglyceride clearance and hypertriglyceridemia.[74] Nitric oxide synthase activity is also reduced, leading to increased vascular tone and hypertension, as well as to increased ROS production.[75]

Gastrointestinal (GI) signaling is also altered in DBCD. The production of incretin hormones that include glucagon-like peptides-1 and peptides-2 is decreased, leading to diminished pancreatic β-cell function, increased hepatic glucose release, and reduced activation of satiety pathways in the hypothalamus.[28] The bacterial speciation and activity of the GI microflora are also affected in DBCD, leading to increased systemic inflammation[76] and potentially driving increased caloric intake and unhealthy dietary choices.[77]

Pancreatic β-cell dysfunction is central to the development and progression of DBCD stage 1 (euglycemic) to stages 2–4 (hyperglycemic).[2] The direct toxicity of FFAs and the reduced incretin and adiponectin signaling contribute to β-cell dysfunction.[28,68] Amyloid deposits within pancreatic islets develop in DBCD and further diminish β-cell activity and advance progression through the DBCD model.[78]

1.6.5 Costs of Type 2 Diabetes

Type 2 diabetes accounts for the greatest share of health expenditures for any chronic disease.[79] The high risks of complications, treatments, testing and screening measures, and emergency room visits contribute to this increase in costs, with end-stage renal disease as the greatest contributor (annual 4- to 6-fold increase per patient),[80] followed by atherosclerotic disease (annual 1.7- to 3-fold increase per patient).[79] Analysis of the effect for specific cardiovascular complications shows median annual costs for patients with T2D who develop coronary artery disease, heart failure, and stroke are higher by 112%, 59%, and 322%, respectively, compared to patients who have these conditions but do not have T2D.[81] Additionally, hospitalization costs in patients with T2D are 3-fold higher than for patients without T2D.[82]

Indirect costs in the USA, which include reduced productivity, lost workdays, mortality, and disability stemming from T2D and its complications, are estimated to be $38 billion annually.[79] Annual costs for microvascular complications, including retinopathy, neuropathy, and renal disease, account for $12 billion, and cardiovascular complications account for $23 billion.[79]

1.6.6 Costs of Prediabetes

Healthcare expenditures for patients with prediabetes are also significant. Annual medical costs for patients with MetS (three of five defining features) are approximately 60% higher than expenditures for patients without MetS.[83,84] Patients with four of five defining features of MetS have an additional 24% increase in healthcare expenditures, mainly due to high rates of complications.[84] An estimate for the direct cost of excessive cardiovascular disease in the USA that stems from insulin resistance development exceeds a total of $1 trillion for the years 2017–2035.[85] Productivity losses from this burden of excess cardiovascular disease in patients with MetS are estimated to be $1.1 trillion per year by 2035.[86]

1.6.7 Worldwide Costs

The European Union estimates an annual cost of €110 billion for excess healthcare expenditures due to MetS and an annual indirect cost of €210 billion through lost productivity.[87] Costs of care for T2D in India, Bangladesh, Pakistan, and Sri Lanka in 2014 exceeded $6.9 billion US, and costs in sub-Saharan Africa were $2.8 billion with an expectation to increase by 61% by 2030.[20] These increased economic costs for DBCD that are universally observed in high-income, middle-income, and low-income countries further highlight the urgency to address this chronic condition. One published economic model of a single lifestyle intervention – increased whole grain consumption – demonstrated a potential cost savings through reduced DBCD burden that amounts to €0.3–1.0 billion over 10 years.[88] A multi-pronged approach to implement an even more comprehensive lifestyle intervention in DBCD is likely to yield greater savings, as well as to improve quality of life and reduce disease severity.[2,28]

1.7   CONCLUSION

The high prevalence, implicated risks, and high cost for each stage of DBCD, as well as associated metabolic risks, such as hypertension, hyperlipidemia, and ABCD, mandate action by individual patients and physicians. Though medical and surgical therapies are generally considered first, a comprehensive lifestyle medicine approach offers opportunities to prevent progression of DBCD and CMBCD with low risk and low cost. Unfortunately, structured lifestyle interventions are seldom implemented in a successful manner. A survey of primary care physicians in the USA representing over 11 million patient visits showed no interventions taken nor suggestions given to over three-quarters of patients who were diagnosed with prediabetes.[89] This immense opportunity carries significant potential for improvement through a prescribed lifestyle intervention.[90] Success in this field can profoundly impact on the lives of a great many patients.[91] For society, lifestyle medicine may be the only practical and cost-effective approach to mitigate the effects of prediabetes, T2D, and the risks of cardiometabolic disease.

Disclosures:
Jeffrey I. Mechanick received honoraria from Abbott Nutrition for lectures and serves on the Advisory Boards for Aveta.Life and Twin Health.

REFERENCES

1. Beran D, Pedersen HB, Robertson J. Noncommunicable Diseases, Access to Essential Medicines and Universal Health Coverage. *Glob Health Action* 2019; **12**(1): 1670014.
2. Mechanick JI, Garber AJ, Grunberger G, Handelsman Y, Garvey WT. Dysglycemia-Based Chronic Disease: An American Association of Clinical Endocrinologists Position Statement. *Endocr Pract* 2018; **24**(11): 995–1011.
3. Lee JT, Hamid F, Pati S, Atun R, Millett C. Impact of Noncommunicable Disease Multimorbidity on Healthcare Utilisation and Out-of-Pocket Expenditures in Middle-Income Countries: Cross Sectional Analysis. *PLoS One* 2015; **10**(7): e0127199.
4. Beulens J, Rutters F, Ryden L, et al. Risk and Management of Pre-Diabetes. *Eur J Prev Cardiol* 2019; **26**(2_suppl): 47–54.
5. Zand A, Ibrahim K, Patham B. Prediabetes: Why Should We Care? *Methodist Debakey Cardiovasc J* 2018; **14**(4): 289–97.

6. Adeva-Andany MM, Martinez-Rodriguez J, Gonzalez-Lucan M, Fernandez-Fernandez C, Castro-Quintela E. Insulin Resistance is a Cardiovascular Risk Factor in Humans. *Diabetes Metab Syndr* 2019; **13**(2): 1449–55.
7. Mezza T, Cinti F, Cefalo CMA, Pontecorvi A, Kulkarni RN, Giaccari A. Beta-Cell Fate in Human Insulin Resistance and Type 2 Diabetes: A Perspective on Islet Plasticity. *Diabetes* 2019; **68**(6): 1121–9.
8. Pandey A, Vaduganathan M, Patel KV, et al. Biomarker-Based Risk Prediction of Incident Heart Failure in Pre-Diabetes and Diabetes. *JACC Heart Fail* 2021; **9**(3): 215–23.
9. Gabriel R, Boukichou Abdelkader N, Acosta T, et al. Early Prevention of Diabetes Microvascular Complications in People with Hyperglycaemia in Europe. ePREDICE randomized trial. Study Protocol, Recruitment and Selected Baseline Data. *PLoS One* 2020; **15**(4): e0231196.
10. American Diabetes Association. 2. Classification and Diagnosis of Diabetes: Standards of Medical Care in Diabetes-2021. *Diabetes Care* 2021; **44**(Suppl 1): S15–S33.
11. Rubin RR, Wadden TA, Bahnson JL, et al. Impact of Intensive Lifestyle Intervention on Depression and Health-Related Quality of Life in Type 2 Diabetes: The Look AHEAD Trial. *Diabetes Care* 2014; **37**(6): 1544–53.
12. Moriconi E, Camajani E, Fabbri A, Lenzi A, Caprio M. Very-Low-Calorie Ketogenic Diet as a Safe and Valuable Tool for Long-Term Glycemic Management in Patients with Obesity and Type 2 Diabetes. *Nutrients* 2021; **13**(3): 758.
13. Triebswetter S, Gutjahr-Lengsfeld LJ, Schmidt KR, Drechsler C, Wanner C, Krane V. Long-Term Survivor Characteristics in Hemodialysis Patients with Type 2 Diabetes. *Am J Nephrol* 2018; **47**(1): 30–9.
14. Grzywacz A, Lubas A, Smoszna J, Niemczyk S. Risk Factors Associated with All-Cause Death Among Dialysis Patients with Diabetes. *Med Sci Monit* 2021; **27**: e930152.
15. Zhang P, Hire D, Espeland MA, et al. Impact of Intensive Lifestyle Intervention on Preference-Based Quality of Life in Type 2 Diabetes: Results from the Look AHEAD Trial. *Obesity (Silver Spring)* 2016; **24**(4): 856–64.
16. Fowler JR, Tucker LA, Bailey BW, LeCheminant JD. Physical Activity and Insulin Resistance in 6,500 NHANES Adults: The Role of Abdominal Obesity. *J Obes* 2020; **2020**: 3848256.
17. Tamayo T, Schipf S, Meisinger C, et al. Regional Differences of Undiagnosed Type 2 Diabetes and Prediabetes Prevalence are Not Explained by Known Risk Factors. *PLoS One* 2014; **9**(11): e113154.
18. Hirode G, Wong RJ. Trends in the Prevalence of Metabolic Syndrome in the United States, 2011–2016. *JAMA* 2020; **323**(24): 2526–8.
19. Ackerman SE, Blackburn OA, Marchildon F, Cohen P. Insights into the Link between Obesity and Cancer. *Curr Obes Rep* 2017; **6**(2): 195–203.
20. Carlsson LMS, Sjoholm K, Jacobson P, et al. Life Expectancy after Bariatric Surgery in the Swedish Obese Subjects Study. *N Engl J Med* 2020; **383**(16): 1535–43.
21. Younossi ZM, Koenig AB, Abdelatif D, Fazel Y, Henry L, Wymer M. Global Epidemiology of Nonalcoholic Fatty Liver Disease-Meta-Analytic Assessment of Prevalence, Incidence, and Outcomes. *Hepatology* 2016; **64**(1): 73–84.
22. Fan W, Philip S, Granowitz C, Toth PP, Wong ND. Prevalence of US Adults with Triglycerides >/= 150 mg/dl: NHANES 2007–2014. *Cardiol Ther* 2020; **9**(1): 207–13.
23. Khattak HK, Hayat F, Pamboukian SV, Hahn HS, Schwartz BP, Stein PK. Obstructive Sleep Apnea in Heart Failure: Review of Prevalence, Treatment with Continuous Positive Airway Pressure, and Prognosis. *Tex Heart Inst J* 2018; **45**(3): 151–61.
24. Writing Group Members, Mozaffarian D, Benjamin EJ, et al. Executive Summary: Heart Disease and Stroke Statistics--2016 Update: A Report From the American Heart Association. *Circulation* 2016; **133**(4): 447–54.

25. Ruiz-Garcia A, Arranz-Martinez E, Lopez-Uriarte B, et al. Prevalence of Hypertriglyceridemia in Adults and Related Cardiometabolic Factors. SIMETAP-HTG Study. *Clin Investig Arterioscler* 2020; **32**(6): 242–55.

26. Gonzalez-Rivas JP, Mechanick JI, Infante-Garcia MM, et al. The Prevalence of Dysglycemia-Based Chronic Disease in a European Population - A New Paradigm to Address Diabetes Burden: A Kardiovize Study. *Endocr Pract* 2021; **27**(5): 455–62.

27. Kulshreshtha A, Vaccarino V, Judd SE, et al. Life's Simple 7 and Risk of Incident Stroke: The Reasons for Geographic and Racial Differences in Stroke Study. *Stroke* 2013; **44**(7): 1909–14.

28. Mechanick JI, Farkouh ME, Newman JD, Garvey WT. Cardiometabolic-Based Chronic Disease, Adiposity and Dysglycemia Drivers: JACC State-of-the-Art Review. *J Am Coll Cardiol* 2020; **75**(5): 525–38.

29. Pavlovska I, Polcrova A, Mechanick JI, et al. Dysglycemia and Abnormal Adiposity Drivers of Cardiometabolic-Based Chronic Disease in the Czech Population: Biological, Behavioral, and Cultural/Social Determinants of Health. *Nutrients* 2021; **13**(7): 2338.

30. GBD 2019 Tobacco Collaborators. Spatial, Temporal, and Demographic Patterns in Prevalence of Smoking Tobacco Use and Attributable Disease Burden in 204 Countries and Territories, 1990–2019: A Systematic Analysis from the Global Burden of Disease Study 2019. *Lancet* 2021; **397**(10292): 2337–60.

31. Messner B, Bernhard D. Smoking and Cardiovascular Disease: Mechanisms of Endothelial Dysfunction and Early Atherogenesis. *Arterioscler Thromb Vasc Biol* 2014; **34**(3): 509–15.

32. Chung-Hall J, Craig L, Gravely S, Sansone N, Fong GT. Impact of the WHO FCTC Over the First Decade: A Global Evidence Review Prepared for the Impact Assessment Expert Group. *Tob Control* 2019; **28**(Suppl 2): s119–s28.

33. GBD 2017 Risk Factor Collaborators. Global, Regional, and National Comparative Risk Assessment of 84 Behavioural, Environmental and Occupational, and Metabolic Risks or Clusters of Risks for 195 Countries and Territories, 1990–2017: A Systematic Analysis for the Global Burden of Disease Study 2017. *Lancet* 2018; **392**(10159): 1923–94.

34. Axley PD, Richardson CT, Singal AK. Epidemiology of Alcohol Consumption and Societal Burden of Alcoholism and Alcoholic Liver Disease. *Clin Liver Dis* 2019; **23** (1): 39–50.

35. World Health Organization. Global Status Report on Alcohol and Health in 2018. 2018. https://www-who-int.eresources.mssm.edu/publications/i/item/97892415656392022

36. Gepner Y, Golan R, Harman-Boehm I, et al. Effects of Initiating Moderate Alcohol Intake on Cardiometabolic Risk in Adults with Type 2 Diabetes: A 2-Year Randomized, Controlled Trial. *Ann Intern Med* 2015; **163**(8): 569–79.

37. Ding C, O'Neill D, Bell S, Stamatakis E, Britton A. Association of Alcohol Consumption with Morbidity and Mortality in Patients with Cardiovascular Disease: Original Data and Meta-Analysis of 48,423 Men and Women. *BMC Med* 2021; **19**(1): 167.

38. Wood AM, Kaptoge S, Butterworth AS, et al. Risk Thresholds for Alcohol Consumption: Combined Analysis of Individual-Participant Data for 599 912 Current Drinkers in 83 Prospective Studies. *Lancet* 2018; **391**(10129): 1513–23.

39. Biddinger KJ, Emdin CA, Haas ME, et al. Association of Habitual Alcohol Intake with Risk of Cardiovascular Disease. *JAMA Netw Open* 2022; **5**(3): e223849.

40. Centers for Disease Control and Prevention (CDC). Vital Signs: Prevalence, Treatment, and Control of High Levels of Low-Density Lipoprotein Cholesterol--United States, 1999–2002 and 2005–2008. *MMWR Morb Mortal Wkly Rep* 2011; **60**(4): 109–14.

41. Kim Y, Nho SJ, Woo G, et al. Trends in the Prevalence and Management of Major Metabolic Risk Factors for Chronic Disease Over 20 Years: Findings from the 1998–2018 Korea National Health and Nutrition Examination Survey. *Epidemiol Health* 2021; **43**: e2021028.

42. Lazar LD, Pletcher MJ, Coxson PG, Bibbins-Domingo K, Goldman L. Cost-Effectiveness of Statin Therapy for Primary Prevention in a Low-Cost Statin Era. *Circulation* 2011; **124**(2): 146–53.

43. Schwarzfuchs D, Golan R, Shai I. Four-Year Follow-Up after Two-Year Dietary Interventions. *N Engl J Med* 2012; **367**(14): 1373–4.

44. Kahleova H, Petersen KF, Shulman GI, et al. Effect of a Low-Fat Vegan Diet on Body Weight, Insulin Sensitivity, Postprandial Metabolism, and Intramyocellular and Hepatocellular Lipid Levels in Overweight Adults: A Randomized Clinical Trial. *JAMA Netw Open* 2020; **3**(11): e2025454.

45. Reaven GM. Relationships among Insulin Resistance, Type 2 Diabetes, Essential Hypertension, and Cardiovascular Disease: Similarities and Differences. *J Clin Hypertens* 2011; **13**(4): 238–43.

46. Wang F, Han L, Hu D. Fasting Insulin, Insulin Resistance and Risk of Hypertension in the General Population: A Meta-Analysis. *Clin Chim Acta* 2017; **464**: 57–63.

47. Stahl CH, Novak M, Lappas G, et al. High-Normal Blood Pressure and Long-Term Risk of Type 2 Diabetes: 35-Year Prospective Population Based Cohort Study of Men. *BMC Cardiovasc Disord* 2012; **12**: 89.

48. Mancusi C, Izzo R, di Gioia G, Losi MA, Barbato E, Morisco C. Insulin Resistance the Hinge Between Hypertension and Type 2 Diabetes. *High Blood Press Cardiovasc Prev* 2020; **27**(6): 515–26.

49. He FJ, Li J, Macgregor GA. Effect of Longer Term Modest Salt Reduction on Blood Pressure: Cochrane Systematic Review and Meta-Analysis of Randomised Trials. *BMJ* 2013; **346**: f1325.

50. GBD 2017 Diet Collaborators. Health Effects of Dietary Risks in 195 Countries, 1990–2017: A Systematic Analysis for the Global Burden of Disease Study 2017. *Lancet* 2019; **393**(10184): 1958–72.

51. Ma Y, He FJ, Sun Q, et al. 24-Hour Urinary Sodium and Potassium Excretion and Cardiovascular Risk. *N Engl J Med* 2022; **386**(3): 252–63.

52. Mechanick JI, Hurley DL, Garvey WT. Adiposity-Based Chronic Disease as a New Diagnostic Term: The American Association of Clinical Endocrinologists and American College of Endocrinology Position Statement. *Endocr Pract* 2017; **23**(3): 372–8.

53. Zheng W, McLerran DF, Rolland B, et al. Association Between Body-Mass Index and Risk of Death in More Than 1 Million Asians. *N Engl J Med* 2011; **364**(8): 719–29.

54. Bluher M. Metabolically Healthy Obesity. *Endocr Rev* 2020; **41**(3): bnaa004.

55. Carbone S, Canada JM, Billingsley HE, Siddiqui MS, Elagizi A, Lavie CJ. Obesity Paradox in Cardiovascular Disease: Where Do We Stand? *Vasc Health Risk Manag* 2019; **15**: 89–100.

56. Tsatsoulis A, Paschou SA. Metabolically Healthy Obesity: Criteria, Epidemiology, Controversies, and Consequences. *Curr Obes Rep* 2020; **9**(2): 109–20.

57. Elias-Lopez D, Vargas-Vazquez A, Mehta R, et al. Natural Course of Metabolically Healthy Phenotype and Risk of Developing Cardiometabolic Diseases: A Three Years Follow-Up Study. *BMC Endocr Disord* 2021; **21**(1): 85.

58. Meigs JB. The Genetic Epidemiology of Type 2 Diabetes: Opportunities for Health Translation. *Curr Diab Rep* 2019; **19**(8): 62.

59. Neel JV. Diabetes Mellitus: A "Thrifty" Genotype Rendered Detrimental by "Progress"? *Am J Hum Genet* 1962; **14**: 353–62.

60. Locke AE, Kahali B, Berndt SI, et al. Genetic Studies of Body Mass Index Yield New Insights for Obesity Biology. *Nature* 2015; **518**(7538): 197–206.

61. Ling C, Ronn T. Epigenetics in Human Obesity and Type 2 Diabetes. *Cell Metab* 2019; **29**(5): 1028–44.

62. Crujeiras AB, Diaz-Lagares A, Moreno-Navarrete JM, et al. Genome-Wide DNA Methylation Pattern in Visceral Adipose Tissue Differentiates Insulin-Resistant from Insulin-Sensitive Obese Subjects. *Transl Res* 2016; **178**: 13–24 e5.

63. Mendelson MM, Marioni RE, Joehanes R, et al. Association of Body Mass Index with DNA Methylation and Gene Expression in Blood Cells and Relations to Cardiometabolic Disease: A Mendelian Randomization Approach. *PLoS Med* 2017; **14**(1): e1002215.

64. Suleyman F. Landmarks in Diabetes Care: A Historical Perspective. *Community Nurse* 1998; **4**(6): 13–6.

65. Di Pino A, DeFronzo RA. Insulin Resistance and Atherosclerosis: Implications for Insulin-Sensitizing Agents. *Endocr Rev* 2019; **40**(6): 1447–67.

66. Kahn CR, Wang G, Lee KY. Altered Adipose Tissue and Adipocyte Function in the Pathogenesis of Metabolic Syndrome. *J Clin Invest* 2019; **129**(10): 3990–4000.

67. Howlader M, Sultana MI, Akter F, Hossain MM. Adiponectin Gene Polymorphisms Associated with Diabetes Mellitus: A descriptive Review. *Heliyon* 2021; **7**(8): e07851.

68. Achari AE, Jain SK. Adiponectin, A Therapeutic Target for Obesity, Diabetes, and Endothelial Dysfunction. *Int J Mol Sci* 2017; **18**(6): 1321.

69. Nicholson T, Church C, Baker DJ, Jones SW. The Role of Adipokines in Skeletal Muscle Inflammation and Insulin Sensitivity. *J Inflamm (Lond)* 2018; **15**: 9.

70. Puurunen VP, Kiviniemi A, Lepojarvi S, et al. Leptin Predicts Short-Term Major Adverse Cardiac Events in Patients with Coronary Artery Disease. *Ann Med* 2017; **49**(5): 448–54.

71. Wu H, Ballantyne CM. Metabolic Inflammation and Insulin Resistance in Obesity. *Circ Res* 2020; **126**(11): 1549–64.

72. Lemmer IL, Willemsen N, Hilal N, Bartelt A. A Guide to Understanding Endoplasmic Reticulum Stress in Metabolic Disorders. *Mol Metab* 2021; **47**: 101169.

73. Pinkas A, Aschner M. Advanced Glycation End-Products and Their Receptors: Related Pathologies, Recent Therapeutic Strategies, and a Potential Model for Future Neurodegeneration Studies. *Chem Res Toxicol* 2016; **29**(5): 707–14.

74. Hirano T. Pathophysiology of Diabetic Dyslipidemia. *J Atheroscler Thromb* 2018; **25**(9): 771–82.

75. Kaur R, Kaur M, Singh J. Endothelial Dysfunction and Platelet Hyperactivity in Type 2 Diabetes Mellitus: Molecular Insights and Therapeutic Strategies. *Cardiovasc Diabetol* 2018; **17**(1): 121.

76. Dabke K, Hendrick G, Devkota S. The Gut Microbiome and Metabolic Syndrome. *J Clin Invest* 2019; **129**(10): 4050–7.

77. Ristori MV, Quagliariello A, Reddel S, et al. Autism, Gastrointestinal Symptoms and Modulation of Gut Microbiota by Nutritional Interventions. *Nutrients* 2019; **11**(11): 2812.

78. Folli F, La Rosa S, Finzi G, et al. Pancreatic Islet of Langerhans' Cytoarchitecture and Ultrastructure in Normal Glucose Tolerance and in Type 2 Diabetes Mellitus. *Diabetes Obes Metab* 2018; **20**(Suppl 2): 137–44.

79. Vaidya V, Gangan N, Sheehan J. Impact of Cardiovascular Complications among Patients with Type 2 Diabetes Mellitus: A Systematic Review. *Expert Rev Pharmacoecon Outcomes Res* 2015; **15**(3): 487–97.

80. Gulumsek E, Keskek SO. Direct Medical Cost of Nephropathy in Patients with Type 2 Diabetes. *Int Urol Nephrol* 2021; **54**(6): 1383–9.

81. Einarson TR, Acs A, Ludwig C, Panton UH. Economic Burden of Cardiovascular Disease in Type 2 Diabetes: A Systematic Review. *Value Health* 2018; **21**(7): 881–90.

82. Stedman M, Lunt M, Davies M, et al. Cost of Hospital Treatment of Type 1 Diabetes (T1DM) and Type 2 Diabetes (T2DM) Compared to the Non-Diabetes Population: A Detailed Economic Evaluation. *BMJ Open* 2020; **10**(5): e033231.

83. Sullivan PW, Ghushchyan V, Wyatt HR, Hill JO. The Medical Cost of Cardiometabolic Risk Factor Clusters in the United States. *Obesity* 2007; **15**(12): 3150–8.

84. Boudreau DM, Malone DC, Raebel MA, et al. Health Care Utilization and Costs by Metabolic Syndrome Risk Factors. *Metab Syndr Relat Disord* 2009; **7**(4): 305–14.

85. Bovolini A, Garcia J, Andrade MA, Duarte JA. Metabolic Syndrome Pathophysiology and Predisposing Factors. *Int J Sports Med* 2021; **42**(3): 199–214.

86. Dunbar SB, Khavjou OA, Bakas T, et al. Projected Costs of Informal Caregiving for Cardiovascular Disease: 2015 to 2035: A Policy Statement From the American Heart Association. *Circulation* 2018; **137**(19): e558–e77.

87. Timmis A, Vardas P, Townsend N, et al. European Society of Cardiology: Cardiovascular Disease Statistics 2021. *Eur Heart J* 2022; **43**(8): 716–99.

88. Martikainen J, Jalkanen K, Heiskanen J, et al. Type 2 Diabetes-Related Health Economic Impact Associated with Increased Whole Grains Consumption among Adults in Finland. *Nutrients* 2021; **13**(10): 3583.

89. Mainous AG, 3rd, Tanner RJ, Baker R. Prediabetes Diagnosis and Treatment in Primary Care. *J Am Board Fam Med* 2016; **29**(2): 283–5.

90. Rippe JM. *Lifestyle Medicine*. London, England: Blackwell Science; 1999.

91. Handelsman Y, Anderson JE, Bakris GL, et al. DCRM Multispecialty Practice Recommendations for the Management of Diabetes, Cardiorenal, and Metabolic Diseases. *J Diabetes Complicat* 2022; **36**(2): 108101.

2 The Evolutionary Biology and Human History of Cardiometabolic Disease

Michael A. Via
Mount Sinai Beth Israel Medical Center
Icahn School of Medicine at Mount Sinai

Jeffrey I. Mechanick
Kravis Center for Cardiovascular Health at Mount Sinai Heart
Icahn School of Medicine at Mount Sinai

CONTENTS

2.1   INTRODUCTION

Evolution, natural selection, adaptive changes in the human genome, epigenome, and other physiological processes interact with environmental and behavioral factors to culminate in a modern human phenotype, broadly regarded in terms of 'health' and 'disease'. The concept of lifestyle medicine is anchored in prevention, but to optimize this process of mitigating or abrogating anticipated pathophysiological events, antecedent mechanistic drivers must be well-understood. From a teleological perspective, scientifically substantiated, relevant events in the distant past need to be

DOI: 10.1201/9781003206637-2

organized along mechanistic lines. Metabolic control mechanisms, some as ancient as the single-celled organism, and others that developed as hormone signal pathways within our more advanced common ancestors, gave rise to energy homeostasis and more complex allostasis in modern humans. These pathways adapted to changing stressors, such as food availability, drought, and predators, to create a robust metabolic and cardiovascular network that improved survival. Technological breakthroughs including the use of stone tools, fire, farming and agricultural advances, transportation, refrigeration, and medical care, among many others, transformed human practices and longevity, eventually determining a modern human culture. In general, the natural interactions among genetics, environment, and behavior have proven beneficial for humans, but technological advances and resultant adverse lifestyles have created a hazardous physiological state without evolutionary precedent. Many of the prevailing hypotheses and theories accounting for evolutionary explanations of health and disease have failed scientific validation, remain unproven, or continue to be controversial. Notwithstanding these limitations, this chapter will survey the key aspects of evolution that impact primary drivers (genetics/epigenetics, environment, and behavior) for cardiometabolic-based chronic disease in order to better understand how lifestyle medicine works.

2.2   NATURAL HISTORY

The forces of evolution and natural selection that drive physiological processes of all living organisms respond to and affect environmental changes that shape a species. Ubiquitous processes, such as glycolysis, are ancient – arising when life on Earth existed only as single-celled organisms, approximately 3.5 billion years BP. Many of the processes that regulate energy metabolism, including insulin signaling, developed within multicellular organisms. Over time, selective processes drove the eventual development of uniquely human characteristics.

Some changes occurred relatively recently on an evolutionary scale. Our last common ancestor separated from the lineage of great apes and primates approximately only 4–5 million years BP. Subsequent developments influenced human behaviors including bipedalism that allowed prehensile hands to grasp food items, changing the diet to possibly include a small amount of meat as well as fruit.[1] A further increase in meat consumption was noted to occur approximately 3 million years BP and is associated with an increase in brain size among *Homo habilis,* the earliest species of the *Homo* genus.[1] Greater meat intake, command of fire, among other changes, drove the development of smaller back molar teeth and larger brains among *Homo erectus* ancestors and eventually the first *Homo sapiens.*

Perhaps the most important factors leading toward modern human lifestyles include these four significant events in the natural history of humans (Figure 2.1):

- **The first appearance of *Homo sapiens*** approximately 200,000 years BP. Physiologically identical (with some exception, described in the dairy section) members of our species lived as hunter-gatherers for the vast majority of human history. *Homo sapiens* made use of fire for cooking and stone

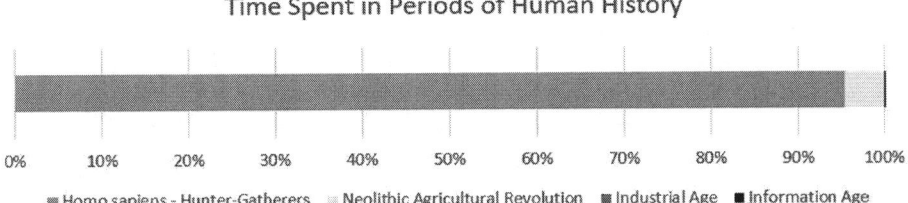

FIGURE 2.1   Visual representation for the amounts of time *Homo sapiens* ancestors followed general lifestyle patterns.

tools, both of which were employed by more distant ancestors in the Homo genus.[1] These technologies significantly impacted lifestyle and dietary contents. For example, through analysis of ancient human fecaliths, seed and grain intake drastically increased in association with use of stone tools.[2] Many of the selective processes in metabolic regulation that led to the high fitness of *H. sapiens* are based on the lifestyles of this period.

- **The Neolithic Agricultural Revolution** approximately 6,000–14,000 years BP. The development of agriculture led to drastic change in human lifestyles. The domestication of animals and plants provided a more stable source of nutrition and drove the development of human settlements with significant effects on daily tasks, dietary contents, and population density.
- **The Industrial Revolution** starting ca. 1850 in Great Britain, quickly spreading to the USA, Western Europe, and eventually worldwide. Changes in this period include the increase in urban populations, wide availability of sugar (sucrose), flour, refrigeration, and increase in sedentary behaviors.
- **The Computer and Information Age** modern human culture is notorious for highly processed foods, sedentary behavior, reduced sleep, and other lifestyle factors associated with non-communicable disease and cardiometabolic risk.

2.3   INFORMATIONAL PHYSIOLOGY – GENETICS, EPIGENETICS, AND MICROFLORA

2.3.1   THE THRIFTY GENE HYPOTHESIS

First introduced in the 1960s, the thrifty gene hypothesis postulates that selective forces during human and pre-human history would optimize the human genome for the conditions of scarcity faced by our hunter-gatherer ancestors, especially affecting genes involved in metabolic regulation.[3] As technologies and human lifestyles have drastically changed, these genomic effects become obsolete, detrimental, and may drive cardiometabolic risk.

Twin and family cohort studies suggest that approximately 45%–70% of the variation in BMI is attributed to heritable traits.[4] However, controlling for shared cultures, environments, and other exposures outside of genes within these studies is difficult and may confound the results.[4] It is known that monogenic syndromes causing obesity are quite rare, leading most authors to suggest the development of obesity in the overwhelming majority of patients with this condition may be attributed to environmental factors in the setting of individual polygenic predisposition.[4]

Over 400 genes have been identified by genome-wide association studies that confer cardiometabolic risk.[5] In spite of these findings, modeling of the data from these studies demonstrates that only 2.7% of the variance in body mass index (BMI) may be explained by genetic variance.[6] This significantly more modest portion of the risk compared to the findings of family and twin studies suggests that non-genetic factors such as environmental and especially lifestyle factors are among the most important in the development of obesity and other manifestations of insulin resistance.[5]

Additionally, 'thrifty' genes within the human genome may be ubiquitous with low variance among populations. One example of this phenomenon is expression of the uricase gene. A warming climate in the Miocene epoch approximately 15–16 million years before present (BP) led to pressures on great ape populations living at that time that faced droughts and food shortages.[7] Mutations in the promoter region and at codon 33 of exon 2 of the uricase gene developed and became dominant in the ancestral great apes living in the Miocene.[7] These same gene variants are present in modern orangutans, gorillas, chimpanzees, and humans, but not in lower primates such as monkeys.[7] Consequent reduced expression of uricase causes a rise in serum uric acid, which allows greater fat storage from the purine depletion that is induced by dietary fructose.[8] By this mechanism, reduced uricase activity leads to more efficient fat storage from ingested fruits.[8] This is believed to confer greater survival during the droughts of the Miocene in which fruit and fructose were scarce, a fitness advantage that may have led to the ubiquitous presence of this thrifty gene among humans as well as other great apes.[1] The present abundance of fructose in western diets imparts a detrimental effect of this previously beneficial gene variant. Dietary choice to reduce fructose intake is the best course to mitigate these vestigial effects of reduced uricase expression. This represents but one example of the potential for maladaptation of modern human lifestyle choices to genomes optimized by natural selection.

2.3.1.1   The Drifty Phenotype

As an alternative or complementary process to the thrifty gene hypothesis, the 'drifty phenotype' hypothesis has been proposed to explain modern human characteristics.[9] Fundamentally, this hypothesis suggests phenotypic change occurred within our human ancestors in association with change in biological niche. Technological developments such as fire and stone tools used by members *of Homo habilis* and *Homo erectus* 2 million years ago may have brought these species to the top of the food chain and suddenly freed these groups of ancient humans from predation.[9] Without predators, this model argues that selective pressures favoring athletic abilities such as speed, stamina, and agility among other characteristics, may diminish, possibly leading to modern sedentary lifestyles.[9] However, this hypothesis overlooks other aspects outside of predator avoidance, such as competition, conflict, hunting, and gathering. Such activities may still provide selective pressure for these same athletic characteristics.[10] Indeed, present-day apex predators in the wild, such as cats, are among the most agile and athletic species.[10] In contrast, the present-day epidemic of obesity among domesticated housecats, with nearly identical genomes to their wild counterparts,[11] suggests the drifty phenotype hypothesis due to the sudden loss of predation may not explain cardiometabolic risk across species.[10]

2.3.2 Epigenetic Change

Mechanisms that regulate gene expression, grouped as epigenetic phenomena, have been recognized to confer cardiometabolic risk.[12] DNA methylation, histone acetylation, and production of noncoding RNA represent the main epigenetic mechanisms. These allow adaptation to environmental change on a scale that occurs within an individual, and, since these changes continue among gametes, epigenetic phenomena influence several generations.

Epigenetic change has been demonstrated to influence risk of insulin resistance both in animal models and in human cohort studies.[12] In patients with obesity and with insulin resistance, hypermethylation of promoter regions for a number of metabolically active genes that include ZF714, COL9A1, MUC2, ADAM4, among others, has been demonstrated.[12] Chromatin methylation and histone acetylation had been demonstrated to regulate P66[SHC], a gene that is highly upregulated within vascular endothelium of visceral fat.[12] These changes are potentially passed to progeny for generations. Since oocytes develop when a female is, herself, *in utero*, epigenetic changes may directly influence at least two generations.[12]

Several other specific epigenetic mechanisms have been identified that influence cardiometabolic health. For example, hypomethylation of the promoter region for insulin-like growth factor 2 (IGF2) was noted up to 60 years later among individuals who were conceived during the Dutch Hunger Winter (1944–1945) and is associated with increased cardiometabolic risk.[13] Another example is the increased risk of childhood obesity among the sons of fathers who smoked starting at age 11, though the specific gene or set of genes to explain this phenomenon has not been identified.[14]

Other examples of epigenetic effects that influence metabolic health involve genes such as leptin, PPARγ, HIF3A, and likely many other genes.[15] In a genome-wide methylation study, approximately 18% of the variance associated with obesity and BMI was attributed to epigenetic change.[16] Transgenerational effects of lifestyle choices highlight the need for the study of optimal lifestyles among reproductive-age individuals to mitigate cardiometabolic risk of subsequent generations.[15]

2.3.2.1 GI Microbiota

The metabolic influence between microorganisms of the GI tract and human hosts has been well-established as a potential cause and consequence of cardiometabolic disease including obesity, insulin resistance, and T2D.[17] Changes in GI bacterial speciation as well as in bacterial gene expression contribute to a complex set of host–microbe interactions and may convey or protect against cardiometabolic risk to the host, as has been demonstrated in numerous studies including animal models, cohort and prospective studies, and fecal transplant studies.[17] In modern humans, a high ratio of Bacteroidetes to Firmicutes bacteria and a reduced GI bacterial diversity are both associated with cardiometabolic risk, while lean individuals demonstrate high amounts of *Lactobacillus*, *Bifidobacterium*, and *Akkermansia* species, as well as a high gene and species diversity.[17]

Genomic studies of human microbiota as well as other bacteria that are associated with animals and plants domesticated during the Neolithic agricultural revolution show rapid and severe genomic alterations during this period.[18] Other contemporary bacteria species outside of these human-associated microbiota do not exhibit similar genomic changes in the same time frame, suggesting a great influence of agriculture on the human GI microbiota.[18] However, it is unclear if this effect alone is detrimental to metabolism, and it appears to manifest a bacterial genomic change rather than a change in speciation.[18]

While somewhat less diverse than gut microbiota, oral microbiota speciation reflects the general speciation of the GI tract and is similarly affected by cardiometabolic risk.[19] Studies of dental enamel, which remarkably preserves oral microbiota in the fossil record, demonstrate only non-pathogenic changes in bacterial speciation after the start of Neolithic agriculture (Figure 2.2, adapted from Adler et al.[20]). Specimens of dental enamel of prehistoric hunter-gatherers were found to be enriched in *Clostridium* sp. and bacteria of the family Ruminococcus. Specimens of Neolithic and Medieval farmers demonstrate increased bacteria taxa including Clostridiales Incertae Sedis, Veillonellaceae family, *Tannerella*, and *Treponema*

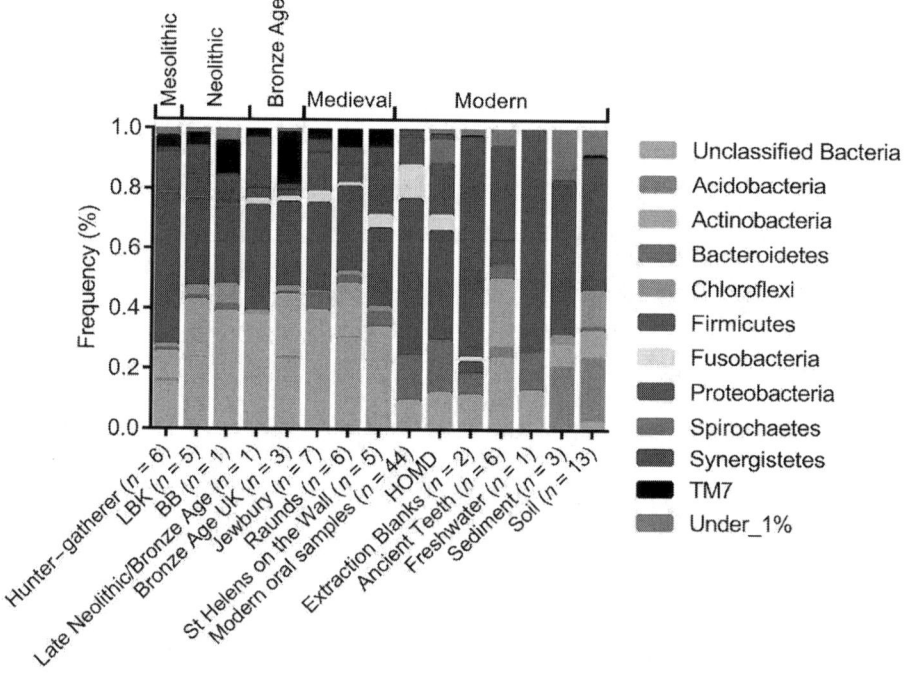

FIGURE 2.2 Reproduced with permission from Adler et al.[20] Bacterial speciation of dental enamel specimens demonstrates change in speciation since the Industrial Revolution. The predominance of Bacteroidetes and the diminished population of Firmicutes among humans of modern times. HOMD, human oral microbiome database.

sp., attributed to increased grain and cereal consumption. These changes are neutral with regard to cardiometabolic risk.[17] In general, GI microbiota speciation during the Neolithic and Medieval periods appear mostly similar to pre-agricultural hunter-gatherers[20] and are also similar to GI microbiota profiles studied in modern-day living hunter-gatherers.[21]

The most significant changes in microbiota are shown in dental enamel specimens of humans that lived after the start of the Industrial Age (Figure 2.2). These modern humans are greatly enriched in Bacteroidetes, diminished in Firmicutes, and show a significant reduction in species diversity.[20] Speciation changes may be attributed to the high carbohydrate, especially high simple sugar intake and reduced fiber content of modern diets.[22] This recent change in GI microbiota implies the Industrial Revolution may have the greatest impact on this driver of cardiometabolic risk among the major historical changes of human lifestyles.

2.4   ENVIRONMENT AND BEHAVIOR

2.4.1   HUNTER-GATHERERS

Careful study of hunter-gatherer people that exist in the present day may give insight to the behaviors and lifestyles of human ancestors who subsisted by using hunting and gathering practices for the vast majority of the time since Homo sapiens first appeared. Undoubtedly, diverse living conditions determined by local environments of prehistoric humans may have necessitated variance in specific behaviors; however, a general understanding of the hunter-gatherer lifestyle provides background to many evolutionary drivers of metabolic regulation and disease. The Hadza tribe, located around the Eyasi Valley of northern Tanzania, is among the most studied groups of modern living hunter-gatherers.[23]

The Hadza diet consists of tubers (7%–20% of calories consumed), berries and baobab fruit (32%–35% of calories consumed), hunted game (35%–40%), and honey (8%–16%).[23] Regular amounts of physical activity are universal, and all Hadza people maintain high levels of physical fitness. On an average day, a Hadza male can travel 6–10 miles on foot, while females travel 4–6 miles. Members of Hadza tribe have a BMI ranging from 18 to 22 kg/m^2, with a 20% body fat among Hadza women and 13% body fat among Hadza men, compared to 38% and 23% body fat among western women and men, respectively.[23] In a metabolic health survey, none of the tribe members were demonstrated to have type 2 diabetes (T2D) or obesity.

Studies of energy expenditure using double-labeled water demonstrate Hadza men spend approximately 2,600 kcal/d, while women spend approximately 1,870 kcal/d.[23] These findings are surprisingly similar to men and women in western cultures, who spend approximately 3,000 and 2,300 kcal/d, respectively, and are identical when corrected for the smaller body size of the Hadza.[23] One may interpret this to suggest that metabolic rate and amount of energy (calories) consumed and utilized by modern humans very closely approximate those of our hunter-gatherer ancestors. However, there is no evidence of insulin resistance, obesity, or T2D among the Hadza.[23] In other words, from these studies, it does not appear that the total number of calories consumed is the culprit in cardiometabolic disease risk. Differences in internal energy allocation and possible malalignment of metabolic regulation with contemporary lifestyles may explain these findings.

These studies are not designed to determine which aspects confer greatest risk; however, their findings emphasize the importance of lifestyle choices in the cardiometabolic health of an individual and provide a basis for hypothesis generation and testing of specific aspects of a hunter-gatherer lifestyle that may be applied in modern humans.

2.4.1.1 Milk and Dairy

Regular consumption of dairy products by adults is a relatively recent practice in human history that became widespread after the domestication of animals during the Neolithic Agricultural Revolution. To metabolize only sugar present in milk, lactose digestion is a requirement of all newborn mammals. Lactose hydrolysis is catalyzed by lactose-phlorizin hydrolase, simply known as lactase, and expression of lactase universally declines after weaning reaching extremely low levels in adult mammals.[24] Humans living after the Neolithic Agricultural Revolution are the single exception.

Approximately one-third of modern adult humans express lactase, with variation in lactase activity ranging from 5% to 100% of that of newborns. Northern European, West African, East African, Middle Eastern, or South Asian ancestry demonstrates among the highest rates of lactase expression, with a single mutation found among European and Asian carriers, while four different mutations are noted within the African populations that express lactase.[25] Rates of adult lactase expression parallel practices of ancestral milk production after animal domestication for consumption of dairy products and occurred approximately 3,000–7,000 years ago by the most current estimate.[25,26] This phenomenon, known as the cultural–historical hypothesis, represents one of the strongest selective pressures faced by the human genome.[26] The rapid incorporation of adult lactase expression is often cited as a prime example by which changes in human behaviors may have induced changes in the human genome.

Newly introduced selective forces following the Neolithic Agricultural Revolution have likely influenced other metabolically important genes, with cardiometabolic implications and potential to influence the definition of a healthy lifestyle.[27] Lactase expression that allows for dairy consumption by adults is the most studied genetic change among humans from this time period.

In addition to genomic changes, it is likely dairy consumption also altered the gastrointestinal (GI) microbiota of ancient humans. Present-day studies demonstrate an increase in the number of colonic bacterial species associated with milk fermentation after introduction of dairy consumption in dairy-naïve humans.[28] Enhanced expression of bacterial lactase is also induced. Many studies demonstrate an association of GI microflora speciation and gene expression with human host cardiometabolic disease.[17] However, it is presently uncertain whether the dairy-induced changes within the human GI microbiome affect cardiometabolic health.[29]

Some authors argue that since regular dairy consumption was not part of our hunter-gatherer ancestors' diet, this practice may be detrimental to human health, including raising the risk of obesity and T2D.[30] However, many studies and systematic reviews have investigated the effects of dietary dairy consumption in modern humans.[31,32] Greater amounts of dairy consumption are associated with reduced weight gain over time, with a 0.4–0.6 kg difference seen between highest and lowest dairy intake quintiles.[32] Dairy intake is also associated with lower rates of obesity in most but not all studies, as well as reduction in fasting glucose by 1–2 mg/dL.[32] As for incidence of T2D, three published studies demonstrate a reduction in risk associated with dairy consumption, while four published studies show no effect, suggesting any potential benefit in risk of T2D may be modest.[32] One explanation for these seemingly conflicting findings may be that the adjustments made for BMI in the studies that show no benefit would inadvertently exclude some of the potential metabolic improvements induced by dairy consumption. In general, these studies show modest beneficial effects of dairy consumption on the risk of obesity, insulin resistance, and T2D.

With regard to risks of cardiovascular events, dairy consumption appears neutral, with no consistently demonstrated effects of benefit or harm among multiple studies.[31,32]

The consumption of milk and dairy products into adulthood represents a clear example of behavior-genomic interaction. Though relatively recent in human history, genomic and microbial changes have been incorporated in current populations. These and potentially other changes have allowed modern humans to safely consume dairy products even though this has not been part of our ancient ancestor's lifestyle.

2.5   A HISTORY OF TYPE 2 DIABETES AND ATHEROSCLEROTIC DISEASE

2.5.1   TYPE 2 DIABETES

The earliest known description of diabetes mellitus was made by ancient Egyptians between 300 and 1500 BCE.[33] A papyrus discovered in the tomb of Thebes describes a 'sugar condition' with severe polyuria. In the second century CE, Galen described diabetes as a wasting condition, while Arateus coined the term 'diabetes' meaning siphon in ancient Greek, referring to the weight loss and polyuria.[34] In his description, Arateus noted diabetes was 'not very common to man', suggesting low prevalence at the time. In the intervening centuries, the clinical description of diabetes included polyuria, wasting, dry skin, and sugar/sweet urine. Observations in children showed near universal mortality from diabetes that occurred relatively quickly, whereas adults who developed diabetes persisted with numerous associated symptoms, mainly skin infections. It may be inferred that many of these early cases refer to type 1 diabetes mellitus (T1D) by the descriptions in children and by an early autopsy report that described a 'shriveled pancreas'.[35] Some cases in adults may have represented T2D, but this is unclear from the ancient descriptions. Though a risk factor for heart disease, T1D results from loss of pancreatic insulin production, often by autoimmune processes, and is independent of both insulin resistance and adiposity.

The prevalence of T2D, which is associated with insulin resistance, was likely to be rare in antiquity and may have been nearly nonexistent among prehistoric humans.[36] No cases of T2D have been observed in studies of present-day hunter-gatherer tribes in pristine conditions, including Pacific islanders, !Kung hunter-gatherers, Central African Pygmies, Australian Aborigines, South African Bantu, the Bimoba, Kusasi, Mamprusi and Peul tribes of east Ghana, the Tsimane of Bolivia, and the Hadza.[23,36,37]

Interestingly, adaptation of a western lifestyle among such isolated groups very commonly leads to a lifestyle-dependent rapid increase in T2D prevalence. One example is the case of the Nauru people that populate an island in the Central Pacific and for millennia subsisted on native fruits, coconuts, and aquaculture.[38] The local discovery and mining of phosphate ore brought sudden wealth to the Nauru starting in 1970. By 1975, the prevalence of T2D was 34%, compared to no observed cases a decade prior.[38] Another example of the high propensity of westernization to lead to T2D is the high prevalence of T2D observed at 50% among the American Pima Indians following adaptation to US culture.[39] Reversibility further highlights lifestyle as the driving factor. In one study that included Australian Aborigines who developed T2D as westernized adults, significant improvement and near resolution of T2D by glucose tolerance testing were demonstrated after resumption of hunter-gatherer behavior for 7 weeks.[40]

In the USA, England, and other western societies, the prevalence of diabetes in general increased in urban and industrial regions during the late decades of the 19th century, coinciding with the start of the Industrial Revolution.[34] Though suspected by some observers, distinction of T1D and T2D was not well-recorded, and at least a portion of possible cases of insulin resistance may represent monogenic forms of diabetes rather than T2D. A definitive diagnosis of T2D was eventually made possible by the development of radioimmunoassays to detect serum insulin in the 1950s. In the earliest nationwide studies of 1958–1960, the prevalence of T2D in the USA was 0.9%.[41] By 2020, only 60 years later, this figure had increased more than ten-fold to 10.5% (Figure 2.3).[41] Globally, the prevalence of T2D has risen by 300% between the years 2000 and 2020, and it is expected to nearly double again by the year 2045.[42] Westernization of cultures around the globe is associated with this meteoric rise. Reversal of this trend with important public health implications may be achieved in part through identification of adverse aspects of modern western lifestyles and through the widespread adoption of healthy choices.

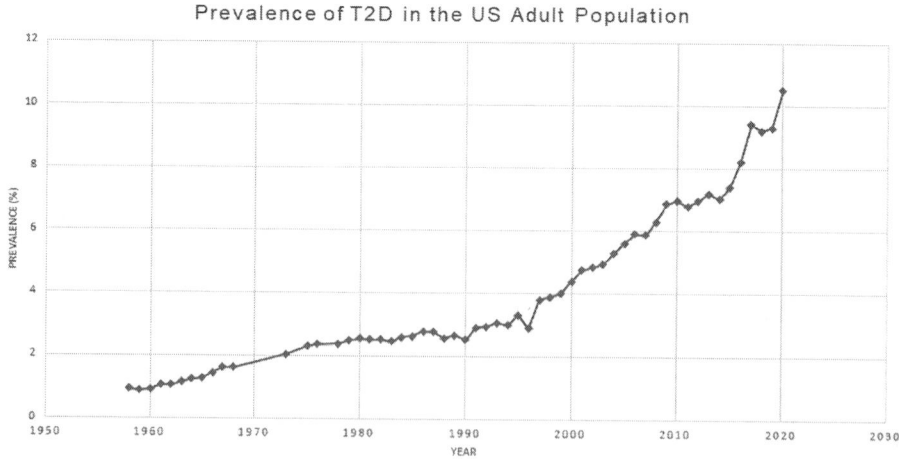

FIGURE 2.3   Prevalence of T2D in the US population. (www.CDC.gov/diabetes/statistics/.[41])

2.5.2 ATHEROSCLEROSIS

Although atherosclerotic disease is the leading cause of death in modern times, with many risk factors such as T2D, obesity, and hypertension that have recently increased in prevalence, atherosclerosis was also commonly present in ancient humans. The Ebers Papyrus (1534 BCE) accurately describes symptoms of angina pectoris.[43] Prior to industrialization, von Haller described the presence of an atheroma within human arteries in 1755.[43] The term atherosclerosis was first used by Marcand more recently in 1904, with reference to the high fat content and 'stiffness' of atheromatous vascular lesions.[43] The prevalence of atherosclerotic heart disease increased as life expectancy increased following industrialization and in association with a reduction in childhood mortality from infectious causes as well as a reduction in mortality from childbirth, allowing a greater portion of women to reach older ages.[44] By 1910, heart disease was the leading cause of mortality in industrialized nations.[44]

Examination of prehistoric anthropologic specimens also demonstrates a high prevalence of calcified arteries. The remains of a 5300-year-old Neolithic man found frozen in the Tyrolean Alps demonstrate such arterial calcifications that represent the oldest known atherosclerotic disease.[45] Atherosclerotic disease has also been described in a number of mummified specimens including remains from ancient Egypt, Peru, Pueblo Native Americans, and the Unangan people of the Aleutian Islands.[46] Approximately 25%–60% of the specimens in each group demonstrate calcified arterial disease, with an overall incidence of 34% of 137 total mummies imaged.[46] The highest prevalence was noted among the mummified specimens that were oldest at time of death.[46] One criticism of the Egyptian cohort is that only the highly affluent Pharaohs and priests were mummified, a group that may have approximated the sedentary lifestyles of modern times with an overabundance of food intake.[47] However, the same cannot be said for the Peruvian and Puebloan mummies that were of subsistence farming populations whose bodies were naturally mummified in the desert conditions. Moreover, the Unangan people were hunter-gatherers without domesticated livestock or agriculture and also commonly demonstrated atherosclerotic disease.

Very few published studies examine living hunter-gatherer populations for the presence of atherosclerosis. One study that evaluated 300 members of the Pygmy tribe of Congo demonstrated the presence of electrocardiogram (ECG) abnormalities in 4% of the group, a similar rate when compared to age- and gender-matched participants of the Framingham Heart Study or to age-matched members of the US Air Force.[48] Though ECG is limited in specificity and sensitivity for coronary atherosclerotic disease, these findings further support the common presence of atherosclerosis among hunter-gatherer lifestyles. In another study of modern-day hunter-gatherers, coronary artery calcium (CAC) scores were measured by non-contrast CT in a cohort of 705 members of the Tsimane tribe, living in Bolivia.[37] In this group, the majority (85%) had CAC score of 0, considered low risk of cardiac atherosclerotic disease, while 89 (13%) had CAC scores between 1 and 100, indicating minimal atherosclerosis, and 20 (3%) had CAC scores greater than 100, indicating moderate atherosclerosis.[37]

The prevalence of elevated CAC scores greater than 100 increased with age and was present in only 1% of Tsimane members age 45–54, 2% of tribe members age 55–64, and 8% of tribe members greater than age 65.[37] Although this represents an approximate five-fold reduction in prevalence of elevated CAC scores compared to westernized populations, these findings indicate atherosclerosis exists in humans following hunter-gatherer lifestyles.

In contrast, non-human primates, including chimpanzees, gorillas, and orangutans, show negligible to no coronary atherosclerosis in necropsy studies.[49] These include specimens obtained from animals that lived in captivity. Additionally, no cases of myocardial infarction among great apes have been reported by zoos or other animal sanctuaries. These findings are especially surprising given the homozygosity of the APOE4 allele in many species of great apes, as well as higher total cholesterol and higher lipoprotein(a) when compared to humans.[49] Each of these lipoprotein markers are highly atherogenic risk factors to humans but apparently not risks in non-human primates.[49] Indeed, atherosclerosis may be inherent to being human. The presence of atherosclerosis among humans in the most pristine metabolic environments suggests that while lifestyle medicine can significantly reduce the risk, atherosclerosis cannot be fully avoided or eradicated in some cases.

2.6   CONCLUSION

Drastic changes in human lifestyles, made possible by progress and technology, drive the development of obesity, insulin resistance, and T2D. The presence of thrifty genes and physiology that was optimized through selective processes to life as a hunter-gatherer may be maladaptive to modern lifestyles. Changes in GI microbiota populations and even changes in human genomes develop in the setting of novel daily human practices. Though radical at the time, the development of agrarian societies and urban living did not appear to affect risk of metabolic disease until thousands of years later, following the Industrial Revolution. Atherosclerosis leading to cardiac disease, which was common throughout human history, has also been exacerbated by practices that are commonplace since the Industrial Revolution. While it must be understood that even the most ideal metabolic lifestyles cannot fully prevent atherosclerosis, a significant reduction in risk can be achieved. The aim of lifestyle medicine is to reduce cardiometabolic risk through adopting healthy practices with an understanding of evolutionary biology of cardiometabolic disease as a guide. Much of the advice that is given in this book and elsewhere is a modern approximation of the lifestyles of our ancestors.

Disclosures:
Jeffrey I. Mechanick received honoraria from Abbott Nutrition for lectures and serves on the Advisory Boards for Aveta.Life and Twin Health.

REFERENCES

1. Andrews P, Johnson RJ. Evolutionary basis for the human diet: consequences for human health. *J Intern Med* 2020; **287**(3): 226–37.
2. Cordain L, Eaton SB, Sebastian A, et al. Origins and evolution of the Western diet: health implications for the 21st century. *Am J Clin Nutr* 2005; **81**(2): 341–54.
3. Neel JV. Diabetes mellitus: a "thrifty" genotype rendered detrimental by "progress"? *Am J Hum Genet* 1962; **14**: 353–62.
4. Stryjecki C, Alyass A, Meyre D. Ethnic and population differences in the genetic predisposition to human obesity. *Obes Rev* 2018; **19**(1): 62–80.
5. Meigs JB. The genetic epidemiology of type 2 diabetes: opportunities for health translation. *Curr Diab Rep* 2019; **19**(8): 62.
6. Locke AE, Kahali B, Berndt SI, et al. Genetic studies of body mass index yield new insights for obesity biology. *Nature* 2015; **518**(7538): 197–206.
7. Oda M, Satta Y, Takenaka O, Takahata N. Loss of urate oxidase activity in hominoids and its evolutionary implications. *Mol Biol Evol* 2002; **19**(5): 640–53.
8. Johnson RJ, Andrews P, Benner SA, Oliver W. Theodore e. Woodward award. The evolution of obesity: insights from the mid-miocene. *Trans Am Clin Climatol Assoc* 2010; **121**: 295–305.
9. Speakman JR. A nonadaptive scenario explaining the genetic predisposition to obesity: the "predation release" hypothesis. *Cell Metab* 2007; **6**(1): 5–12.
10. Voss JD, Goodson MS, Leon JC. Phenotype diffusion and one health: a proposed framework for investigating the plurality of obesity epidemics across many species. *Zoonoses Public Health* 2018; **65**(3): 279–90.
11. Kim S, Cho YS, Kim HM, et al. Comparison of carnivore, omnivore, and herbivore mammalian genomes with a new leopard assembly. *Genome Biol* 2016; **17**(1): 211.
12. Crujeiras AB, Diaz-Lagares A, Moreno-Navarrete JM, et al. Genome-wide DNA methylation pattern in visceral adipose tissue differentiates insulin-resistant from insulin-sensitive obese subjects. *Transl Res* 2016; **178**: 13–24.
13. Heijmans BT, Tobi EW, Stein AD, et al. Persistent epigenetic differences associated with prenatal exposure to famine in humans. *Proc Natl Acad Sci U S A* 2008; **105**(44): 17046–9.
14. Pembrey ME, Bygren LO, Kaati G, et al. Sex-specific, male-line transgenerational responses in humans. *Eur J Hum Genet* 2006; **14**(2): 159–66.
15. Lima RS, de Assis Silva Gomes J, Moreira PR. An overview about DNA methylation in childhood obesity: characteristics of the studies and main findings. *J Cell Biochem* 2020; **121**(5–6): 3042–57.
16. Mendelson MM, Marioni RE, Joehanes R, et al. Association of body mass index with DNA methylation and gene expression in blood cells and relations to cardiometabolic disease: a Mendelian randomization approach. *PLoS Med* 2017; **14**(1): e1002215.
17. Hills RD, Jr., Pontefract BA, Mishcon HR, Black CA, Sutton SC, Theberge CR. Gut microbiome: profound implications for diet and disease. *Nutrients* 2019; **11**(7): 1613.
18. Mira A, Pushker R, Rodriguez-Valera F. The Neolithic revolution of bacterial genomes. *Trends Microbiol* 2006; **14**(5): 200–6.
19. Singh H, Torralba MG, Moncera KJ, et al. Gastro-intestinal and oral microbiome signatures associated with healthy aging. *Geroscience* 2019; **41**(6): 907–21.
20. Adler CJ, Dobney K, Weyrich LS, et al. Sequencing ancient calcified dental plaque shows changes in oral microbiota with dietary shifts of the Neolithic and Industrial revolutions. *Nat Genet* 2013; **45**(4): 450–55.
21. Schnorr SL, Candela M, Rampelli S, et al. Gut microbiome of the Hadza hunter-gatherers. *Nat Commun* 2014; **5**: 3654.

22. Hujoel P. Dietary carbohydrates and dental-systemic diseases. *J Dent Res* 2009; **88**(6): 490–502.
23. Pontzer H, Raichlen DA, Wood BM, et al. Energy expenditure and activity among Hadza hunter-gatherers. *Am J Hum Biol* 2015; **27**(5): 628–37.
24. Flatz G. Genetics of lactose digestion in humans. *Adv Hum Genet* 1987; **16**: 1–77.
25. Segurel L, Bon C. On the evolution of lactase persistence in humans. *Annu Rev Genomics Hum Genet* 2017; **18**: 297–319.
26. Tishkoff SA, Reed FA, Ranciaro A, et al. Convergent adaptation of human lactase persistence in Africa and Europe. *Nat Genet* 2007; **39**(1): 31–40.
27. O'Brien MJ, Bentley RA. Genes, culture, and the human niche: an overview. *Evol Anthropol* 2021; **30**(1): 40–9.
28. Shuai M, Zuo LS, Miao Z, et al. Multi-omics analyses reveal relationships among dairy consumption, gut microbiota and cardiometabolic health. *EBioMedicine* 2021; **66**: 103284.
29. Bastiaanssen TFS, Cryan JF. Dairy alters the microbiome, are we but skimming the surface? *EBioMedicine* 2021; **68**: 103417.
30. Melnik BC. The pathogenic role of persistent milk signaling in mTORC1- and milk-microRNA-driven type 2 diabetes mellitus. *Curr Diabetes Rev* 2015; **11**(1): 46–62.
31. Fontecha J, Calvo MV, Juarez M, Gil A, Martinez-Vizcaino V. Milk and dairy product consumption and cardiovascular diseases: an overview of systematic reviews and meta-analyses. *Adv Nutr* 2019; **10**(suppl_2): S164–S89.
32. Kratz M, Baars T, Guyenet S. The relationship between high-fat dairy consumption and obesity, cardiovascular, and metabolic disease. *Eur J Nutr* 2013; **52**(1): 1–24.
33. Majumdar SK. Glimpses of the history of insulin. *Bull Indian Inst Hist Med Hyderabad* 2001; **31**(1): 57–70.
34. Suleyman F. Landmarks in diabetes care: a historical perspective. *Community Nurse* 1998; **4**(6): 13–6.
35. King KM, Rubin G. A history of diabetes: from antiquity to discovering insulin. *Br J Nurs* 2003; **12**(18): 1091–5.
36. Gurven MD, Trumble BC, Stieglitz J, et al. Cardiovascular disease and type 2 diabetes in evolutionary perspective: a critical role for helminths? *Evol Med Public Health* 2016; **2016**(1): 338–57.
37. Kaplan H, Thompson RC, Trumble BC, et al. Coronary atherosclerosis in indigenous South American Tsimane: a cross-sectional cohort study. *Lancet* 2017; **389**(10080): 1730–9.
38. Zimmet P, Taft P, Guinea A, Guthrie W, Thoma K. The high prevalence of diabetes mellitus on a Central Pacific Island. *Diabetologia* 1977; **13**(2): 111–5.
39. Bennett PH, Burch TA, Miller M. Diabetes mellitus in American (Pima) Indians. *Lancet* 1971; **2**(7716): 125–8.
40. O'Dea K. Marked improvement in carbohydrate and lipid metabolism in diabetic Australian aborigines after temporary reversion to traditional lifestyle. *Diabetes* 1984; **33**(6): 596–603.
41. CDC. http://www.cdc.gov/diabetes/statistics/. Diabetes Data and Statistics (accessed 2023).
42. International Diabetes Federation. https://diabetesatlas.org/. International Diabetes Fund Diabetes Atlas (accessed 2023).
43. Minelli S, Minelli P, Montinari MR. Reflections on atherosclerosis: lesson from the past and future research directions. *J Multidiscip Healthc* 2020; **13**: 621–33.
44. Guyer B, Freedman MA, Strobino DM, Sondik EJ. Annual summary of vital statistics: trends in the health of Americans during the 20th century. *Pediatrics* 2000; **106**(6): 1307–17.
45. Murphy WA, Jr., Nedden DZ, Gostner P, Knapp R, Recheis W, Seidler H. The iceman: discovery and imaging. *Radiology* 2003; **226**(3): 614–29.
46. Clarke EM, Thompson RC, Allam AH, et al. Is atherosclerosis fundamental to human aging? Lessons from ancient mummies. *J Cardiol* 2014; **63**(5): 329–34.

47. Allam AH, Mandour Ali MA, Wann LS, et al. Atherosclerosis in ancient and modern Egyptians: the Horus study. *Glob Heart* 2014; **9**(2): 197–202.
48. Mann GV, Roels OA, Price DL, Merrill JM. Cardiovascular disease in African Pygmies: a survey of the health status, serum lipids and diet of Pygmies in Congo. *J Chronic Dis* 1962; **15**: 341–71.
49. Varki N, Anderson D, Herndon JG, et al. Heart disease is common in humans and chimpanzees, but is caused by different pathological processes. *Evol Appl* 2009; **2**(1): 101–12.

3 The Role of Cardiac Energetics in Cardiometabolic-Based Chronic Disease

Qiuyu Sun and Gary D. Lopaschuk
University of Alberta

CONTENTS

DOI: 10.1201/9781003206637-3

3.1   BACKGROUND

Cardiovascular disease (CVD) is one of the leading causes of death worldwide. Of importance, CVD is not a disease on its own but rather a consequence of other underlying conditions such as type 2 diabetes (T2D) and obesity. The contribution of T2D and obesity to CVD was recently conceptualized as a cardiometabolic-based chronic disease (CMBCD) [1]. To further categorize this, obesity characterized by abnormal adiposity is termed adiposity-based chronic disease (ABCD) [2], and this diagnostic term has been adopted by the American Association of Clinical Endocrinologists and the European Association for the study of obesity [2]. On the other hand, the pathological process led by dysregulated glycemic control is termed dysglycemia-based chronic disease (DBCD) [3]. These terms are created essentially intending to clarify the confusion related to CMBCD, which could either stem from ABCD or DBCD.

    T2D and obesity are two major drivers of CVD. The common denominator between the two risk factors is insulin resistance. Insulin is an anabolic hormone that plays a crucial role in maintaining a balanced metabolic state of the body. Depending on tissue types/organs, insulin has specific physiological and metabolic effects. For example, insulin can stimulate glucose uptake in the skeletal muscle whereas it inhibits lipolysis in adipose tissues. Insulin resistance is a clinical condition where the regulatory effect of insulin on glucose and lipid metabolism is either partially impaired or lost, which leads to dysregulated glycemic control and elevated release of free fatty acids and pro-inflammatory cytokines. Even though insulin resistance can be considered an adaptive response of the body to accommodate situations like starvation and pregnancy [4], in most cases insulin resistance is a strong driver for metabolic diseases, including but not limited to T2D and obesity [5]. The dysregulated balance between glucose and fatty acid metabolism is a significant driver for adverse cardiac remodeling as well as attenuated cardiac function. How altered cardiac energy metabolism plays a role in the formation of CVD and its relevance in lifestyle intervention, pharmacotherapy, and surgical operations are the focus of this review.

3.2 CARDIAC ENERGY METABOLISM

3.2.1 CARDIAC ENERGY METABOLISM IN NORMAL HEARTS

The heart requires a large amount of energy input to sustain contractile function. The form of energy that is used by the heart is adenosine 5'-triphosphate (ATP). Despite having a high energy demand, the heart has essentially no ATP reserves to support its function. To put things into perspective, if ATP was not replenished, the heart would run out of ATP in just a few seconds [6]. As a result, a continuous generation of ATP is paramount for the heart to maintain a continuous and forceful contraction. To meet this goal, the heart relies on a variety of substrates for energy production, including fatty acids, glucose, lactate, ketones, and amino acids. Mitochondrial oxidative phosphorylation constitutes the majority of ATP production in the heart (approximately 95%). As its name implies, this process requires a large amount of oxygen. Hence, disruptions in oxygen supply to the heart will compromise energy production, leading to impaired cardiac function. The two main energy substrates utilized by the mitochondria are fatty acids and glucose, although ketones, amino acids, and other types of carbohydrates can also participate in mitochondrial oxidative phosphorylation to a lesser extent. All these energy substrates generate acetyl-coenzyme A (CoA) during this process. Acetyl-CoA will then feed into the tricarboxylic acid (TCA) cycle to produce reduced equivalents to support the action of the electron transport chain (ETC) for ATP synthesis.

Among all oxidative substrates, fatty acid ß-oxidation contributes to approximately 40%–60% of the overall cardiac ATP production [7] (Figure 3.1). Hence, fatty acids are regarded the major source of fuel for the heart. Fatty acids that enter the myocardium can be either from circulating free fatty acids bound to albumin or from hydrolyzed fatty acids residing in chylomicrons and very-low-density lipoproteins. Fatty acids can enter the myocardium via the fatty acid transporter (CD36) and/or fatty acid–binding proteins (FABP). Following their uptake, fatty acids must be "activated" before entering the mitochondrial oxidation process. Fatty acids are first esterified to fatty acyl-CoA, followed by the transfer of the fatty acids to carnitine by carnitine palmitoyltransferase 1 (CPT1) to form a long-chain acylcarnitine. Long-chain acylcarnitine is then transported into the mitochondria and converted back into fatty acyl-CoA. Fatty acid β-oxidation produces acetyl-CoA, which feeds into the TCA cycle and subsequent ATP production by the ETC.

Glucose is the second major source of fuel for the heart and provides around 20%–40% of the overall cardiac ATP production. Glucose enters the cardiomyocyte via glucose transporter 4 (GLUT4) or glucose transporter 1 (GLUT1). The translocation of glucose by GLUT4 is insulin-dependent, with insulin regulating the trafficking of GLUT4 from intracellular stores to the cell membrane. Of importance, glucose metabolism occurs in two separate phases. In the first phase, glycolysis converts glucose to pyruvate. This process produces less than 10% of the total ATP production in the heart [7]. However, it is important to recognize that glycolysis can occur in

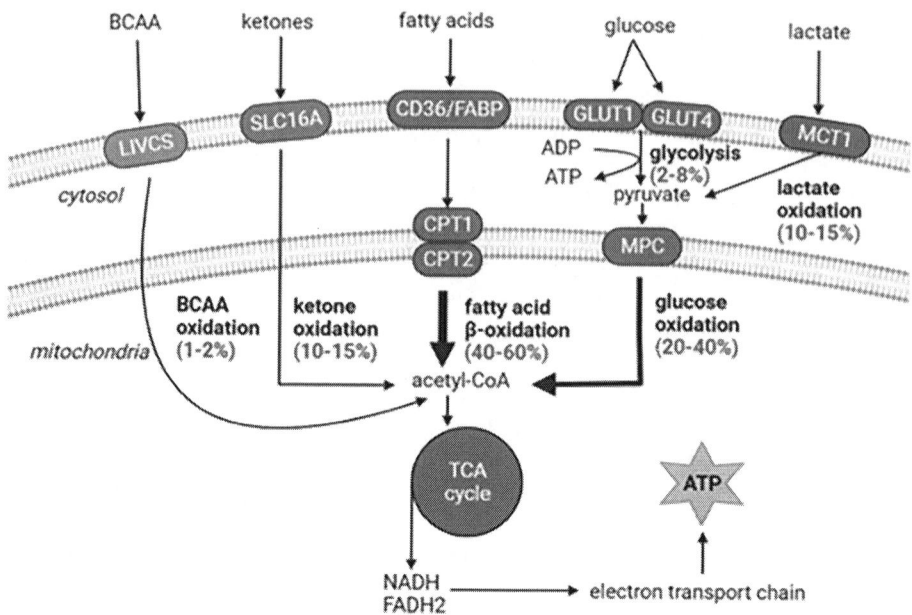

FIGURE 3.1 Cardiac energy metabolism in the normal heart. The heart uses various energy substrates for ATP production, including fatty acids, glucose, ketones, lactate, and amino acids such as BCAA. The bracketed numbers in red represent the approximate contribution of this pathway to overall ATP production. Abbreviations: ATP, adenosine triphosphate; BCAAs, branched-chain amino acids; CD36, fatty acid transporter; CPT1/2, carnitine palmitoyltransferase 1/2; FADH2, flavin adenine dinucleotide; GLUT1/4, glucose transporter 1/4; LIVCS, branched-chain amino acid:cation symporter; MCT1, monocarboxylate transporter 1; MPC, mitochondrial pyruvate carrier; NADH, nicotinamide adenine dinucleotide (NAD) + hydrogen (H); SLC16A, monocarboxylate transporters; TCA, tricarboxylic acid cycle.

the absence of oxygen since the ATP produced during this process does not require oxygen consumption. Due to this unique characteristic, glycolysis can be viewed as a backup source for cardiac energy production when oxygen cannot be delivered sufficiently, such as in heart failure or ischemic heart disease. The second phase of glucose metabolism is glucose oxidation, which occurs in the mitochondria and converts pyruvate to acetyl-CoA. Pyruvate that enters the mitochondria is mainly generated from glucose by glycolysis, or to a lesser extent, from lactate.

In addition to fatty acids and glucose, ketone bodies are increasingly being recognized as an important contributor to energy production in the heart, where approximately 15%–20% of total cardiac ATP production can be attributed to ketone oxidation [8]. Ketone bodies are endogenously produced mainly by the liver under conditions of low circulating levels of glucose, such as during dieting, prolonged exercise, or fasting. There are three main forms of ketone bodies: acetoacetate (AcAc), β-hydroxybutyrate (βOHB), and acetone. Among these, βOHB is the major circulating ketone body. Interestingly, ketone bodies can become a major source of fuel for the heart as they can be readily oxidized when available at high concentrations [9].

Mitochondrial oxidation of amino acids is also a source of ATP in the heart. However, they contribute only modestly to ATP production in the heart. For instance, oxidation of branched-chain amino acids (BCAAs), namely leucine, isoleucine, and valine, accounts for less than 2% of the total cardiac ATP production [10]. Despite this, the BCAAs and their metabolites play an essential role as signaling molecules to regulate overall cardiac energy metabolism.

The normal heart is metabolically flexible as it can switch back and forth between the oxidation of fatty acids and other energy substrates, such as glucose, depending on the circumstances (e.g., workload and substrate availability) [11]. This metabolic flexibility ensures that the heart produces the necessary amount of ATP to maintain contractility under a wide range of situations. As such, when describing the percentage of ATP production by individual substrates, it is most often described in a range, as this number could fluctuate dramatically depending on the state of the heart. One example of such metabolic flexibility is that glucose oxidation rates will decrease dramatically in response to an increase in fatty acid ß-oxidation rates and *vice versa* [12]. Another example is that ketone oxidation is increased in the failing heart, which is seen as an adaptive response, as ketone oxidation provides an additional source of energy for the failing heart [13].

3.2.2 Cardiac Energy Metabolism in Obesity

Obesity is defined as body mass index (BMI) over an ethnicity-based threshold (e.g., 30 kg/m² for Caucasians), and overweight is defined as BMI between the range of normal and obesity. With reference to the definition of ABCD, obesity corresponds to stage 3 ABCD. ABCD is a complex chronic progressive disease that is characterized by an abnormality in the amount and distribution of adiposity [2]. Of interest, there is a lack of strict correlation between obesity and the risk of developing CVD. Patients with obesity can sometimes possess normal insulin sensitivity with no increase in the risk of developing CVD [14]. This is supported by the NHANES cohort, where 1/5 of U.S. patients who are overweight or obese do not have metabolic syndrome [15]. In addition, only about 11% of the population with insulin resistance can be explained by increased BMI [16]. In fact, patients with normal weight can also sometimes have metabolic syndrome.

Even though the mechanistic link between cardiac dysfunction and obesity is not fully understood, alterations in cardiac energy metabolism in response to obesity could offer some explanations for the development of obesity-induced cardiomyopathies [17]. One of the most widely used rodent models is the diet-induced obesity model. The use of a high caloric intake, mostly from fat, leads to an increase in fat mass, total weight gain, and insulin resistance. Genetically modified animal models, such as the *ob/ob* and *db/db* mouse, are also frequently used. Most studies report an increase in fatty acid ß-oxidation in the heart with a concurrent decrease in glucose oxidation and glycolysis in these obesity models (Figure 3.2) [17]. This shift in metabolic fuel preference is also accompanied by impaired cardiac mechanical efficiency due to the increased contribution of fatty acids to overall energy production [17]. In accordance with the observations seen in preclinical animal models, human studies using positron emission tomography (PET) and¹¹C-palmitate imaging also show an

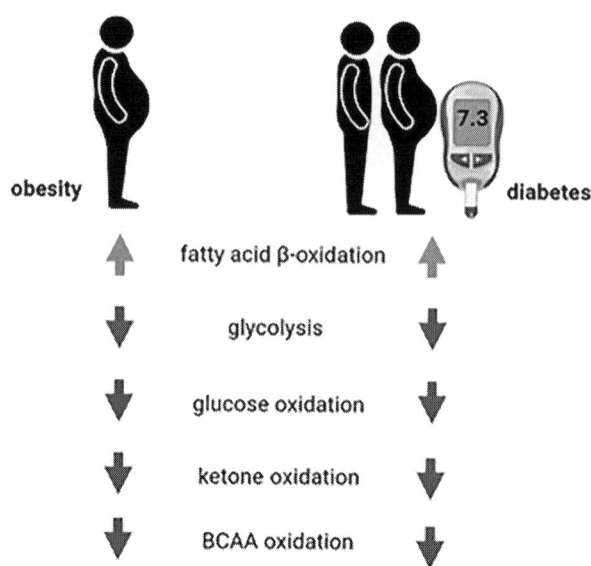

FIGURE 3.2 Alterations of cardiac energy metabolism in obesity and type 2 diabetes (T2D). In both obesity and T2D, there is an increased reliance on fatty acid β-oxidation for cardiac ATP production and a concomitant suppression of glycolysis, glucose oxidation, ketone oxidation, and BCAA oxidation. The imbalance between fatty acid and glucose oxidation contributes to the development of cardiac dysfunction and adverse left ventricular remodeling. The read of the glucometer has the unit of mmol/L and is reflective of fasting blood glucose levels. A fasting blood sugar level less than 5.6 mmol/L is normal. A fasting blood sugar level 7 mmol/L or higher indicates the state of T2D. Abbreviation: ATP, adenosine triphosphate; BCAAs, branched-chain amino acids.

increase in the uptake and oxidation of fatty acids in female patients with obesity [18]. Moreover, circulating levels of free fatty acids and triacylglycerol (TAG) are higher in patients with obesity than their lean counterparts, which is more prominent in females [19]. This increased availability of fatty acids to the heart contributes to the heart utilizing more fatty acids as an energy substrate, resulting in a simultaneous inhibition of glucose oxidation.

3.2.3 CARDIAC ENERGY METABOLISM IN TYPE 2 DIABETES

In T2D, the metabolic flexibility of the heart is impaired and there is a greater reliance on fatty acid ß-oxidation for ATP production [20–22]. Simultaneously, there is an overall decrease in glucose transport, glycolysis, and glucose oxidation. The expression levels for both glucose transporters (GLUT1 and GLUT4) are decreased [23]. Insulin resistance contributes to impaired glucose uptake, as the translocation of the GLUT4 transporter to the cell membrane is insulin dependent. Moreover, phosphofructokinase 1 (PFK1) and pyruvate dehydrogenase (PDH), which are the rate-limiting enzymes for glycolysis and glucose oxidation respectively, are allosterically inhibited by high levels of citrate and NADH/NAD+ ratios [24–26]. This occurs, in part, because of the increase in circulating fatty acids and increased fatty acid ß-oxidation rates. Increased plasma levels of free fatty acids are attributed to insulin resistance in the adipose tissues. The inhibitory action of insulin on lipolysis is lost, leading to an increase in the breakdown of fat storage, which releases more free fatty acids into circulation. As a result, fatty acids become more available to the heart, enabling an increase in both the uptake and ß-oxidation of fatty acids in the heart. Fatty acid uptake into the myocardium is regulated by the fatty acid transporters located on the cell membrane. In T2D, there is an upregulation of key enzymes involved in fatty acid uptake and handlings, such as CD36 and FABP [27–29].

The increase in fatty acid uptake does not fully explain the increased reliance on fatty acid ß-oxidation for cardiac ATP production in the heart of patients with T2D. A complex reprogramming of the key proteins involved in fatty acid metabolism through various transcriptional, post-translational, and allosteric processes also occurs [30]. At the transcriptional level, there are increases in the expression of peroxisome proliferator-activated receptor-α (PPARα) and estrogen-related receptor-γ (ERRγ) [31,32]. PPARα is a key transcriptional regulator for proteins involved in fatty acid ß-oxidation. The expression of PPARα is found to be increased in murine diabetic hearts [33]. Increases in PPARα activate the expression of genes involved in fatty acid metabolism, such as mitochondrial CPT1, acyl-coenzyme A synthetase (ACS), and long-chain acyl-CoA dehydrogenase (LCAD) [34,35]. In addition to its direct effect of enhancing cardiac fatty acid ß-oxidation, PPARα also regulates glucose oxidation indirectly by stimulating the expression of pyruvate dehydrogenase kinase 4 (PDK4), an enzyme that phosphorylates and inhibits the action of PDH, thus suppressing glucose oxidation. Overexpression of cardiac ERRγ also recapitulates key characteristics of the heart in T2D mice, and the expression of PPARα is also under the control of ERRγ [36]. As such, there exists a potential ERRγ-PPARα axis for reprogramming substrate utilization in the heart of T2D.

At an allosteric level, malonyl-CoA plays an important role in accelerated cardiac fatty acid ß-oxidation. It allosterically inhibits mitochondrial fatty acid uptake via CPT1. The level of malonyl-CoA depends on the balance between its synthesis by acetyl-CoA carboxylase (ACC) and its degradation by malonyl-CoA decarboxylase (MCD) [37]. In both streptozotocin-treated T1D mice and diet-induced obese T2D mice, there is a decrease in the levels of malonyl-CoA due to the increased expression and activity of MCD [38,39]. Upregulation of PPARα can explain the elevated expression of MCD and the decrease in the levels of malonyl-CoA in T2D [40]. As a result, the inhibition of malonyl-CoA on CPT1 is lifted, rendering more fatty acids to be taken up into the mitochondria for further ß-oxidation.

3.2.4 THE IMPACT OF HIGH CARDIAC FATTY ACID β-OXIDATION ON CARDIAC FUNCTION

The increased reliance of the heart on fatty acids as an energy source, observed in both obesity and T2D, has many deleterious effects. One is the lowering of cardiac efficiency, as fatty acid ß-oxidation is less oxygen-efficient than glucose. To generate ATP by the process of oxidative phosphorylation, fatty acids consume more oxygen molecules compared to glucose. As a result, increased dependence on fatty acid ß-oxidation for ATP production requires more oxygen, resulting in the heart working less efficiently (cardiac work/oxygen consumed). Studies on T2D animal models, the *ob/ob* mice, have shown that the heart can require as much as 30% more oxygen for generating the same or even less contractile force compared to normal control mice [41]. On top of that, cardiac efficiency is compromised due to the increased cycling of fatty acids through cardiac TAG. This is because the process of TAG synthesis requires energy input to convert fatty acids to fatty acyl-CoAs. In addition to reducing cardiac efficiency, the marked increase of using fatty acids for energy production could impair cellular ATP shuttling, as long-chain acyl-CoA derivatives inhibit the ADP/ATP carrier protein (AAC), which transports ATP from mitochondria to cytosol [42]. Finally, increases in fatty acid ß-oxidation rates can induce mitochondrial uncoupling, leading to the loss of membrane potential through upregulation of uncoupling proteins (UCPs) 2 and 3 [43].

3.3 MOLECULAR MECHANISMS THAT CONTRIBUTE TO THE ALTERED CARDIAC ENERGETICS

3.3.1 Epigenetics-Mediated Dysregulation of Gene Expression

The pathogenesis for both obesity and T2D is complex and multifactorial, with genetic, lifestyle, and environmental factors all contributing and being intertwined with one another. Similarly, modulation of epigenetics could account for a large range of non-genetic factors such as aging, diet, sex, and environmental stress. Hence, many studies have begun to investigate the role of epigenetics in cardiometabolic diseases [44]. Epigenetic status is represented as alterations in chromatin conformation and accessibility in response to DNA methylation, histone modification, and non-coding RNA-associated gene silencing. DNA methylation occurs via methyltransferases that covalently anchor a methyl group to the nucleotide. The chromatin structure becomes more condensed, and DNA is less available for transcription, leading to either the silencing or suppression of the targeted gene. Histone modifications affect the binding affinity of other transcription-regulating proteins to the DNA strand, which can occur through the form of phosphorylation, acetylation, or methylation. Last but not least, non-coding RNAs exert epigenetic modulation through assembling with the Argonaute proteins to form the RNA-induced silencing complexes [45], as well as inducing gene silencing through the mechanism of RNA-directed DNA methylation (RdDM) [46].

Genome-wide DNA methylation analysis of patients with dilated cardiomyopathy found significant changes in DNA methylation in the myocardium [47]. In accordance with this, differential DNA methylation is also observed in patients with ischemic heart disease [48]. In obesity, liver function is paramount as it is the main site carrying out both fatty acid β-oxidation and fatty acid synthesis. A high-fat diet can induce widespread chromatin remodeling in the liver, as evidenced by the differential expression of more than 300 genes [49]. Another study shows an increase in the expression of hepatic histone deacetylase 6 (HDAC6) and histone demethylases Kdm3b, Kdm5b, and Kdm5c in response to a high-fat diet feeding [50], suggesting that altered gene expression observed with high-fat feeding could be modulated by changes occurred in histone-modifying enzymes.

The effects brought by epigenetics are long-lasting. In animals, after blood glucose levels are normalized post streptozotocin injection, there remain changes in the miRNA landscape of the heart, suggesting persistent effects of diabetes on cardiac function [51]. In compliance with this, human clinical trials on patients with T1D show that the effect of intense glycemic control could persist for decades, as evidenced by the lowering of diabetic complications in the short term as well as the reduced chances of developing both micro- and macrovascular complications decades after the initial treatment [52]. Similarly, studies in patients with T2D also show improved patient outcomes that are long-lasting after the initial intensive glycemic control [53].

3.3.2 Post-Translational Modification

Extensive studies and literature have pinpointed the differential expression of key enzymes involved in cardiac energy metabolism that induce the disproportional utilization between fatty acids and glucose in T2D and obesity [54]. At the early stage of heart failure, where there are no present changes of key enzymes involved in metabolic pathways at the transcriptional level, transcriptomic and metabolomic analyses still reveal dramatic alterations in the levels of metabolites [55]. These early changes can be, in part, explained by potential post-translational modifications (PTMs), which enable rapid modulation of protein function. Several types of PTMs have been shown to occur, including acetylation, phosphorylation, ubiquitylation, succinylation, malonation, methylation, and O-GlcNAcylation. The focus of this section will be on acetylation, but other types of PTMs are also crucial for regulating cardiac energy metabolism in both healthy and pathological states.

Acetylation of proteins is carried out by acetyltransferases, whose action is dependent on the level of mitochondrial acetyl-CoA. Deacetylation of proteins is governed by the availability of nicotinamide adenine dinucleotide (NAD^+), a cofactor for deacetylase enzymes that removes the acetylation from targeted proteins. Even though it is generally accepted that lysine acetylation of enzymes involved in fatty acid β-oxidation, such as LCAD, contributes to the dysregulated cardiac metabolism, there is no consensus as to the precise effects of this acetylation on the actual rates of fatty acid β-oxidation. While some studies suggest that acetylation stimulates fatty acid β-oxidation [56], others propose that acetylation has an inhibitory effect [57]. For instance, sirtuin 3 (SIRT3) is a NAD^+-dependent deacetylase. In SIRT3 knockout mice, fatty acid β-oxidation is impaired in the liver with a simultaneous reduction of LCAD enzymatic activity, suggesting that removal of SIRT3 deacetylase activity suppresses fatty acid β-oxidation rates in the liver [57]. However, this is unlikely to be the case for the heart, as in diabetes- and obesity-induced cardiomyopathy, SIRT3 is downregulated, yet the rate of cardiac fatty acid β-oxidation is increased [58]. Animals fed with a high-fat diet for 16 weeks show downregulation of SIRT3, as well as an increase in both the LCAD and 3-hydroxy acyl-CoA dehydrogenase (β-HAD) acetylation states [56]. Both enzymes are key proteins involved in fatty acid β-oxidation in the heart. In addition to SIRT3, other acetyltransferases such as general control of amino acid synthesis 5 like-1 (GCN5L1) also play a role in stimulating fatty acid oxidation by increasing acetylation on

LCAD [59]. The trifunctional protein complex subunit α is another enzyme for fatty acid β-oxidation and its acetylation status is found to be positively correlated with the rate of fatty acid β-oxidation [60].

In both T2D and obesity, mitochondrial oxidative phosphorylation capacity is impaired. Flux through the ETC is suppressed due to a deficiency of complex I. As a result, the NAD^+ to NADH ratio is decreased, thus limiting the deacetylase activity of SIRT3 since the activity of SIRT3 is dependent on the availability of the cofactor, NAD^+. A recently discovered chemical agent, namely honokiol, demonstrates SIRT3-activating capability, and it was reported that honokiol can ameliorate cardiac hypertrophy in preclinical animal models [61].

3.3.3 Cardiac Insulin Resistance

Insulin resistance is a prominent clinical symptom diagnosed in patients with CMBCD. Insulin resistance is defined as the impaired signaling action of insulin in regulating metabolism in targeted organs. Evidence from epidemiological studies shows that insulin resistance is a predictor of heart failure, as supported by the positive correlation between the risk of congestive heart failure with the presence of insulin resistance [62]. The insulin signaling pathway involves a series of interactions among the insulin receptor, insulin, insulin receptor substrate (IRS)-1/2, phosphoinositide 3-kinase (PI3K), and protein kinase B (PKB/Akt), which ultimately regulates glucose and fatty acid metabolism through various intracellular mechanisms. At the level of adipose tissues, insulin inhibits lipolysis to limit circulating free fatty acids. At the level of the heart, insulin resistance is manifested as a decreased uptake and utilization of glucose and a simultaneous increase in the uptake and oxidation of fatty acids [63]. As insulin regulates the translocation of GLUT4 and CD36 to the myocyte sarcolemma, insulin resistance renders CD36 being preferentially localized to the sarcolemma, while GLUT4 is internalized to intracellular locations. This is supported by a study showing that the expression levels of GLUT4 are lower in insulin-resistant hearts [23]. Furthermore, the activities of two crucial proteins involved in glycolysis and glucose oxidation, PFK-1 and PDH respectively, are found to be suppressed in insulin-resistant hearts [24,26]. Of importance, insulin has additional regulatory functions by stimulating glucose oxidation directly through enhancing mitochondrial Akt activity [64]. This direct stimulation of glucose oxidation is attenuated in insulin-resistant hearts.

Accumulation of lipid metabolites in the myocardium can negatively impact insulin signaling. Lipid intermediates, such as diacylglycerols and ceramides, can activate cascades of kinases that inhibit the activities of key enzymes involved in insulin signaling, including phosphorylation of IRS-1 and Akt inhibition. Mitochondrial dysfunction observed in diabetes and obesity can also render excessive ROS production, reduced mitochondrial membrane potential, and abnormal mitochondrial biogenesis [65]. ROS has a number of damaging effects on myocardial function. ROS can dissipate mitochondrial membrane potential by inducing the opening of the mitochondrial permeability transition pore (mPTP). Cardiac ATP production is then impaired due to the loss of mitochondrial membrane potential. Interestingly, ROS production can also be self-amplifying, meaning that the more mitochondrial ROS there is, the more ROS will be released. This release of ROS further perpetuated the development of insulin resistance. Furthermore, cardiac inflammation, characterized by a higher prevalence of pro-inflammatory cytokines like tumor necrosis factor-α (TNF-α), also contributes to the inhibition of insulin action, partially through activating c-Jun NH2-terminal kinases (JNK) [66]. JNK induces inhibitory phosphorylation of IRS-1 at Ser307, which compromises insulin-stimulated tyrosine phosphorylation of IRS-1, thus leading to insulin resistance [67].

3.3.4 LIPOTOXICITY

Cardiac lipotoxicity describes the accumulation or overload of unmetabolized lipids inside cardiomyocytes. This is observed in the heart in both T2D and obesity [68]. This lipid overload occurs preceding the onset of left ventricular dysfunction, suggesting the potential to be targeted for therapy. Lipotoxicity is not the result of decreased oxidation of fatty acids, as cardiac fatty acid ß-oxidation occurs at an accelerated rate in obesity and T2D [18]. However, a buildup of lipids occurs within the cytosol primarily because the rates of fatty acid uptake exceed that of its oxidation. This is due to both the increase in fatty acid supply to the heart, as well as the upregulation of proteins involved in fatty acid uptake (CD36) and fatty acid activation (acyl-CoA synthetase) [69,70]. As a result, fatty acids that are not oxidized are converted to potentially toxic lipid intermediates, such as long-chain acyl-CoAs, diacylglycerols, ceramides, and TAG. The accumulation of lipid intermediates can have several adverse effects on cardiac function. For example, the accumulation of ceramides and diacylglycerols promotes apoptosis of cardiomyocytes and activates protein kinase C (PKC), which in turn impairs β-adrenergic signaling and compromises heart contractility. Activation of PKC in response to lipotoxicity also impairs insulin signaling via phosphorylation of IRS1 at its inhibitory site Ser1101 [71].

3.3.5 GLUCOTOXICITY

Accumulation of glucose and its metabolites in the heart has the potential of inducing left ventricular adverse remodeling. Glucotoxicity can occur under the situation of an uncoupling between glycolysis and glucose oxidation, resulting in increased accumulation of glucose and glycolytic intermediates in the heart. This is problematic because this glucose and/or its metabolites can enter other glucose metabolic pathways, such as the hexosamine biosynthetic pathway (HBP), polyol pathway, pentose phosphate pathway, advanced glycation end product pathway, mannose and galactosamine synthetic pathways, and one-carbon metabolism pathways; products of which have been linked to the activation of downstream signaling pathways that may contribute to adverse left ventricular remodeling [72]. Accumulation of these glucose metabolites (e.g., HBP metabolites) is closely related to the development of heart failure [73]. The glycolytic intermediate, fructose-6-phosphate, can be re-routed from the glycolysis pathway to the HBP by the enzymatic action of L-glutamine:D-fructose-6-phosphate amidotransferase (GFAT), which converts fructose-6-phosphate into glucosamine-6-phosphate. The HBP synthesizes the substrate for O-linked N-acetylglucosamine (O-GlcNAc) modification. O-GlcNAc modification is a reversible PTM, and excessive

O-GlcNAcylation (by genetic modulation on enzymes involved in O-GlcNAc) is found in patients with progressive dilated cardiomyopathy and aortic stenosis [74,75].

3.3.6 CARDIAC INFLAMMATION

Systemic inflammation is a prominent symptom of obesity, as macrophages can accumulate within the adipose tissues, and the number of macrophages increases with increasing obesity [76]. This is supported by studies on patients with obesity showing a higher expression of pro-inflammatory proteins, such as TNF-α and IL-6, in adipose tissues compared to their lean counterparts [77]. Clinical evidence shows that BMI positively correlates with systemic inflammation and oxidative stress, independent of glycemic control [78]. Accelerated infiltration of pro-inflammatory cytokines into the myocardium can lead to adverse myocardial remodeling, myocyte hypertrophy, and apoptosis. Through modulating the endothelium, pro-inflammatory cytokines also induce the formation of cardiac fibrosis, thus decreasing the contractility of the heart. Of interest, the NOD-like receptor family pyrin domain containing 3 (NLRP3) inflammasome is a key player underpinning metabolic and hemodynamic dysfunction in diabetes [79]. Increased levels of plasma-free fatty acids are observed in patients with either obesity or diabetes and can activate NLRP3 inflammasomes via ROS-mediated pathways, leading to impairment of insulin signaling and glucose intolerance [80]. Although NLRP3 inflammasome has been implicated in the development of cardiac dysfunction [81], the exact underlying mechanism of adverse myocardial remodeling is not yet completely understood.

3.4 LIFESTYLE INTERVENTIONS AND SURGICAL PROCEDURES FOR TREATING OBESITY AND T2D

3.4.1 CALORIC RESTRICTION

Caloric restriction is defined as a reduction of caloric intake by 10%–40% without compromising the intake of proteins and micronutrients. McCay et al. [82] first established the beneficial effect of caloric restriction on both extending the lifespan and health span. Of importance, there is growing evidence from animal studies and human clinical trials showing that caloric restriction can effectively attenuate the risk of developing CVD, and this risk reduction is in addition to the effect of weight loss [83,84]. Although the reduction in body weight partially contributes to CV health, this is secondary to the metabolic alterations induced by caloric restriction (Table 3.1 and Figure 3.3). One study shows that a 50% caloric restriction for 3 months attenuates cardiac dysfunction post-ischemia/reperfusion injury in rats [85]. Similarly, in obese mice, an improvement in left ventricular ejection fraction with a concomitant reduction in cardiac hypertrophy is seen with only 8 weeks of a 40% caloric restriction [86].

Several clinical trials have shown positive results of caloric restriction on cardiac function in patients with heart failure and obesity, where caloric restriction caused an increase in left ventricular ejection fraction, improvement in both systolic and diastolic function, reduction in left ventricular mass, and higher cardiac efficiency [85].

TABLE 3.1

Effects of Lifestyle Interventions on Cardiovascular Health

	Class of Therapy	Main Effects	Source
Caloric restriction	Lifestyle intervention	Reduced body weight Improved insulin resistance Restored metabolic flexibility of the heart Reduced TAG levels in cardiomyocytes	[87] [88] [59]
Physical activity	Lifestyle intervention	Decreased cardiac glycolytic rates Increased cardiac glucose oxidation rates Increased transcriptional levels of insulin-dependent glucose transporters GLUT4 Increased activities of glucose oxidation enzymes, such as pyruvate dehydrogenase	[89] [90] [91]
Ketogenic diets	Lifestyle intervention	Improved insulin resistance Lowered A1c and plasma TAG Reduced blood pressure Reduced body weight Additional source of fuel for the heart	[92] [93] [94]
Bariatric procedure	Surgical operation	Enhanced insulin sensitivity Altered bile acid concentrations Altered enteric gut hormones Increased metabolic activity of brown adipose tissues Altered intestinal glucose metabolism Modified composition of gut microbiota	[95]

The major systemic and cardiometabolic effects of each lifestyle intervention as well as surgical procedure are listed in the table.

Abbreviations: GLUT4, glucose transporter 4; A1c, glycated hemoglobin; TAG: triacylglycerol.

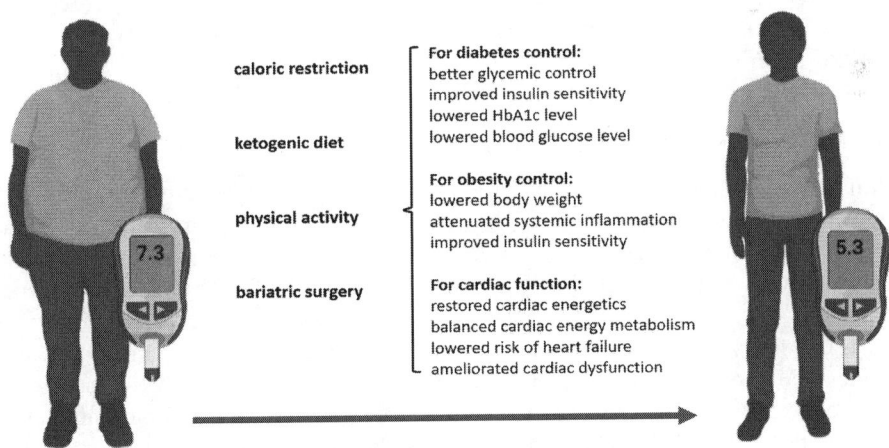

FIGURE 3.3 Lifestyle and surgical approaches for treating type 2 diabetes (T2D) and obesity. The read of the glucometer has the unit of mmol/L and is reflective of fasting blood glucose levels. A fasting blood sugar level less than 5.6 mmol/L is normal. A fasting blood sugar level 7 mmol/L or higher indicates the state of T2D.

Furthermore, long-term sustained weight loss in patients with heart failure and obesity also shows a reduction in arrhythmia burden and preservation of sinus rhythm [96]. The rate of heart failure re-hospitalization decreases with the use of a nutritional strategy aimed at the reduction of weight in patients with chronic heart failure [97]. As a result, caloric restriction without malnutrition may effectively induce weight loss in patients with heart failure and obesity, with a significant improvement in cardiac function. However, prolonged caloric restriction may adversely impact cardiac function since the deficiency of energy substrate could limit mitochondrial ATP production. For example, insufficient carbohydrate ingestion for 30 weeks in mice resulted in impaired contractility and reduced ventricular mass [98]. During starvation, the heart responds to this situation by increasing protein and fat catabolism with the hope of replenishing the void of energy [99]. This leads to loss of cellular volume and atrophy, which can be observed in many essential organs such as the brain, liver, kidney, skeletal muscle, and heart. In particular, weight loss induced by a low-carbohydrate diet can lead to a high risk of developing CVD, as cardiac fatty acid β-oxidation rates increase to compensate for limited glucose metabolism. This impairs cardiac efficiency and leads to contractile dysfunction. In extreme cases, such as patients with anorexia nervosa with chronic and severe starvation, prominent interstitial fibrosis is observed, which is attributable to the development of rhythm disturbances [100]. As a result, a well-planned caloric restriction regimen is necessary to ensure proper weight loss without the risk of malnutrition or energy deficiency.

Nutrition plays an important role in regulating blood energy substrates, which in turn influences insulin sensitivity in various tissues. This is particularly important in the heart, as insulin is responsible for maintaining the balance between fatty acid and glucose metabolism. Caloric restriction can improve insulin resistance in overweight patients, restoring the metabolic flexibility of the heart [59]. In patients with coronary artery disease without heart failure, one year of caloric restriction effectively lowered plasma insulin levels, suggesting improved insulin sensitivity [87]. Similarly, in patients with metabolic syndrome, caloric restriction improves insulin sensitivity, in addition to reductions in CVD risk [101].

3.4.2 PHYSICAL ACTIVITY

Maintaining a physically active lifestyle brings many health benefits that contribute to lowering CVD risks and improving physiological health. Improvements in cardiac performance could, in part, be due to the effect of exercise on inducing physiological hypertrophy of the heart [102]. There are two types of cardiac hypertrophy: pathological hypertrophy which develops due to adverse cardiac remodeling under various stress conditions such as high blood pressure and physiological hypertrophy which is an adaptive response to compensate for higher cardiac output with enhanced contractile function. The differences between pathological and physiological hypertrophy lie at both molecular and structural levels. Physical exercise, such as endurance training, has the potential to transform pathological cardiac hypertrophy into a physiological state. This includes important transformations in cardiac energy metabolism. Glucose oxidation rates are increased in hearts hypertrophied by physical exercise, while glycolytic rates are decreased [89]. The mRNA levels of insulin-dependent glucose transporters, such as GLUT4, are elevated in rats undergoing exercise training [90]. Additionally, the activity of glucose oxidation enzymes, such as PDH, is also increased. *Ex vivo* working heart perfusion of exercise-adapted rat hearts also shows reduced glycolytic rates with a simultaneous increase in glucose oxidation [91].

3.5 PHARMACOLOGICAL APPROACHES FOR TREATING OBESITY AND T2D

Lifestyle interventions that target cardiac energetics are generally implemented first, as part of primordial (preventing CVD risk), primary (preventing CVD), and secondary (preventing CVD progression) prevention tactics. However, a discussion of pharmacotherapy here serves two purposes: first, to further demonstrate the feasibility of targeting cardiac energetics, especially in secondary and tertiary (preventing suffering and mortality due to CVD), and second, to provide a real-life context wherein lifestyle and pharmacotherapeutic modalities are commonly used together and are not mutually exclusive (Table 3.2 and Figure 3.4).

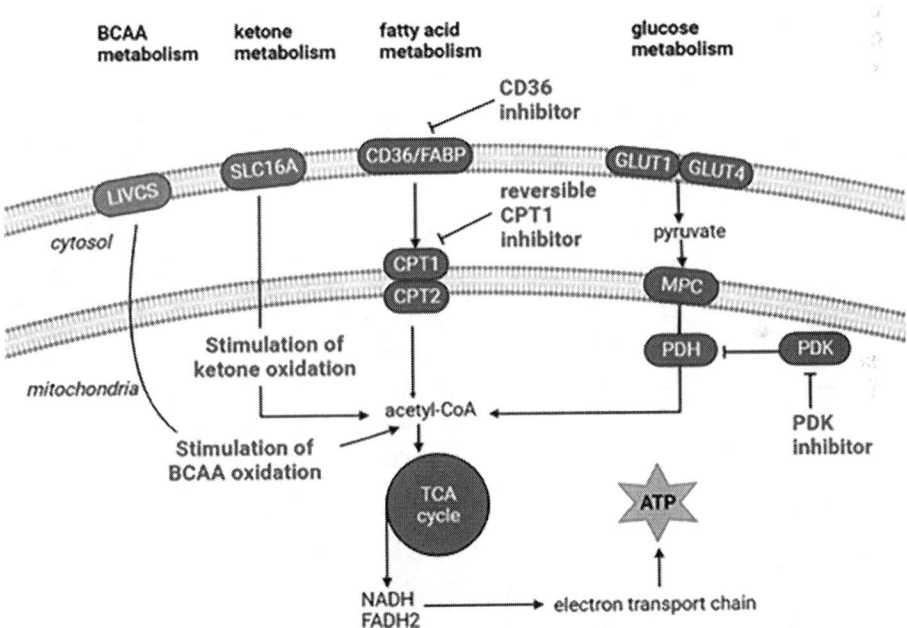

FIGURE 3.4 Potential pharmacological approaches for treating obesity- and type 2 diabetes (T2D)-induced cardiomyopathy. Red bolded letters represent potential approaches for improving the cardiometabolic state of the heart. Abbreviations: ATP, adenosine triphosphate; BCAA, branched-chain amino acids; CD36, fatty acid transporter; CPT1/2, carnitine palmitoyltransferase 1/2; FABP, fatty acid–binding protein; FADH$_2$, flavin adenine dinucleotide; GLUT1/4, glucose transporter 1/4; LIVCS, branched-chain amino acid:cation symporter; MPC, mitochondrial pyruvate carrier; NADH, nicotinamide adenine dinucleotide (NAD)+hydrogen (H); PDH, pyruvate dehydrogenase; PDK, PDH kinase; SLC16A, monocarboxylate transporters.

TABLE 3.2

Effects of Pharmacotherapy on Cardiac Energetics

Medications	Class of Therapy	Molecular Effect	Potential Cardiometabolic Effect	Main Effect	Source
Metformin	Antihyperglycemic drug	AMPK activator	Stimulation of fatty acid β-oxidation	Adverse	[103]
SGLT2 inhibitors	Antihyperglycemic drugs Lipid-lowering drugs	Inhibitor of SGLT2	Increased circulating levels of ketone bodies Increased cardiac energy production	Beneficial	[104]
GLP-1 receptor agonists	Antihyperglycemic drugs	Agonist of GLP-1 receptors	Peripheral stimulation of insulin and glucagon secretion, indirect stimulation of cardiac glucose oxidation, suppression of fatty acid β-oxidation	Beneficial	[105]
DPP4 inhibitors	Antihyperglycemic drugs	DPP4 inhibitors	Stimulation of glucose and fatty acid uptake	Adverse	[104]
TZDs	Antihyperglycemic drugs	PPARγ agonist	Stimulation of fatty acid β-oxidation	Adverse	[106]
Glitazars	Antihyperglycemic drugs	Dual PPARα and PPARγ agonists	Stimulation of fatty acid β-oxidation Inhibition of glucose oxidation	Adverse	[107]
IPE	Lipid-lowering drugs	Hepatic modulation of lipid metabolism and lipid synthesis	Indirect suppression of cardiac fatty acid β-oxidation through lowering circulating fatty acids	Beneficial	[108]
Statins	Lipid-lowering drugs	HMG-CoA reductase inhibitors Enhancement of PGC-1α and activity	Stimulation of mitochondrial biogenesis	Beneficial	[109]
Fibrates	Lipid-lowering drugs	PPARα activator	Enhancement of circulating levels of ketone bodies	Beneficial	[110]
Nicotinic acid	Lipid-lowering drugs	Activator of G-protein-coupled receptor HM74A	De novo NAD+ synthesis Reduction of TAG synthesis	Beneficial	[111]

The cellular mechanisms and the potential cardiometabolic effect of each medication are provided.

Abbreviations: DPP4, dipeptidyl peptidase 4; GLP-1, glucagon-like peptide-1; HMG-CoA, β-Hydroxy β-methylglutaryl-CoA; IPE, icosapent ethyl; PGC-1α, peroxisome proliferator-activated receptor-gamma coactivator; PPARα, peroxisome proliferator-activated receptor-α; SGLT2, sodium-glucose cotransporter 2; TAG, triacylglycerol; TZD, thiazolidinediones.

3.5.1 ANTIHYPERGLYCEMIC DRUGS

Antihyperglycemic drugs lower plasma glucose levels and are commonly used in patients with T2D. However, there is not a direct equivalence of their antihyperglycemic effects to their cardioprotective effects. Some antihyperglycemic drugs, such as SGLT2 inhibitors, have statistically significant effects on CVD risk reduction, despite only having moderate antihyperglycemic effects [112]. While others, such as thiazolidinediones, are more potent at lowering blood glucose levels, yet are associated with increased risks of CV events [113].

3.5.1.1 Metformin

Metformin is the first-line pharmacological therapy for treating/preventing T2D according to published guidelines [114,115]. The main effects of metformin are to inhibit hepatic gluconeogenesis and oppose the action of glucagon, but many other effects have been proposed that altogether contribute to its antihyperglycemic action. Even though metformin improves myocardial energy metabolism and decreases inflammation, systematic reviews and meta-analysis show no demonstrable benefit on heart failure development [116,103]. In cardiomyocytes, metformin potentially activates the action of AMP-activated protein kinase (AMPK), which leads to phosphorylation and inhibition of ACC [117]. Levels of malonyl-CoA are decreased such that the inhibition of fatty acid uptake into the mitochondria is impaired. This could lead to an increase in cardiac fatty acid β-oxidation, which may partially explain the absence of cardioprotective effects by metformin. That being said, animal studies have shown that metformin can improve systolic cardiac function in mice after myocardial infarction by upregulating the expression of SIRT3 and the activity of PGC-1α [118]. Whether metformin could be clinically relevant for treating heart failure by modulating cardiac energy metabolism through activating AMPK is debatable, as studies were done in isolated hearts showing that the AMPK-activating potential of metformin has used non-physiologically relevant concentrations of metformin [117]. That being said, the potential stimulating effect on fatty acid β-oxidation via metformin might be undesirable for cardiac function; thus, its usage in patients with T2D should be interpreted with caution [119].

3.5.1.2 Sodium-Glucose Cotransporter 2 Inhibitors

Sodium-glucose cotransporter 2 inhibitors (SGLT2is) are antihyperglycemic agents that lower plasma glucose levels primarily by inhibiting glucose and sodium reabsorption in the kidneys. To date, there are four SGLT2is that are approved for clinical use: empagliflozin, dapagliflozin, ertugliflozin, and canagliflozin. Of interest, results from several large-scale clinical trials have demonstrated that SGLT2is reduce the overall CV risk, rate of mortality, and rate of hospitalization of heart failure in patients with T2D at high risk of CVD [120], in both patients with heart failure and reduced ejection fraction (HFrEF) with and without T2D [121] and in patients with heart failure with preserved ejection fraction (HFpEF) with and without T2D [122]. The underlying mechanisms to address their associated CV benefits are nicely discussed in the state-of-the-art review by Verma and McMurray [123]. In essence, the cardioprotective effects of SGLT2is can be explained by the following mechanisms:

attenuating cardiac fibrosis, improving cardiac hemodynamics, reducing inflammation (e.g., via the NLRP3 inflammasome), improving ventricular-loading conditions, improving cardiac metabolism, inhibiting myocardial Na^+/H^+ exchange, and altering epicardial adipose tissue mass [101]. SGLT2is can also modulate cardiac energy metabolism through increased ketone oxidation, which leads to an additional source of energy for ATP production [104].

3.5.1.3   Glucagon-Like Peptide-1 Receptor Agonists

Glucagon-like peptide-1 receptor agonists (GLP-1Ras) are used for improving glycemic control in patients with T2D. GLP-1Ras have demonstrated improved CV outcomes in several major clinical trials [124,125]. Meta-analysis of long-acting GLP-1Ras, namely liraglutide, semaglutide, and exenatide long-acting release, shows a prominent reduction in major adverse cardiovascular events (MACE) and non-fatal strokes [126]. Similarly, the double-blind, randomized placebo-controlled Researching Cardiovascular Events with a Weekly Incretin in Diabetes trial also suggests the protective effects of dulaglutide on CV outcomes [127]. The expression of glucagon-like peptide 1 receptors is mostly found in atrial cardiac myocytes and vascular smooth muscle cells and is virtually undetectable within ventricular cardiac myocytes [128,129]. Therefore, the cardioprotection exerted by GLP-Ras is likely mediated through peripheral actions. GLP-1Ras act on the pancreas to stimulate insulin secretion while simultaneously limiting glucagon secretion, which could indirectly affect cardiac energy metabolism through the actions of insulin and glucagon on modulating cardiac glucose oxidation and fatty acid β-oxidation, respectively. This is supported by the observation that GLP-1Ras treatment protects the heart against myocardial infarction induced by permanent left anterior descending coronary artery ligation in mice with atrial-specific glucagon-like peptide 1 receptor deletion, emphasizing that it is the peripheral effect of GLP-1Ras that provide cardioprotective effects [105]. However, this does not rule out the possibility of GLP-1Ras directly modulating cardiac energy metabolism, as a number of studies have demonstrated that the application of native glucagon-like peptide 1 to isolated working hearts can increase the rate of glucose uptake, mimicking the action of insulin [130,131].

3.5.1.4   Dipeptidyl Peptidase 4 Inhibitors

Dipeptidyl peptidase 4 inhibitors (DPP4is) improve glycemic control by preventing the breakdown of native glucagon-like peptide 1. The inhibition of dipeptidyl peptidase 4 preserves the stimulatory action of glucagon-like peptide 1 on pancreatic insulin secretion and concurrent suppressive action on glucagon secretion. Nevertheless, a recent cohort study comparing SGLT2is to DPP4is shows that SGLT2is was associated with a marked lowering of risks for heart failure, myocardial infarction, and stroke as opposed to DPP4is, which failed to demonstrate superiority in CV outcome trials [132,133]. Moreover, several clinical trials have even indicated that one of the DPP4is – saxagliptin – is associated with a significantly increased risk of heart failure [134]. Myocardial energy substrate analysis showed that DPP4is treatment significantly increases glucose uptake as well as fatty acid uptake [104], which may offer explanation to the absence of cardioprotection or worsening of cardiac function exerted by DPPis.

3.5.1.5   Thiazolidinediones

Thiazolidinediones (TZDs) are a class of PPARγ-specific agonists. TZDs function by improving the metabolic control in patients with T2D, thus enabling better insulin sensitivity. However, TZDs are known for causing fluid retention and increasing the risk of developing congestive heart failure [135]. In addition, several major randomized clinical trials have shown that treatment with TZDs can increase the new onset of heart failure, as well as increase the risk of heart failure hospitalization [136]. The question arises as to whether TZDs have direct or indirect effects on cardiac energy metabolism. Studies on rodents demonstrate that the application of pioglitazone can effectively reduce myocardial infarct size through direct stimulation of cardiac PPARγ, PI3K, Akt, and endothelial nitric oxide synthase pathways [107]. However, similar results were not found in isolated cell studies, as direct administration of TZDs to cardiomyocytes did not activate genes involved in fatty acid β-oxidation, suggesting that PPARγ-activating actions of TZDs are more peripheral than directly cardiac [137].

3.5.1.6   Glitazars

Glitazars are dual PPARα and PPARγ agonists. Even though it has been shown that glitazars can improve glycemic control and lipid metabolism in patients with T2D, most investigations of the glitazars have been discontinued due to promoting significant major CV events. Glitazars were found to worsen congestive heart failure when given to patients with T2D and increase the risk of developing heart failure [138]. A possible explanation for the worsening of cardiac function by glitazars is the potential lipotoxicity driven by PPARγ- and PPARα-induced activation of fatty acid uptake and oxidation. Saroglitazar is the only glitazar that is still in clinical development. In a randomized, double-blinded phase III study, treatment of patients with T2D with saroglitazar improved glycemic control and ameliorated lipid parameters, with a significant reduction of CVD risk [139]. Whether saroglitazar mediates these CV effects through the peripheral activation of PPARα and PPARγ, or whether they directly modulate cardiac energy metabolism through stimulating PPARα and PPARγ, remains to be determined. It is worth noting that saroglitazar has been approved in India since 2013 for use in patients with diabetic dyslipidemia and hypertriglyceridemia that cannot be controlled by statin therapy. Since January 2020, saroglitazar has been approved as an add-on therapy to metformin for T2D in India. Shortly afterward, it also received approval as a therapy for non-alcoholic steatohepatitis.

3.5.2   Lipid-Lowering Drugs

Icosapent ethyl (IPE) is an ultra-purified type of omega-3 fatty acid, namely eicosapentaenoic acid (EPA), which is derived from marine oil. Most recently, IPE has been approved as an adjunctive therapy for patients with CVD or diabetes. Of importance, IPE showed a reduction in CV risk that is independent of the TAG-lowering effect, as evidenced by the results from the REDUCE-IT trial [140]. REDUCE-IT was a phase III, double-blinded, randomized, and placebo-controlled trial that recruited patients with established CVD and patients with T2D that are at high risk of developing CVD. Over the span of 5 years of follow-up, the study showed that an intake of IPE (4 g per day) had a 25% relative risk reduction with respect to first primary endpoint events which include CV death, non-fatal myocardial infarction, non-fatal stroke, coronary revascularization, and unstable angina. Secondary analysis of the REDUCE-IT trial shows that, in addition to reducing the risk of primary endpoint events, IPE also reduced the risk of subsequent development of MACE [141]. Sub-analysis of REDUCE-IT also showed that IPE significantly decreased the incidence rate of cardiac arrest and sudden cardiac death. Of interest, the 25% of relative risk reduction of the primary endpoints is much higher when compared with the only 20% reduction of TAG, suggesting that IPE conveys cardioprotective effects beyond lowering TAG. Even though REDUCE-IT produced promising results for the use of IPE as a therapeutic approach to reduce CV risk, the exact mechanisms remain unclear. With the data collected so far, it is believed that IPE is converted to EPA by lipase, which then enters the circulation in the form of chylomicrons. EPA and its downstream metabolites contribute to the anti-inflammatory, anti-thrombotic, and plaque stabilization effects that all together lower CV events [108].

3.5.2.1 Statins

Statins are cholesterol-lowering drugs that have been used extensively in patients to prevent or lower the risk of strokes and heart attacks. Besides the effectiveness of statins in reducing plasma cholesterol, they also have pleiotropic effects, including but not limited to improving endothelial cell function, decreasing platelet aggregation, decreasing inflammation, increasing neovascularization of ischemic tissues, increasing plaque stability, and increasing endothelial progenitor cells [142]. Statins are useful in reducing the risk of CV events as a primary prevention [143]. Similarly, statins can lower the incidence of MI as a secondary prevention method for those who have established heart disease [144]. However, one of the side effects of statins is an increased risk of developing diabetes, as both insulin production and sensitivity are impaired in a dose-dependent manner. Interestingly, statins can activate PGC-1α and stimulate gene expression of acyl-CoA oxidase, CPT1a, and PDK4, leading to an elevation of fatty acid β-oxidation and simultaneous suppression of glucose oxidation in the liver [145]. Whether statins can directly regulate energy metabolism in cardiomyocytes by activating PGC1-α is unclear.

3.5.2.2 Fibrates

Fibrates activate PPARα, a transcription factor that regulates lipid metabolism in the liver, adipose tissues, kidneys, heart, and skeletal muscle. Fibrates stimulate fatty acid ß-oxidation by regulating gene expression of key enzymes involved in fatty acid utilization, which is beneficial in lowering plasma lipid levels. However, the use of fibrates should be considered with caution, as the expression of PPARα is upregulated in diabetic cardiomyopathy [35]. Activation of PPARα can induce metabolic derangements in the heart by stimulating genes involved in fatty acid utilization, while simultaneously suppressing genes involved in glucose metabolism. These direct perturbations on cardiac glucose and fatty acid oxidation may predispose the heart to cardiac dysfunction.

3.5.2.3 Nicotinic Acid

Nicotinic acid can lower plasma cholesterol by acting on the orphan receptor HM74A to reduce TAG synthesis in the liver, inhibit lipolysis of TAG in adipose tissues, and increase the formation of high-density lipoprotein. The study has suggested that nicotinic acid can lower the risk of atherosclerosis progression and CVD [111]. The use of nicotinic acid could potentially benefit cardiac function by stimulating the *de novo* synthesis of NAD^+, such that the activity of deacetylases, such as SIRT3, is stimulated. Decreasing acetylation could potentially lower fatty acid ß-oxidation, thus restoring the balance between glucose and fatty acid oxidation in the heart. However, it should be acknowledged that in cardiomyocytes, NAD^+ is mainly generated through the salvage pathways that recycle nicotinamide mononucleotide by NAD-consuming enzymes. As such, the significance of nicotinic acid in directly stimulating cardiac *de novo* NAD^+ synthesis in improving cardiac function is unclear.

3.5.3 DRUGS THAT INHIBIT FATTY ACID β-OXIDATION

3.5.3.1 CPT1 Inhibitors

One possible approach to suppress the escalated fatty acid β-oxidation is to inhibit CPT1, a key enzyme involved in mitochondrial fatty acid uptake (Figure 3.4). There have been two clinically approved CPT1 inhibitors for treating heart failure: etomoxir and perhexiline. Both etomoxir and perhexiline have been shown to improve cardiac function in patients with heart failure [146,147]. Consistent with this, perhexiline also improves cardiac energetics in patients with symptomatic hypertrophic cardiomyopathy. Nonetheless, neither etomoxir nor perhexiline offers clinical significance due to the potential hepatotoxicity and peripheral neuropathy. One possible explanation for these toxicities, as well as their limitation in moving forward, is that both etomoxir and perhexiline are irreversible CPT1 inhibitors. Sustained or permanent inhibition of CPT1 is undesirable as the fatty acid β-oxidation contributes to a heavy portion of total cardiac ATP production. Hence, excessive inhibition of fatty acid transport into the mitochondria would impair cardiac energetics.

3.5.3.2 Fatty Acid ß-Oxidation Inhibitors

Trimetazidine directly suppresses fatty acid β-oxidation by inhibiting long-chain 3-ketoacyl-CoA thiolase, the last enzyme of fatty acid β-oxidation. It is primarily used as an anti-anginal agent by switching myocardial substrate utilization from fatty acid β-oxidation to glucose oxidation [148]. A small clinical trial shows that trimetazidine improves left ventricular ejection fraction and cardiac diastolic function in patients with heart failure, with simultaneous improvement in the quality of life and exercise capacity [149]. The positive effects of trimetazidine are accompanied by the preservation of cardiac high-energy phosphates [150].

3.5.4 DRUGS THAT STIMULATE GLUCOSE OXIDATION

As cardiac glucose oxidation is suppressed in T2D and obesity, stimulating glucose oxidation could be a potential approach for correcting cardiac energetics. PDH is the rate-limiting enzyme for mitochondrial glucose oxidation that converts pyruvate to acetyl-CoA. The activity of PDH is modulated by PDH kinase (PDK), which can phosphorylate and inhibit the action of PDH. Dichloroacetate (DCA) is a PDK inhibitor that increases myocardial glucose oxidation by preventing the inhibitory action of PDK [151]. Experimental studies showed that DCA improves the functional recovery of the heart post-ischemia and re-establishes the coupling of glucose oxidation and glycolysis, thus preventing ion accumulation and adverse remodeling of the heart [152]. In addition, DCA improves heart function in heart failure by increasing energy reserves [153]. Clinical data support the experimental studies, as patients with coronary heart disease have enhanced myocardial efficiency and higher stroke volume with intravenous DCA administration [154]. Acute DCA administration also improves heart function in patients with heart failure, potentially by skewing the heart toward glucose oxidation [155]. However, the short half-life and poor pharmacokinetic properties of DCA limit its clinical usefulness.

3.5.5   POTENTIAL FUTURE THERAPEUTIC APPROACHES

3.5.5.1   Inhibition of Myocardial Fatty Acid Uptake

Inhibition of fatty acid uptake at the level of sarcolemma is promising because it not only limits fatty acid β-oxidation but could also impede the occurrence of lipotoxicity from an early step. Therefore, inhibition of fatty acid uptake at the sarcolemma could reverse the cardiac metabolic dysregulation observed in T2D and obesity. One of the most important transporters for sarcolemma fatty acid uptake is CD36 (Figure 3.4). CD36 accounts for approximately 50% of the fatty acids transported into the myocardium [156]. One molecule that can inhibit CD36 is sulfo-N-succinimidyl-oleate (SSO). The use of SSO in experimental studies indicates its effectiveness in suppressing fatty acid uptake with a secondary effect of increasing glucose oxidation in post-ischemic hearts [157]. Whether this could be applied to humans has yet to be determined.

3.5.5.2   Reversible CPT1 Inhibition

As discussed, fatty acid transport inhibition of CPT1 inhibition could potentially decrease fatty acid ß-oxidation in obesity and T2D. However, existing CPT1 inhibitors have limited clinical applicability as they irreversibly inhibit CPT1. Irreversible inhibition of fatty acid β-oxidation is less than desirable since fatty acids are a major source of fuel for the heart and the use of irreversible CPT1 inhibitors may impose the risk of cardiac energy shortage. With that in mind, a reversible CPT1 inhibitor could avoid this problem. However, data on reversible CPT1 inhibitors use in CMBCD is lacking.

Another approach to reversibly inhibit CPT1 is to raise myocardial levels of malonyl-CoA, a potent endogenous inhibitor of CPT1. This can be achieved by inhibiting MCD, which degrades malonyl-CoA to acetyl-CoA. Therefore, inhibition of MCD could be a potential way for increasing cardiac levels of malonyl-CoA, thus reversibly suppressing fatty acid uptake into the mitochondria. Experimental studies in ischemia/reperfusion and heart failure animal models have shown that MCD inhibitors can improve functional recovery during ischemia/reperfusion, reduce the infarct size, and decrease the severity of heart failure [7,158]. These benefits of MCD inhibitors can be explained by the primary effect of decreasing fatty acid β-oxidation, as well as the secondary effect of increasing glucose oxidation.

3.5.5.3 Potent Stimulators of Glucose Oxidation

As discussed, inhibition of PDK is a promising approach for stimulating cardiac glucose oxidation and treating T2D and obesity. However, more potent PDK inhibitors are needed, with better pharmacokinetics than DCA. While newer PDK inhibitors have been developed, the clinical applicability of these newer PDK inhibitors in treating CMBCD has yet to be determined.

3.5.5.4 Stimulation of Ketone Oxidation

Ketone bodies are an important contributor to energy production in the heart and with oxidation may provide an additional source of fuel for the energetically deprived heart. An increase in ketone oxidation in heart failure also appears to be an adaptive process [159,160]. This is supported by clinical data where an acute intravenous infusion of ketone bodies improves cardiac function in patients with heart failure [159]. However, it should be recognized that even though ketone bodies can be readily used by the heart, ketone bodies are not the most efficient source of energy, as the P/O ratio (phosphate/oxygen ratio) for glucose is higher than that for ketone bodies [9]. That being said, increasing ketone body supply to the heart still has the potential as a metabolic-modulating approach for treating heart diseases.

There are several established ways to increase circulating ketone bodies, such as using ketone esters, SGLTis, or implementing ketogenic diets. Even though the administration of ketone esters has the potential in treating heart failure [161], its applicability for chronic use is still unknown. On the other hand, the use of SGLT2is is a promising approach to increase the plasma levels of ketone bodies and stimulate cardiac ketone oxidation. SGLT2is can stimulate hepatic ketogenesis, thereby increasing circulating levels of ketone bodies, leading to increased cardiac ketone oxidation and improved cardiac energy metabolism.

Another approach to increase circulating ketone levels is through administering a ketogenic diet, a diet composed of a high amount of fat and protein but with minimal carbohydrates. However, ketogenic diets *per se* are not well tolerated in patients with heart failure [162]. That being said, clinical studies have shown that a ketogenic diet can improve insulin resistance, as well as cardiac function and metabolism in patients with T2D. A recently published systematic review summarized a total of nine studies with 734 patients with T2D regarding the efficacy of ketogenic diets. It showed that a short-term ketogenic diet could lower the Hemoglobin (A1c) as well as plasma TAG [92]. A systematic review that analyzed the efficacy of a very-low-calorie ketogenic diet in patients with obesity showed a reduction in BMI, a lowering of plasma TAG and cholesterol, an improved glucose tolerance, as well as reduced systolic and diastolic blood pressure, thus suggesting benefits in the management of obesity [93].

Despite the potential benefits of enhancing cardiac ketone oxidation, using a ketogenic diet as a way to increase ketone supply to the heart is questionable, as studies have found minimal benefits on cardiac function in heart failure [159]. One possible explanation for this might be that ketogenic diets are composed of a high amount of fat. The resulting elevated circulating fatty acids could potentially induce higher uptake and oxidation of fatty acids in the heart. Another major concern with ketogenic diets is the risk of inducing ketosis. Interestingly, the level of circulating ketone body concentrations does not always correlate with that of the myocardial ketone oxidation rate. While ketogenic diets could raise circulating ketone levels, a chronic ketotic environment may elicit compensatory changes in the heart to adjust to the surplus of circulating ketone bodies [163].

3.5.5.5 Stimulation of BCAA Oxidation

Even though BCAA oxidation only accounts for 1%–2% of total cardiac ATP production, BCAAs are important signaling molecules. There is a strong positive relationship between the level of circulating BCAAs and whole-body insulin resistance in both T1D and T2D. By activating the mammalian/mechanistic target of rapamycin, BCAAs impair insulin signaling by phosphorylating IRS1 via p70S6 kinase [164]. In the failing heart, BCAA accumulation in the myocardium is significant, which is in part due to impaired BCAA oxidation [165]. The accumulation of branched-chain α-keto acids (BCKAs), the by-products of BCAAs, also contributes to cardiac insulin resistance [166]. In animal models of heart failure with pressure overload and post-myocardial infarction injury, lowering BCAA and BCKA levels by stimulating BCAA oxidation is cardioprotective, as evidenced by improved heart function and reduced infarct size [165,167]. Therefore, pharmacological approaches that aim to stimulate cardiac BCAA oxidation to restore cardiac function should be investigated in future studies.

3.6   BARIATRIC PROCEDURES

Bariatric surgery has been used in the clinical setting to induce weight loss and glycemic control in patients with severe obesity with or without poorly controlled T2D. Dietary and/or exercise interventions are difficult to sustain over time, and many patients regain the weight after a few months. As such, bariatric surgery may be useful and more applicable for long-term weight loss. The study shows that around 80% of patients can be resolved of obesity- and/or diabetes-related complications following surgery, emphasizing its effectiveness [168]. Of importance, bariatric surgery can improve cardiac function, ameliorate left ventricular hypertrophy, and lower the left ventricular mass. A large clinical trial analyzing the long-term, approximately 15 years, CV benefits of bariatric surgery in patients with severe obesity showed a significant reduction in the incidence of CV deaths and frequency of myocardial infarction or stroke [169]. The follow-up STAMPEDE trial suggests that for patients with T2D, bariatric surgery plus intensive medical therapy has a much greater reduction in A1c levels than in patients who received intensive medical therapy alone [170,171].

Interestingly, the cardioprotective effects of bariatric surgery are independent of weight loss. Several proposed mechanisms include, but are not limited to, enhanced insulin sensitivity, altered bile acid concentrations, altered enteric gut hormone and microbiota, increased metabolic activity of brown adipose tissues, and improved intestinal glucose metabolism [95]. These metabolic alterations induced by bariatric surgery occur almost instantaneously after surgery, which together assist in improving insulin sensitivity and glucose metabolism. Modification of cardiac energy metabolism by bariatric surgery may also play an important role. Using 1H nuclear magnetic resonance spectroscopy and ultra-performance liquid chromatography–mass spectroscopy, global metabolite alterations induced by bariatric surgery were characterized in male Wistar rats undergoing the Roux-en-Y gastric operation [172]. This study found a global enhancement of cardiac energy metabolism, emphasizing that the cardioprotective effects of bariatric surgery can be partially attributed to the improvement in cardiac energetics.

3.7   CONCLUDING REMARKS

Altered cardiac energy metabolism plays an indispensable role in the development of cardiac dysfunction induced by either obesity or T2D. Both metabolic drivers for CVD share the common denominator: insulin resistance. Understanding the metabolic disturbances that occur at the level of the heart can offer insights into both the pathogenesis of CMBCD, as well as identifying novel therapeutic strategies, particularly in lifestyle medicine. In obesity and T2D, the heart shows increased fatty acid β-oxidation rates, with concurrent suppression of glucose oxidation rates. These disturbances of cardiac metabolism are attributed to the combinational effects of various cellular mechanisms. Targeting cardiac energy metabolism and optimizing the metabolic profile of the heart are potential approaches to reverse and/or prevent the occurrence of cardiac dysfunction induced by metabolic drivers such as obesity and T2D.

REFERENCES

1. Mechanick JI, Farkouh ME, Newman JD, Garvey WT: Cardiometabolic-based chronic disease, adiposity and dysglycemia drivers: JACC state-of-the-art review. *Journal of the American College of Cardiology* 2020, 75(5):525–538.
2. Mechanick JI, Hurley DL, Garvey WT: Adiposity-based chronic disease as a new diagnostic term: the American Association of Clinical Endocrinologists and American College of Endocrinology position statement. *Endocrine Practice* 2017, 23(3):372–378.
3. Mechanick JI, Garber AJ, Grunberger G, Handelsman Y, Garvey WT: Dysglycemia-based chronic disease: an American Association of Clinical Endocrinologists position statement. *Endocrine Practice* 2018, 24(11):995–1011.
4. Catalano PM: Obesity, insulin resistance and pregnancy outcome. *Reproduction* 2010, 140(3):365.
5. Gast KB, Tjeerdema N, Stijnen T, Smit JW, Dekkers OM: Insulin resistance and risk of incident cardiovascular events in adults without diabetes: meta-analysis. *PLoS One* 2012, 7(12):e52036.
6. Lopaschuk GD, Ussher JR, Folmes CD, Jaswal JS, Stanley WC: Myocardial fatty acid metabolism in health and disease. *Physiological Reviews* 2010, 90(1):207–258.
7. Allard M, Schonekess B, Henning S, English D, Lopaschuk GD: Contribution of oxidative metabolism and glycolysis to ATP production in hypertrophied hearts. *American Journal of Physiology-Heart and Circulatory Physiology* 1994, 267(2):H742–H750.
8. Karwi QG, Biswas D, Pulinilkunnil T, Lopaschuk GD: Myocardial ketones metabolism in heart failure. *Journal of Cardiac Failure* 2020, 26(11):998–1005.

9. Ho KL, Karwi QG, Wagg C, Zhang L, Vo K, Altamimi T, Uddin GM, Ussher JR, Lopaschuk GD: Ketones can become the major fuel source for the heart but do not increase cardiac efficiency. *Cardiovascular Research* 2021, 117(4):1178–1187.

10. Fillmore N, Wagg CS, Zhang L, Fukushima A, Lopaschuk GD: Cardiac branched-chain amino acid oxidation is reduced during insulin resistance in the heart. *American Journal of Physiology-Endocrinology and Metabolism* 2018, 315(5):E1046–E1052.

11. Karwi QG, Uddin GM, Ho KL, Lopaschuk GD: Loss of metabolic flexibility in the failing heart. *Frontiers in Cardiovascular Medicine* 2018, 5:68.

12. Ruderman N, Chisholm D, Pi-Sunyer X, Schneider S: The metabolically obese, normal-weight individual revisited. *Diabetes* 1998, 47(5):699–713.

13. Ho KL, Zhang L, Wagg C, Al Batran R, Gopal K, Levasseur J, Leone T, Dyck JR, Ussher JR, Muoio DM: Increased ketone body oxidation provides additional energy for the failing heart without improving cardiac efficiency. *Cardiovascular Research* 2019, 115(11):1606–1616.

14. Guo F, Moellering DR, Garvey WT: The progression of cardiometabolic disease: validation of a new cardiometabolic disease staging system applicable to obesity. *Obesity* 2014, 22(1):110–118.

15. Guo F, Garvey WT: Trends in cardiovascular health metrics in obese adults: National Health and Nutrition Examination Survey (NHANES), 1988–2014. *Journal of the American Heart Association* 2016, 5(7):e003619.

16. Lara-Castro C, Garvey WT: Diet, insulin resistance, and obesity: zoning in on data for Atkins dieters living in South Beach. *The Journal of Clinical Endocrinology & Metabolism* 2004, 89(9):4197–4205.

17. Lopaschuk GD, Folmes CD, Stanley WC: Cardiac energy metabolism in obesity. *Circulation Research* 2007, 101(4):335–347.

18. Peterson LR, Herrero P, Schechtman KB, Racette SB, Waggoner AD, Kisrieva-Ware Z, Dence C, Klein S, Marsala J, Meyer T: Effect of obesity and insulin resistance on myocardial substrate metabolism and efficiency in young women. *Circulation* 2004, 109(18):2191–2196.

19. Koutsari C, Jensen MD: Thematic review series: patient-oriented research. Free fatty acid metabolism in human obesity. *Journal of Lipid Research* 2006, 47(8):1643–1650.

20. Karwi QG, Ho KL, Pherwani S, Ketema EB, Sun QY, Lopaschuk GD: Concurrent diabetes and heart failure: interplay and novel therapeutic approaches. *Cardiovascular Research* 2021;118(3):686–715.

21. Peterson LR, Saeed IM, McGill JB, Herrero P, Schechtman KB, Gunawardena R, Recklein CL, Coggan AR, DeMoss AJ, Dence CS: Sex and type 2 diabetes: obesity-independent effects on left ventricular substrate metabolism and relaxation in humans. *Obesity* 2012, 20(4):802–810.

22. Rijzewijk LJ, van der Meer RW, Lamb HJ, de Jong HW, Lubberink M, Romijn JA, Bax JJ, de Roos A, Twisk JW, Heine RJ: Altered myocardial substrate metabolism and decreased diastolic function in nonischemic human diabetic cardiomyopathy: studies with cardiac positron emission tomography and magnetic resonance imaging. *Journal of the American College of Cardiology* 2009, 54(16):1524–1532.

23. Camps M, Castello A, Munoz P, Monfar M, Testar X, Palacin M, Zorzano A: Effect of diabetes and fasting on GLUT-4 (muscle/fat) glucose-transporter expression in insulin-sensitive tissues. Heterogeneous response in heart, red and white muscle. *Biochemical Journal* 1992, 282(3):765–772.

24. Bockus LB, Matsuzaki S, Vadvalkar SS, Young ZT, Giorgione JR, Newhardt MF, Kinter M, Humphries KM: Cardiac insulin signaling regulates glycolysis through phosphofructokinase 2 content and activity. *Journal of the American Heart Association* 2017, 6(12):e007159.

25. Randle P, Garland P, Hales C, Newsholme E: The glucose fatty-acid cycle its role in insulin sensitivity and the metabolic disturbances of diabetes mellitus. *The Lancet* 1963, 281(7285):785–789.

26. Wall SR, Lopaschuk GD: Glucose oxidation rates in fatty acid-perfused isolated working hearts from diabetic rats. *Biochimica et Biophysica Acta (BBA)-Lipids and Lipid Metabolism* 1989, 1006(1):97–103.

27. Luiken JJ, Arumugam Y, Dyck DJ, Bell RC, Pelsers MM, Turcotte LP, Tandon NN, Glatz JF, Bonen A: Increased rates of fatty acid uptake and plasmalemmal fatty acid transporters in obese Zucker rats. *Journal of Biological Chemistry* 2001, 276(44):40567–40573.

28. Carley A, Atkinson L, Bonen A, Harper M-E, Kunnathu S, Lopaschuk G, Severson D: Mechanisms responsible for enhanced fatty acid utilization by perfused hearts from type 2 diabetic db/db mice. *Archives of Physiology and Biochemistry* 2007, 113(2):65–75.

29. Coort SL, Hasselbaink DM, Koonen DP, Willems J, Coumans WA, Chabowski A, van der Vusse GJ, Bonen A, Glatz JF, Luiken JJ: Enhanced sarcolemmal FAT/CD36 content and triacylglycerol storage in cardiac myocytes from obese zucker rats. *Diabetes* 2004, 53(7):1655–1663.

30. Karwi QG, Sun Q, Lopaschuk GD: The contribution of cardiac fatty acid oxidation to diabetic cardiomyopathy severity. *Cells* 2021, 10(11):3259.

31. Finck BN, Lehman JJ, Leone TC, Welch MJ, Bennett MJ, Kovacs A, Han X, Gross RW, Kozak R, Lopaschuk GD: The cardiac phenotype induced by PPARα overexpression mimics that caused by diabetes mellitus. *The Journal of Clinical Investigation* 2002, 109(1):121–130.

32. Lasheras J, Vilà M, Zamora M, Riu E, Pardo R, Poncelas M, Cases I, Ruiz-Meana M, Hernández C, Feliu JE: Gene expression profiling in hearts of diabetic mice uncovers a potential role of estrogen-related receptor γ in diabetic cardiomyopathy. *Molecular and Cellular Endocrinology* 2016, 430:77–88.

33. Finck BN, Han X, Courtois M, Aimond F, Nerbonne JM, Kovacs A, Gross RW, Kelly DP: A critical role for PPARα-mediated lipotoxicity in the pathogenesis of diabetic cardiomyopathy: modulation by dietary fat content. *Proceedings of the National Academy of Sciences* 2003, 100(3):1226–1231.

34. Gilde AJ, van der Lee KA, Willemsen PH, Chinetti G, van der Leij FR, van der Vusse GJ, Staels B, van Bilsen M: Peroxisome proliferator-activated receptor (PPAR) α and PPARβ/δ, but not PPARγ, modulate the expression of genes involved in cardiac lipid metabolism. *Circulation Research* 2003, 92(5):518–524.

35. Buchanan J, Mazumder PK, Hu P, Chakrabarti G, Roberts MW, Yun UJ, Cooksey RC, Litwin SE, Abel ED: Reduced cardiac efficiency and altered substrate metabolism precedes the onset of hyperglycemia and contractile dysfunction in two mouse models of insulin resistance and obesity. *Endocrinology* 2005, 146(12):5341–5349.

36. Huss JM, Torra IP, Staels B, Giguere V, Kelly DP: Estrogen-related receptor α directs peroxisome proliferator-activated receptor α signaling in the transcriptional control of energy metabolism in cardiac and skeletal muscle. *Molecular and Cellular Biology* 2004, 24(20):9079–9091.

37. Dyck JR, Lopaschuk GD: Malonyl CoA control of fatty acid oxidation in the ischemic heart. *Journal of Molecular and Cellular Cardiology* 2002, 34(9):1099–1109.

38. Sakamoto J, Barr RL, Kavanagh KM, Lopaschuk GD: Contribution of malonyl-CoA decarboxylase to the high fatty acid oxidation rates seen in the diabetic heart. *American Journal of Physiology-Heart and Circulatory Physiology* 2000, 278(4):H1196–H1204.

39. Young ME, Goodwin GW, Ying J, Guthrie P, Wilson CR, Laws FA, Taegtmeyer H: Regulation of cardiac and skeletal muscle malonyl-CoA decarboxylase by fatty acids. *American Journal of Physiology-Endocrinology and Metabolism* 2001, 280(3): E471–E479.

40. Campbell FM, Kozak R, Wagner A, Altarejos JY, Dyck JR, Belke DD, Severson DL, Kelly DP, Lopaschuk GD: A role for peroxisome proliferator-activated receptor α (PPARα) in the control of cardiac malonyl-CoA levels: reduced fatty acid oxidation rates and increased glucose oxidation rates in the hearts of mice lacking PPARα are associated with higher concentrations of malonyl-CoA and reduced expression of malonyl-CoA decarboxylase. *Journal of Biological Chemistry* 2002, 277(6):4098–4103.

41. Mazumder PK, O'Neill BT, Roberts MW, Buchanan J, Yun UJ, Cooksey RC, Boudina S, Abel ED: Impaired cardiac efficiency and increased fatty acid oxidation in insulin-resistant *ob/ob* mouse hearts. *Diabetes* 2004, 53(9):2366–2374.

42. Woldegiorgis G, Yousufzai S, Shrago E: Studies on the interaction of palmitoyl coenzyme A with the adenine nucleotide translocase. *Journal of Biological Chemistry* 1982, 257(24):14783–14787.

43. Vettor R, Fabris R, Serra R, Lombardi A, Tonello C, Granzotto M, Marzolo M, Carruba M, Ricquier D, Federspil G: Changes in FAT/CD36, UCP2, UCP3 and GLUT4 gene expression during lipid infusion in rat skeletal and heart muscle. *International Journal of Obesity* 2002, 26(6):838–847.

44. Costantino S, Mohammed SA, Ambrosini S, Paneni F: Epigenetic processing in cardiometabolic disease. *Atherosclerosis* 2019, 281:150–158.

45. Holoch D, Moazed D: RNA-mediated epigenetic regulation of gene expression. *Nature Reviews Genetics* 2015, 16(2):71–84.

46. Matzke MA, Mosher RA: RNA-directed DNA methylation: an epigenetic pathway of increasing complexity. *Nature Reviews Genetics* 2014, 15(6):394–408.

47. Meder B, Haas J, Sedaghat-Hamedani F, Kayvanpour E, Frese K, Lai A, Nietsch R, Scheiner C, Mester S, Bordalo DM: Epigenome-wide association study identifies cardiac gene patterning and a novel class of biomarkers for heart failure. *Circulation* 2017, 136(16):1528–1544.

48. Pepin ME, Ha C-M, Crossman DK, Litovsky SH, Varambally S, Barchue JP, Pamboukian SV, Diakos NA, Drakos SG, Pogwizd SM: Genome-wide DNA methylation encodes cardiac transcriptional reprogramming in human ischemic heart failure. *Laboratory Investigation* 2019, 99(3):371–386.

49. Leung A, Parks BW, Du J, Trac C, Setten R, Chen Y, Brown K, Lusis AJ, Natarajan R, Schones DE: Open chromatin profiling in mice livers reveals unique chromatin variations induced by high fat diet. *Journal of Biological Chemistry* 2014, 289(34):23557–23567.

50. Knutson SK, Chyla BJ, Amann JM, Bhaskara S, Huppert SS, Hiebert SW: Liver-specific deletion of histone deacetylase 3 disrupts metabolic transcriptional networks. *The EMBO Journal* 2008, 27(7):1017–1028.

51. Martin-Mateos R, De Assuncao TM, Arab JP, Jalan-Sakrikar N, Yaqoob U, Greuter T, Verma VK, Mathison AJ, Cao S, Lomberk G: Enhancer of zeste homologue 2 inhibition attenuates TGF-β dependent hepatic stellate cell activation and liver fibrosis. *Cellular and Molecular Gastroenterology and Hepatology* 2019, 7(1):197–209.

52. Control D, Trial C: Intensive diabetes treatment and cardiovascular outcomes in type 1 diabetes: the DCCT/EDIC study 30-year follow-up. *Diabetes Care* 2016, 39(5):686–693.

53. Agrawal L, Azad N, Bahn GD, Ge L, Reaven PD, Hayward RA, Reda DJ, Emanuele NV: Long-term follow-up of intensive glycaemic control on renal outcomes in the Veterans Affairs Diabetes Trial (VADT). *Diabetologia* 2018, 61(2):295–299.

54. Karwi QG, Jörg AR, Lopaschuk GD: Allosteric, transcriptional and post-translational control of mitochondrial energy metabolism. *Biochemical Journal* 2019, 476(12):1695–1712.

55. Lai L, Leone TC, Keller MP, Martin OJ, Broman AT, Nigro J, Kapoor K, Koves TR, Stevens R, Ilkayeva OR: Energy metabolic reprogramming in the hypertrophied and early stage failing heart: a multisystems approach. *Circulation: Heart Failure* 2014, 7(6):1022–1031.

56. Alrob OA, Sankaralingam S, Ma C, Wagg CS, Fillmore N, Jaswal JS, Sack MN, Lehner R, Gupta MP, Michelakis ED: Obesity-induced lysine acetylation increases cardiac fatty acid oxidation and impairs insulin signalling. *Cardiovascular Research* 2014, 103(4):485–497.

57. Hirschey MD, Shimazu T, Goetzman E, Jing E, Schwer B, Lombard DB, Grueter CA, Harris C, Biddinger S, Ilkayeva OR: SIRT3 regulates mitochondrial fatty-acid oxidation by reversible enzyme deacetylation. *Nature* 2010, 464(7285):121–125.

58. Fukushima A, Lopaschuk GD: Acetylation control of cardiac fatty acid β-oxidation and energy metabolism in obesity, diabetes, and heart failure. *Biochimica et Biophysica Acta (BBA)-Molecular Basis of Disease* 2016, 1862(12):2211–2220.

59. Sankaralingam S, Alrob OA, Zhang L, Jaswal JS, Wagg CS, Fukushima A, Padwal RS, Johnstone DE, Sharma AM, Lopaschuk GD: Lowering body weight in obese mice with diastolic heart failure improves cardiac insulin sensitivity and function: implications for the obesity paradox. *Diabetes* 2015, 64(5):1643–1657.

60. Vazquez EJ, Berthiaume JM, Kamath V, Achike O, Buchanan E, Montano MM, Chandler MP, Miyagi M, Rosca MG: Mitochondrial complex I defect and increased fatty acid oxidation enhance protein lysine acetylation in the diabetic heart. *Cardiovascular Research* 2015, 107(4):453–465.

61. Pillai VB, Samant S, Sundaresan NR, Raghuraman H, Kim G, Bonner MY, Arbiser JL, Walker DI, Jones DP, Gius D: Honokiol blocks and reverses cardiac hypertrophy in mice by activating mitochondrial Sirt3. *Nature Communications* 2015, 6(1):1–16.

62. Ingelsson E, Sundström J, Ärnlöv J, Zethelius B, Lind L: Insulin resistance and risk of congestive heart failure. *JAMA* 2005, 294(3):334–341.

63. Ussher JR, Koves TR, Jaswal JS, Zhang L, Ilkayeva O, Dyck JR, Muoio DM, Lopaschuk GD: Insulin-stimulated cardiac glucose oxidation is increased in high-fat diet–induced obese mice lacking malonyl CoA decarboxylase. *Diabetes* 2009, 58(8):1766–1775.

64. Karwi QG, Wagg CS, Altamimi TR, Uddin GM, Ho KL, Darwesh AM, Seubert JM, Lopaschuk GD: Insulin directly stimulates mitochondrial glucose oxidation in the heart. *Cardiovascular Diabetology* 2020, 19(1):1–14.

65. Saotome M, Ikoma T, Hasan P, Maekawa Y: Cardiac insulin resistance in heart failure: the role of mitochondrial dynamics. *International Journal of Molecular Sciences* 2019, 20(14):3552.

66. Condorelli G, Morisco C, Latronico MV, Claudio PP, Dent P, Tsichlis P, Condorelli G, Frati G, Drusco A, Croce CM: TNF-α signal transduction in rat neonatal cardiac myocytes: definition of pathways generating from the TNF-α receptor. *The FASEB Journal* 2002, 16(13):1732–1737.

67. Aguirre V, Uchida T, Yenush L, Davis R, White MF: The c-Jun NH2-terminal kinase promotes insulin resistance during association with insulin receptor substrate-1 and phosphorylation of Ser307. *Journal of Biological Chemistry* 2000, 275(12):9047–9054.

68. Zlobine I, Gopal K, Ussher JR: Lipotoxicity in obesity and diabetes-related cardiac dysfunction. *Biochimica et Biophysica Acta (BBA)-Molecular and Cell Biology of Lipids* 2016, 1861(10):1555–1568.

69. Ouwens D, Diamant M, Fodor M, Habets D, Pelsers M, El Hasnaoui M, Dang Z, Van den Brom C, Vlasblom R, Rietdijk A: Cardiac contractile dysfunction in insulin-resistant rats fed a high-fat diet is associated with elevated CD36-mediated fatty acid uptake and esterification. *Diabetologia* 2007, 50(9):1938–1948.

70. Forcheron F, Basset A, Abdallah P, Del Carmine P, Gadot N, Beylot M: Diabetic cardiomyopathy: effects of fenofibrate and metformin in an experimental model–the Zucker diabetic rat. *Cardiovascular Diabetology* 2009, 8(1):1–13.

71. Li Y, Soos TJ, Li X, Wu J, DeGennaro M, Sun X, Littman DR, Birnbaum MJ, Polakiewicz RD: Protein kinase C θ inhibits insulin signaling by phosphorylating IRS1 at Ser1101. *Journal of Biological Chemistry* 2004, 279(44):45304–45307.

72. Lopaschuk GD, Karwi QG, Tian R, Wende AR, Abel ED: Cardiac energy metabolism in heart failure. *Circulation Research* 2021, 128(10):1487–1513.

73. Zhang Y, Taufalele PV, Cochran JD, Robillard-Frayne I, Marx JM, Soto J, Rauckhorst AJ, Tayyari F, Pewa AD, Gray LR: Mitochondrial pyruvate carriers are required for myocardial stress adaptation. *Nature Metabolism* 2020, 2(11):1248–1264.

74. Umapathi P, Mesubi OO, Banerjee PS, Abrol N, Wang Q, Luczak ED, Wu Y, Granger JM, Wei A-C, Reyes Gaido OE: Excessive O-GlcNAcylation causes heart failure and sudden death. *Circulation* 2021, 143(17):1687–1703.

75. Lunde IG, Aronsen JM, Kvaløy H, Qvigstad E, Sjaastad I, Tønnessen T, Christensen G, Grønning-Wang LM, Carlson CR: Cardiac O-GlcNAc signaling is increased in hypertrophy and heart failure. *Physiological Genomics* 2012, 44(2):162–172.

76. Wang Z, Nakayama T: Inflammation, a link between obesity and cardiovascular disease. *Mediators of Inflammation* 2010, 2010:535918.

77. Fried SK, Bunkin DA, Greenberg AS: Omental and subcutaneous adipose tissues of obese subjects release interleukin-6: depot difference and regulation by glucocorticoid. *The Journal of Clinical Endocrinology & Metabolism* 1998, 83(3):847–850.

78. Keaney Jr JF, Larson MG, Vasan RS, Wilson PW, Lipinska I, Corey D, Massaro JM, Sutherland P, Vita JA, Benjamin EJ: Obesity and systemic oxidative stress: clinical correlates of oxidative stress in the Framingham Study. *Arteriosclerosis, Thrombosis, and Vascular Biology* 2003, 23(3):434–439.

79. Sharma A, Tate M, Mathew G, Vince JE, Ritchie RH, De Haan JB: Oxidative stress and NLRP3-inflammasome activity as significant drivers of diabetic cardiovascular complications: therapeutic implications. *Frontiers in Physiology* 2018, 9:114.

80. Lee H-M, Kim J-J, Kim HJ, Shong M, Ku BJ, Jo E-K: Upregulated NLRP3 inflammasome activation in patients with type 2 diabetes. *Diabetes* 2013, 62(1):194–204.

81. Butts B, Gary RA, Dunbar SB, Butler J: The importance of NLRP3 inflammasome in heart failure. *Journal of Cardiac Failure* 2015, 21(7):586–593.

82. McCay CM, Crowell MF, Maynard LA: The effect of retarded growth upon the length of life span and upon the ultimate body size: one figure. *The Journal of Nutrition* 1935, 10(1):63–79.

83. Takatsu M, Nakashima C, Takahashi K, Murase T, Hattori T, Ito H, Murohara T, Nagata K: Calorie restriction attenuates cardiac remodeling and diastolic dysfunction in a rat model of metabolic syndrome. *Hypertension* 2013, 62(5):957–965.

84. Waldman M, Cohen K, Yadin D, Nudelman V, Gorfil D, Laniado-Schwartzman M, Kornwoski R, Aravot D, Abraham NG, Arad M: Regulation of diabetic cardiomyopathy by caloric restriction is mediated by intracellular signaling pathways involving 'SIRT1 and PGC-1α'. *Cardiovascular Diabetology* 2018, 17(1):1–12.

85. Bianchi VE: Caloric restriction in heart failure: a systematic review. *Clinical Nutrition ESPEN* 2020, 38:50–60.

86. Karwi QG, Zhang L, Altamimi TR, Wagg CS, Patel V, Uddin GM, Joerg AR, Padwal RS, Johnstone DE, Sharma A: Weight loss enhances cardiac energy metabolism and function in heart failure associated with obesity. *Diabetes, Obesity and Metabolism* 2019, 21(8):1944–1955.

87. Ellsworth DL, Mamula KA, Blackburn HL, McDyer FA, Jellema GL, van Laar R, Costantino NS, Engler RJ, Vernalis MN: Importance of substantial weight loss for altering gene expression during cardiovascular lifestyle modification. *Obesity* 2015, 23(6):1312–1319.

88. Hammer S, Snel M, Lamb HJ, Jazet IM, van der Meer RW, Pijl H, Meinders EA, Romijn JA, de Roos A, Smit JW: Prolonged caloric restriction in obese patients with type 2 diabetes mellitus decreases myocardial triglyceride content and improves myocardial function. *Journal of the American College of Cardiology* 2008, 52(12):1006–1012.

89. Xiang K, Qin Z, Zhang H, Liu X: Energy metabolism in exercise-induced physiologic cardiac hypertrophy. *Frontiers in Pharmacology* 2020, 11:1133.
90. Vettor R, Valerio A, Ragni M, Trevellin E, Granzotto M, Olivieri M, Tedesco L, Ruocco C, Fossati A, Fabris R: Exercise training boosts eNOS-dependent mitochondrial biogenesis in mouse heart: role in adaptation of glucose metabolism. *American Journal of Physiology-Endocrinology and Metabolism* 2014, 306(5):E519–E528.
91. Burelle Y, Wambolt RB, Grist M, Parsons HL, Chow JC, Antler C, Bonen A, Keller A, Dunaway GA, Popov KM: Regular exercise is associated with a protective metabolic phenotype in the rat heart. *American Journal of Physiology-Heart and Circulatory Physiology* 2004, 287(3):H1055–H1063.
92. Meng Y, Bai H, Wang S, Li Z, Wang Q, Chen L: Efficacy of low carbohydrate diet for type 2 diabetes mellitus management: a systematic review and meta-analysis of randomized controlled trials. *Diabetes Research and Clinical Practice* 2017, 131:124–131.
93. Castellana M, Conte E, Cignarelli A, Perrini S, Giustina A, Giovanella L, Giorgino F, Trimboli P: Efficacy and safety of very low calorie ketogenic diet (VLCKD) in patients with overweight and obesity: a systematic review and meta-analysis. *Reviews in Endocrine and Metabolic Disorders* 2020, 21(1):5–16.
94. Lopaschuk GD, Karwi QG, Ho KL, Pherwani S, Ketema EB: Ketone metabolism in the failing heart. *Biochimica et Biophysica Acta (BBA)-Molecular and Cell Biology of Lipids* 2020, 1865(12):158813.
95. Batterham RL, Cummings DE: Mechanisms of diabetes improvement following bariatric/metabolic surgery. *Diabetes Care* 2016, 39(6):893–901.
96. Pathak RK, Middeldorp ME, Meredith M, Mehta AB, Mahajan R, Wong CX, Twomey D, Elliott AD, Kalman JM, Abhayaratna WP: Long-term effect of goal-directed weight management in an atrial fibrillation cohort: a long-term follow-up study (LEGACY). *Journal of the American College of Cardiology* 2015, 65(20):2159–2169.
97. Wang X-H, Qiu J-B, Ju Y, Chen G-C, Yang J-H, Pang J-H, Zhao X: Reduction of heart failure rehospitalization using a weight management education intervention. *Journal of Cardiovascular Nursing* 2014, 29(6):528–534.
98. Zheng Q, Zhao K, Han X, Huff AF, Cui Q, Babcock SA, Yu S, Zhang Y: Inhibition of AMPK accentuates prolonged caloric restriction-induced change in cardiac contractile function through disruption of compensatory autophagy. *Biochimica et Biophysica Acta (BBA)-Molecular Basis of Disease* 2015, 1852(2):332–342.
99. Casiero D, Frishman WH: Cardiovascular complications of eating disorders. *Cardiology in Review* 2006, 14(5):227–231.
100. Lamzabi I, Syed S, Reddy VB, Jain R, Harbhajanka A, Arunkumar P: Myocardial changes in a patient with anorexia nervosa: a case report and review of literature. *American Journal of Clinical Pathology* 2015, 143(5):734–737.
101. von Bibra H, Ströhle A, Sutton MSJ, Worm N: Dietary therapy in heart failure with preserved ejection fraction and/or left ventricular diastolic dysfunction in patients with metabolic syndrome. *International Journal of Cardiology* 2017, 234:7–15.
102. Woodiwiss AJ, Norton GR: Exercise-induced cardiac hypertrophy is associated with an increased myocardial compliance. *Journal of Applied Physiology* 1995, 78(4):1303–1311.
103. Dludla PV, Nyambuya TM, Johnson R, Silvestri S, Orlando P, Mazibuko-Mbeje SE, Gabuza KB, Mxinwa V, Mokgalaboni K, Tiano L: Metformin and heart failure–related outcomes in patients with or without diabetes: a systematic review of randomized controlled trials. *Heart Failure Reviews* 2021, 26(6):1437–1445.
104. Verma S, Rawat S, Ho KL, Wagg CS, Zhang L, Teoh H, Dyck JE, Uddin GM, Oudit GY, Mayoux E: Empagliflozin increases cardiac energy production in diabetes: novel translational insights into the heart failure benefits of SGLT2 inhibitors. *JACC: Basic to Translational Science* 2018, 3(5):575–587.

105. Ussher JR, Baggio LL, Campbell JE, Mulvihill EE, Kim M, Kabir MG, Cao X, Baranek BM, Stoffers DA, Seeley RJ: Inactivation of the cardiomyocyte glucagon-like peptide-1 receptor (GLP-1R) unmasks cardiomyocyte-independent GLP-1R-mediated cardioprotection. *Molecular Metabolism* 2014, 3(5):507–517.

106. Yasuda S, Kobayashi H, Iwasa M, Kawamura I, Sumi S, Narentuoya B, Yamaki T, Ushikoshi H, Nishigaki K, Nagashima K: Antidiabetic drug pioglitazone protects the heart via activation of PPAR-γ receptors, PI3-kinase, Akt, and eNOS pathway in a rabbit model of myocardial infarction. *American Journal of Physiology-Heart and Circulatory Physiology* 2009, 296(5):H1558–H1565.

107. Lincoff AM, Tardif J-C, Schwartz GG, Nicholls SJ, Rydén L, Neal B, Malmberg K, Wedel H, Buse JB, Henry RR: Effect of aleglitazar on cardiovascular outcomes after acute coronary syndrome in patients with type 2 diabetes mellitus: the AleCardio randomized clinical trial. *JAMA* 2014, 311(15):1515–1525.

108. Jia X, Koh S, Al Rifai M, Blumenthal RS, Virani SS: Spotlight on icosapent ethyl for cardiovascular risk reduction: evidence to date. *Vascular Health and Risk Management* 2020, 16:1.

109. Bouitbir J, Charles A-L, Echaniz-Laguna A, Kindo M, Daussin F, Auwerx J, Piquard F, Geny B, Zoll J: Opposite effects of statins on mitochondria of cardiac and skeletal muscles: a 'mitohormesis' mechanism involving reactive oxygen species and PGC-1. *European Heart Journal* 2012, 33(11):1397–1407.

110. Kim NH, Kim SG: Fibrates revisited: potential role in cardiovascular risk reduction. *Diabetes & Metabolism Journal* 2020, 44(2):213–221.

111. Bruckert E, Labreuche J, Amarenco P: Meta-analysis of the effect of nicotinic acid alone or in combination on cardiovascular events and atherosclerosis. *Atherosclerosis* 2010, 210(2):353–361.

112. Ferrannini E, Mark M, Mayoux E: CV protection in the EMPA-REG OUTCOME trial: a "thrifty substrate" hypothesis. *Diabetes Care* 2016, 39(7):1108–1114.

113. Lago RM, Singh PP, Nesto RW: Congestive heart failure and cardiovascular death in patients with prediabetes and type 2 diabetes given thiazolidinediones: a meta-analysis of randomised clinical trials. *The Lancet* 2007, 370(9593):1129–1136.

114. Garber AJ, Handelsman Y, Grunberger G, Einhorn D, Abrahamson MJ, Barzilay JI, Blonde L, Bush MA, DeFronzo RA, Garber JR: Consensus statement by the American Association of Clinical Endocrinologists and American College of Endocrinology on the comprehensive type 2 diabetes management algorithm–2020 executive summary. *Endocrine Practice* 2020, 26(1):107–139.

115. Davies MJ, D'Alessio DA, Fradkin J, Kernan WN, Mathieu C, Mingrone G, Rossing P, Tsapas A, Wexler DJ, Buse JB: Management of hyperglycemia in type 2 diabetes, 2018. A consensus report by the American Diabetes Association (ADA) and the European Association for the Study of Diabetes (EASD). *Diabetes Care* 2018, 41(12):2669–2701.

116. Packer M: Is metformin beneficial for heart failure in patients with type 2 diabetes? *Diabetes Research and Clinical Practice* 2018, 136:168–170.

117. Zhang L, He H, Balschi JA: Metformin and phenformin activate AMP-activated protein kinase in the heart by increasing cytosolic AMP concentration. *American Journal of Physiology-Heart and Circulatory Physiology* 2007, 293(1):H457–H466.

118. Sun D, Yang F: Metformin improves cardiac function in mice with heart failure after myocardial infarction by regulating mitochondrial energy metabolism. *Biochemical and Biophysical Research Communications* 2017, 486(2):329–335.

119. Crowley MJ, Diamantidis CJ, McDuffie JR, Cameron CB, Stanifer JW, Mock CK, Wang X, Tang S, Nagi A, Kosinski AS: Clinical outcomes of metformin use in populations with chronic kidney disease, congestive heart failure, or chronic liver disease: a systematic review. *Annals of Internal Medicine* 2017, 166(3):191–200.

120. Fitchett D, Zinman B, Wanner C, Lachin JM, Hantel S, Salsali A, Johansen OE, Woerle HJ, Broedl UC, Inzucchi SE: Heart failure outcomes with empagliflozin in patients with type 2 diabetes at high cardiovascular risk: results of the EMPA-REG OUTCOME® trial. *European Heart Journal* 2016, 37(19):1526–1534.
121. Kosiborod MN, Jhund PS, Docherty KF, Diez M, Petrie MC, Verma S, Nicolau JC, Merkely B, Kitakaze M, DeMets DL: Effects of dapagliflozin on symptoms, function, and quality of life in patients with heart failure and reduced ejection fraction: results from the DAPA-HF trial. *Circulation* 2020, 141(2):90–99.
122. Packer M, Butler J, Zannad F, Filippatos G, Ferreira JP, Pocock SJ, Carson P, Anand I, Doehner W, Haass M: Effect of empagliflozin on worsening heart failure events in patients with heart failure and preserved ejection fraction: EMPEROR-preserved trial. *Circulation* 2021, 144(16):1284–1294.
123. Verma S, McMurray JJ: SGLT2 inhibitors and mechanisms of cardiovascular benefit: a state-of-the-art review. *Diabetologia* 2018, 61(10):2108–2117.
124. Marso SP, Bain SC, Consoli A, Eliaschewitz FG, Jódar E, Leiter LA, Lingvay I, Rosenstock J, Seufert J, Warren ML: Semaglutide and cardiovascular outcomes in patients with type 2 diabetes. *New England Journal of Medicine* 2016, 375:1834–1844.
125. Marso SP, Daniels GH, Brown-Frandsen K, Kristensen P, Mann JF, Nauck MA, Nissen SE, Pocock S, Poulter NR, Ravn LS: Liraglutide and cardiovascular outcomes in type 2 diabetes. *New England Journal of Medicine* 2016, 375(4):311–322.
126. Jia X, Alam M, Ye Y, Bajaj M, Birnbaum Y: GLP-1 receptor agonists and cardiovascular disease: a meta-analysis of recent cardiac outcome trials. *Cardiovascular Drugs and Therapy* 2018, 32(1):65–72.
127. Gerstein HC, Colhoun HM, Dagenais GR, Diaz R, Lakshmanan M, Pais P, Probstfield J, Riesmeyer JS, Riddle MC, Rydén L: Dulaglutide and cardiovascular outcomes in type 2 diabetes (REWIND): a double-blind, randomised placebo-controlled trial. *The Lancet* 2019, 394(10193):121–130.
128. Kim M, Platt MJ, Shibasaki T, Quaggin SE, Backx PH, Seino S, Simpson JA, Drucker DJ: GLP-1 receptor activation and Epac2 link atrial natriuretic peptide secretion to control of blood pressure. *Nature Medicine* 2013, 19(5):567–575.
129. Richards P, Parker HE, Adriaenssens AE, Hodgson JM, Cork SC, Trapp S, Gribble FM, Reimann F: Identification and characterization of GLP-1 receptor–expressing cells using a new transgenic mouse model. *Diabetes* 2014, 63(4):1224–1233.
130. Zhao T, Parikh P, Bhashyam S, Bolukoglu H, Poornima I, Shen Y-T, Shannon RP: Direct effects of glucagon-like peptide-1 on myocardial contractility and glucose uptake in normal and postischemic isolated rat hearts. *Journal of Pharmacology and Experimental Therapeutics* 2006, 317(3):1106–1113.
131. Ban K, Noyan-Ashraf MH, Hoefer J, Bolz S-S, Drucker DJ, Husain M: Cardioprotective and vasodilatory actions of glucagon-like peptide 1 receptor are mediated through both glucagon-like peptide 1 receptor–dependent and–independent pathways. *Circulation* 2008, 117(18):2340–2350.
132. Kohsaka S, Lam CS, Kim DJ, Cavender MA, Norhammar A, Jørgensen ME, Birkeland KI, Holl RW, Franch-Nadal J, Tangri N: Risk of cardiovascular events and death associated with initiation of SGLT2 inhibitors compared with DPP-4 inhibitors: an analysis from the CVD-REAL 2 multinational cohort study. *The Lancet Diabetes & Endocrinology* 2020, 8(7):606–615.
133. Mechanick JI, Farkouh ME, Newman JD, Garvey WT: Cardiometabolic-based chronic disease, addressing knowledge and clinical practice gaps: JACC state-of-the-art review. *Journal of the American College of Cardiology* 2020, 75(5):539–555.
134. Kongwatcharapong J, Dilokthornsakul P, Nathisuwan S, Phrommintikul A, Chaiyakunapruk N: Effect of dipeptidyl peptidase-4 inhibitors on heart failure: a meta-analysis of randomized clinical trials. *International Journal of Cardiology* 2016, 211:88–95.

135. Delea TE, Edelsberg JS, Hagiwara M, Oster G, Phillips LS: Use of thiazolidinediones and risk of heart failure in people with type 2 diabetes: a retrospective cohort study. *Diabetes Care* 2003, 26(11):2983–2989.
136. Loke YK, Kwok CS, Singh S: Comparative cardiovascular effects of thiazolidinediones: systematic review and meta-analysis of observational studies. *BMJ* 2011, 342:d1309.
137. Madrazo JA, Kelly DP: The PPAR trio: regulators of myocardial energy metabolism in health and disease. *Journal of Molecular and Cellular Cardiology* 2008, 44(6): 968–975.
138. Kendall DM, Rubin CJ, Mohideen P, Ledeine J-M, Belder R, Gross J, Norwood P, O'Mahony M, Sall K, Sloan G: Improvement of glycemic control, triglycerides, and HDL cholesterol levels with muraglitazar, a dual (α/γ) peroxisome proliferator–activated receptor activator, in patients with type 2 diabetes inadequately controlled with metformin monotherapy: a double-blind, randomized, pioglitazone-comparative study. *Diabetes Care* 2006, 29(5):1016–1023.
139. Krishnappa M, Patil K, Parmar K, Trivedi P, Mody N, Shah C, Faldu K, Maroo S, Parmar D: Effect of saroglitazar 2 mg and 4 mg on glycemic control, lipid profile and cardiovascular disease risk in patients with type 2 diabetes mellitus: a 56-week, randomized, double blind, phase 3 study (PRESS XII study). *Cardiovascular Diabetology* 2020, 19(1):1–13.
140. Bhatt DL, Steg PG, Miller M, Brinton EA, Jacobson TA, Ketchum SB, Doyle Jr RT, Juliano RA, Jiao L, Granowitz C: Cardiovascular risk reduction with icosapent ethyl for hypertriglyceridemia. *New England Journal of Medicine* 2019, 380(1):11–22.
141. Bhatt DL, Steg PG, Miller M, Brinton EA, Jacobson TA, Ketchum SB, Doyle RT, Juliano RA, Jiao L, Granowitz C: Effects of icosapent ethyl on total ischemic events: from REDUCE-IT. *Journal of the American College of Cardiology* 2019, 73(22):2791–2802.
142. Oesterle A, Laufs U, Liao JK: Pleiotropic effects of statins on the cardiovascular system. *Circulation Research* 2017, 120(1):229–243.
143. Taylor F, Ward K, Moore TH, Burke M, Smith GD, Casas JP, Ebrahim S: Statins for the primary prevention of cardiovascular disease. *Cochrane Database of Systematic Reviews* 2011, (1):CD004816.
144. Afilalo J, Duque G, Steele R, Jukema JW, de Craen AJ, Eisenberg MJ: Statins for secondary prevention in elderly patients: a hierarchical Bayesian meta-analysis. *Journal of the American College of Cardiology* 2008, 51(1):37–45.
145. Wang W, Wong C-W: Statins enhance peroxisome proliferator-activated receptor γ coactivator-1α activity to regulate energy metabolism. *Journal of Molecular Medicine* 2010, 88(3):309–317.
146. Holubarsch CJ, Rohrbach M, Karrasch M, Boehm E, Polonski L, Ponikowski P, Rhein S: A double-blind randomized multicentre clinical trial to evaluate the efficacy and safety of two doses of etomoxir in comparison with placebo in patients with moderate congestive heart failure: the ERGO (etomoxir for the recovery of glucose oxidation) study. *Clinical Science* 2007, 113(4):205–212.
147. Lee L, Campbell R, Scheuermann-Freestone M, Taylor R, Gunaruwan P, Williams L, Ashrafian H, Horowitz J, Fraser AG, Clarke K: Metabolic modulation with perhexiline in chronic heart failure: a randomized, controlled trial of short-term use of a novel treatment. *Circulation* 2005, 112(21):3280–3288.
148. Ussher JR, Fillmore N, Keung W, Mori J, Beker DL, Wagg CS, Jaswal JS, Lopaschuk GD: Trimetazidine therapy prevents obesity-induced cardiomyopathy in mice. *Canadian Journal of Cardiology* 2014, 30(8):940–944.
149. Fragasso G, Palloshi A, Puccetti P, Silipigni C, Rossodivita A, Pala M, Calori G, Alfieri O, Margonato A: A randomized clinical trial of trimetazidine, a partial free fatty acid oxidation inhibitor, in patients with heart failure. *Journal of the American College of Cardiology* 2006, 48(5):992–998.

150. Fragasso G, Perseghin G, De Cobelli F, Esposito A, Palloshi A, Lattuada G, Scifo P, Calori G, Del Maschio A, Margonato A: Effects of metabolic modulation by trimetazidine on left ventricular function and phosphocreatine/adenosine triphosphate ratio in patients with heart failure. *European Heart Journal* 2006, 27(8):942–948.

151. Stacpoole PW: The pharmacology of dichloroacetate. *Metabolism* 1989, 38(11): 1124–1144.

152. Liu Q, Docherty JC, Rendell JC, Clanachan AS, Lopaschuk GD: High levels of fatty acids delay the recoveryof intracellular pH and cardiac efficiency inpost-ischemic hearts by inhibiting glucose oxidation. *Journal of the American College of Cardiology* 2002, 39(4):718–725.

153. Kato T, Niizuma S, Inuzuka Y, Kawashima T, Okuda J, Tamaki Y, Iwanaga Y, Narazaki M, Matsuda T, Soga T: Analysis of metabolic remodeling in compensated left ventricular hypertrophy and heart failure. *Circulation: Heart Failure* 2010, 3(3):420–430.

154. Wargovich TJ, MacDonald RG, Hill JA, Feldman RL, Stacpoole PW, Pepine CJ: Myocardial metabolic and hemodynamic effects of dichloroacetate in coronary artery disease. *The American Journal of Cardiology* 1988, 61(1):65–70.

155. Lopaschuk GD, Wambolt R, Barr R: An imbalance between glycolysis and glucose oxidation is a possible explanation for the detrimental effects of high levels of fatty acids during aerobic reperfusion of ischemic hearts. *Journal of Pharmacology and Experimental Therapeutics* 1993, 264(1):135–144.

156. Goldberg IJ, Eckel RH, Abumrad NA: Regulation of fatty acid uptake into tissues: lipoprotein lipase-and CD36-mediated pathways. *Journal of Lipid Research* 2009, 50:S86–S90.

157. Coort SL, Willems J, Coumans WA, Van Der Vusse GJ, Bonen A, Glatz JF, Luiken JJ: Sulfo-N-succinimidyl esters of long chain fatty acids specifically inhibit fatty acid translocase (FAT/CD36)-mediated cellular fatty acid uptake. *Molecular and Cellular Biochemistry* 2002, 239(1):213–219.

158. Dyck JR, Cheng J-F, Stanley WC, Barr R, Chandler MP, Brown S, Wallace D, Arrhenius T, Harmon C, Yang G: Malonyl coenzyme a decarboxylase inhibition protects the ischemic heart by inhibiting fatty acid oxidation and stimulating glucose oxidation. *Circulation Research* 2004, 94(9):e78–e84.

159. Horton JL, Davidson MT, Kurishima C, Vega RB, Powers JC, Matsuura TR, Petucci C, Lewandowski ED, Crawford PA, Muoio DM: The failing heart utilizes 3-hydroxybutyrate as a metabolic stress defense. *JCI Insight* 2019, 4(4):e124079.

160. Uchihashi M, Hoshino A, Okawa Y, Ariyoshi M, Kaimoto S, Tateishi S, Ono K, Yamanaka R, Hato D, Fushimura Y: Cardiac-specific Bdh1 overexpression ameliorates oxidative stress and cardiac remodeling in pressure overload–induced heart failure. *Circulation: Heart Failure* 2017, 10(12):e004417.

161. Yurista SR, Matsuura TR, Silljé HH, Nijholt KT, McDaid KS, Shewale SV, Leone TC, Newman JC, Verdin E, van Veldhuisen DJ: Ketone ester treatment improves cardiac function and reduces pathologic remodeling in preclinical models of heart failure. *Circulation: Heart Failure* 2021, 14(1):e007684.

162. Kosinski C, Jornayvaz FR: Effects of ketogenic diets on cardiovascular risk factors: evidence from animal and human studies. *Nutrients* 2017, 9(5):517.

163. Wentz AE, d'Avignon DA, Weber ML, Cotter DG, Doherty JM, Kerns R, Nagarajan R, Reddy N, Sambandam N, Crawford PA: Adaptation of myocardial substrate metabolism to a ketogenic nutrient environment. *Journal of Biological Chemistry* 2010, 285(32):24447–24456.

164. Newgard CB, An J, Bain JR, Muehlbauer MJ, Stevens RD, Lien LF, Haqq AM, Shah SH, Arlotto M, Slentz CA: A branched-chain amino acid-related metabolic signature that differentiates obese and lean humans and contributes to insulin resistance. *Cell Metabolism* 2009, 9(4):311–326.

165. Wang W, Zhang F, Xia Y, Zhao S, Yan W, Wang H, Lee Y, Li C, Zhang L, Lian K: Defective branched chain amino acid catabolism contributes to cardiac dysfunction and remodeling following myocardial infarction. *American Journal of Physiology-Heart and Circulatory Physiology* 2016, 311(5):H1160–H1169.

166. Uddin GM, Karwi QG, Pherwani S, Gopal K, Wagg CS, Biswas D, Atnasious M, Wu Y, Wu G, Zhang L: Deletion of BCATm increases insulin-stimulated glucose oxidation in the heart. *Metabolism* 2021, 124:154871.

167. Sun H, Olson KC, Gao C, Prosdocimo DA, Zhou M, Wang Z, Jeyaraj D, Youn J-Y, Ren S, Liu Y: Catabolic defect of branched-chain amino acids promotes heart failure. *Circulation* 2016, 133(21):2038–2049.

168. Buchwald H, Estok R, Fahrbach K, Banel D, Jensen MD, Pories WJ, Bantle JP, Sledge I: Weight and type 2 diabetes after bariatric surgery: systematic review and meta-analysis. *The American Journal of Medicine* 2009, 122(3):248–256.

169. Sjöström L, Peltonen M, Jacobson P, Sjöström CD, Karason K, Wedel H, Ahlin S, Anveden Å, Bengtsson C, Bergmark G: Bariatric surgery and long-term cardiovascular events. *JAMA* 2012, 307(1):56–65.

170. Schauer PR, Bhatt DL, Kirwan JP, Wolski K, Brethauer SA, Navaneethan SD, Aminian A, Pothier CE, Kim ES, Nissen SE: Bariatric surgery versus intensive medical therapy for diabetes—3-year outcomes. *New England Journal of Medicine* 2014, 370(21):2002–2013.

171. Schauer PR, Bhatt DL, Kirwan JP, Wolski K, Aminian A, Brethauer SA, Navaneethan SD, Singh RP, Pothier CE, Nissen SE: Bariatric surgery versus intensive medical therapy for diabetes—5-year outcomes. *New England Journal of Medicine* 2017, 376:641–651.

172. Ashrafian H, Li JV, Spagou K, Harling L, Masson P, Darzi A, Nicholson JK, Holmes E, Athanasiou T: Bariatric surgery modulates circulating and cardiac metabolites. *Journal of Proteome Research* 2014, 13(2):570–580.

4 Endocrine-Disrupting Chemicals

Keerthana Haridas and Michael A. Via
Icahn School of Medicine at Mount Sinai

Jeffrey I. Mechanick
Kravis Center for Cardiovascular Health at Mount Sinai Heart
Icahn School of Medicine at Mount Sinai

CONTENTS

DOI: 10.1201/9781003206637-4

ABBREVIATIONS

AGE	Advanced glycation end product
AhR	Aryl hydrocarbon receptor
AR	Androgen receptor
AZT	Atrazine
BMI	Body mass index
BPA	Bisphenol A
cAMP	Cyclic adenosine monophosphate
DDE	Dichlorodiphenyldichloroethylene
DDT	Dichlorodiphenyltrichloroethane
DEHP	Di(2-ethylhexyl)phthalate
DES	Diethylstilbestrol
EDC	Endocrine-Disrupting Chemical
EDSP	Endocrine Disruptor Screening Program

EPA	Environment Protection Agency
ER	Estrogen receptor
IL	Interleukin
IRS	Insulin receptor substrate
KC	Key characteristic
LDL	low-density lipoprotein
NCD	Non-communicable disease
NHANES	National Health and Nutrition Examination Survey
NIEHS	National Institute of Environmental Health Sciences
OC	Organochlorine
PAH	Polycyclic aromatic hydrocarbon
PAD	Peripheral arterial disease
PCB	Polychlorinated biphenyl
PCBDE	Polybrominated diphenyl ethers
PFA	Perfluoroalkyl substances
PFOA	Perfluorooctanoic acid
POP	Persistent organic pollutant
PPAR	Peroxisome proliferator-activated receptor
PXR	Pregnane X Receptor
ROS	Reactive oxygen species
SREBP1C	Sterol regulatory element-binding protein 1C
T1D	Type 1 diabetes
T2D	Type 2 diabetes
TBBPA	Tetrabromobisphenol A
TBT	Tributyltin
TCDD	Tetrachlorodibenzodioxin
TRH	Thyrotropin-Releasing Hormone

4.1 INTRODUCTION

The endocrine system facilitates and regulates virtually all homeostatic and allostatic metabolic processes through the secretion of hormones in response to internal and external signals. Homeostatic mechanisms resist change and maintain biological oscillators like temperature and pH in a very narrow range. Allostatic mechanisms confer stability through change by enabling complex pathways to adjust set points for adaptation to endogenous or exogenous stressors. In addition to "healthy" chemicals that nurture these biological processes and must be replenished through the diet (e.g., nutrients), endocrine-disrupting chemicals (EDC) are "unhealthy" chemicals from the environment, consumed as part of food or incidental to living, that subvert or otherwise compromise these biological processes [1]. This chapter will focus on EDC that augment cardiometabolic risk with the intent to formulate evidence-based recommendations that can mitigate or even eliminate these adverse effects.

The framework for the discovery of endocrine-disrupting chemicals was first laid down by Hertz in 1958, who proposed that chemicals used to feed livestock could result in adverse health outcomes in humans who consumed them [2,3]. In 1962, Carson, in the book "Silent Spring" wrote of the potential effects of compounds, widely used in the wake of the Industrial Revolution, in their ability to alter external ecosystems and the internal milieu of animals and humans [4]. The decade that followed witnessed the establishment of the National Institute of Environmental Health Sciences and the Environment Protection Agency (EPA) where the concept of EDC began to be widely discussed. Compounds within industrial waste were discovered to alter hormone-signaling pathways integral to maintaining normal homeostatic, metabolic, and reproductive functions [3].

An EDC is defined by the U.S. EPA as "an exogenous agent that interferes with the synthesis, secretion, transport, metabolism, binding action, or elimination of natural blood-borne hormones that are present in the body and are responsible for homeostasis, reproduction, and developmental processes" [5]. An operational working definition of an EDC was put forward about 5 years later by the Endocrine Society, describing it as an exogenous chemical, or a mixture of chemicals that interferes with any aspect of hormone action [6]. It is thus a compound or a mixture of compounds, either natural or synthetic, which through inappropriate environmental exposures possesses the ability to alter the internal hormonal milieu [3]. Over 1,000 chemicals have been deemed fit to fall into this class of compounds. This class includes highly heterogeneous chemicals (Table 4.1).

4.2   COMMON ENDOCRINE-DISRUPTING CHEMICALS

4.2.1   BISPHENOL A

Bisphenol A (BPA), first synthesized in 1891, is used in manufacturing and packaging toys and other commodities. BPA resins are found in the lining of many canned foods and beverages and may leak into food or water under conditions of high heat, physical manipulation, or repetitive use [7]. Due to the ubiquitous nature of BPA leading to frequent exposure, 93% of Americans were noted to have a measurable amount of this EDC in their urine. In addition, BPA has been detected in the breast milk of some women [8]. The U.S. EPA has set the safe level of exposure to BPA at 50 µg/kg/d, whereas that of the European Food Safety Authority is set to 4 µg/kg/d. However, evidence supports the toxic effects of BPA in mammals with exposure to even lower levels [5–8].

4.2.2   PHTHALATES

Phthalates and phthalate esters like mono-n-benzyl phthalate, mono-[2-ethyl-5-hydroxylhexyl] phthalate, mono-[2-ethyl-5-oxohexyl] phthalate, and monoethyl phthalate, first used in the 1920s, include a large group of compounds used as liquid plasticizers found in cosmetics, plastics, coatings, vinyl flooring, and medical tubing. They can leach into the environment since they are not chemically bound to plastics. Phthalates have been detected in human serum, urine, and milk samples with the estimated daily exposure to a major phthalate, di(2-ethylhexyl)phthalate (DEHP), ranging from 3 to 30 µg/kg/d [9].

TABLE 4.1

Cardiometabolic Effects of EDC

EDC Class	Source	Cardiometabolic Effect
Bisphenol A	Plastic and polycarbonate production, food and beverage linings, packaging, toys, DVD, dental materials, thermal paper	Insulin resistance, increased glucagon secretion, obesity, atherosclerosis
Phthalates	Plastic production, cosmetics, perfumes, adhesives, paints, food containers and wrappers, toys, medical tubing	Insulin resistance, decreased insulin secretion, obesity, atherosclerosis
Polychlorinated biphenyls, polybrominated diphenyl esters	Electrical equipment and insulation, plasticizers, copy paper, ink, adhesives, flame retardants, paints	Insulin resistance, obesity, atherosclerosis
Dioxins	By-products of combustion of wastes and manufacture of herbicides, disinfectants	Decreased insulin secretion, insulin resistance, atherosclerosis
PFOAs	Non-stick cookware, packaging material, paints, varnishes, waterproof clothing	Insulin resistance, obesity
DDT, DDE	Insecticides	Obesity, atherosclerosis, insulin resistance
Organotins	Agricultural products – fungicides, wood and paper mills, breweries, cooling systems	Obesity, insulin resistance, atherosclerosis

4.2.3 ATRAZINE

Atrazine (2-chloro-4-ethylamino-6-isopropylamino-s-triazine) (ATR) is a broad-spectrum herbicide used on a variety of commercial crops as well as in parks, farms, and golf courses. However, ATR and its metabolites are commonly reported contaminants in groundwater, surface water, and drinking water [10].

4.2.4 POLYCHLORINATED BIPHENYLS AND POLYBROMINATED DIPHENYL ETHERS

This class of compounds contains paired phenolic rings and variable degrees of halogenation. Chlorinated forms (polychlorinated biphenyls [PCBs]) were in use from the 1920s until they were banned by the U.S. EPA in 1979, after which their brominated congeners replaced them. They found use in plasticizers, adhesives, carbonless copy paper, paints, and inks. They are highly resistant to breakdown and have a high propensity to bioaccumulate in the environment. Consequently, polybrominated diphenyl ethers (PCBDEs) belong to a class of compounds known as persistent organic pollutants (POP). North Americans constitute the largest user of PCBDEs and have the highest blood levels, compared to other regions of the world [11,12].

4.2.5   DICHLORODIPHENYLTRICHLOROETHANE AND DICHLORODIPHENYLDICHLOROETHYLENE

Dichlorodiphenyltrichloroethane (DDT) is a synthetic industrial and household insecticide that causes a range of metabolic and carcinogenic adverse effects. It was banned in the United States in 1972 after years of extensive use as a result of these toxicities [13]. A worldwide ban was instituted in 2001, though DDT use continues in some areas. Dichlorodiphenyldichloroethylene (DDE) is a metabolite of DDT with similar toxic effects [6].

Persistent Organic Pollutant is a term, that includes in its umbrella, a vast number of compounds like DDT, PCB, PBDEs, aldrin, and other aromatic hydrocarbons that are toxic and resistant to degradation and possess long half-lives [14]. They accumulate in fatty tissues of animals and humans, with concentrations increasing at successive levels of the food chain due to biomagnification [14].

4.3   BODY BURDEN AND LIPOPHILICITY OF EDC

EDC, such as BPA and phthalates, are not highly lipophilic, so they do not accumulate in adipose tissue and largely remain in circulation upon significant exposure. Levels of these compounds detected in serum or urine are considered reflective of their "body burden," which is defined as the total amount of an EDC that is present in the human body at a given point in time.

On the contrary, halogenated polyphenyls, such as PCB, PCBDE, and DDT and its congeners, are highly lipophilic. These compounds are primarily stored in adipose tissues, especially white adipose tissue, and only a fraction is released into circulation, more so during times of rapid weight loss [6]. It is important to note that measured levels of these compounds in serum or urine are unreliable indicators of the true whole-body burden in humans and animals [6]. To some degree, lipophilicity functions as a protective mechanism since it decreases the amount of EDC entering circulation at a given time and potentially decreases the degree of interaction with receptors, second messengers, or downstream targets.

White adipose tissue storage leads to EDC transmission through successive rungs of the food chain. Accumulation continues even after the completion of the life cycle of the exposed host, establishing many lipophilic EDC as POP [15]. Some of these compounds have been detected in so-called "pristine" environments at remote distances from the site where EDC were produced, used, or released due to water and air currents and through movements of migratory animals. The concentration of EDC in consecutive levels of the food chain increases through the phenomenon of biomagnification, which has important ramifications on the health, not just of human beings, but multiple plant and animal species in various ecosystems [5].

4.4   OUTCOMES OF EXPOSURE

There are five basic factors that determine the outcomes of exposure [5].

1. **Intensity of Exposure**: A combination of the duration of exposure and the concentration of the specific EDC determine the cumulative dose of exposure and may predict the range of disruption produced in homeostatic and allostatic mechanisms.

2. **Age at Exposure**: "The developmental basis of health and disease" hypothesis posits that fetal and perinatal exposures to environmental insults, including harmful compounds, may lead to the late manifestation of disease or dysfunction in offspring [16]. This occurs by virtue of their effects on structural and functional development, as well as by alteration of gene expression. Thus, a variable period of latency may exist between exposure to the EDC and the manifestation of its adverse effect.

3. **Transmissibility through Germlines**: Effects of exposure may not be limited to the host generation but may be transmitted to subsequent generations through genetic as well as epigenetic alterations [17–19]. An epigenetic change refers to a change in a non-coding region of DNA that alters gene expression. An example of this transgenerational genetic and epigenetic inheritance phenomenon may be seen through the effects of diethylstilbestrol (DES), which are known to persist into the next (F2) generation, i.e., the grandsons of women who took DES during pregnancy are at increased risk of genital defects, including hypospadias and cryptorchidism [20]. The F3 generation, with no direct exposure to DES, has also been noted to experience consequences of exposure of the antecedent generation [20,21]. Studies show that vinclozolin is associated with decreased spermatogenic capacity and benzopyrene with the occurrence of lung adenomas, both in F3 generations [17,18].

4. **Exposure to More Than One Harmful Compound**: While each EDC may exert its own harmful effect, combinations of EDC can exert synergistic effects, leading to a greater degree of dysfunction than predicted by the sum total of combined exposures [6].

5. **Non-Traditional Dose-Response Curves**: Due to the influence of receptor and ligand characteristics in hormone action, complex non-monotonic U-shaped and inverted U-shaped dose-response curves have been known to occur in the actions of hormones, neurotransmitters, and EDC [3,5]. To this end, multiple-dose studies have described a non-monotonic relationship between prenatal and perinatal BPA exposure and metabolic alterations, such as increased weight, insulin resistance, and glucose tolerance [22]. Furthermore, smaller doses of EDC may exert greater harmful effects than higher doses [3].

4.5 MECHANISM OF ACTION

A certain degree of correlation is thought to exist between the structure of EDC and their mechanism of action [5,6]. For example, dioxins, polyphenols, and pesticides have a phenolic moiety that is thought to mimic natural steroid hormones, facilitating interaction with steroid hormone receptors. Structural characteristics are also thought to mediate the disruption of thyroid hormone function. Endocrine-disrupting chemicals can also interfere with the rhythm of hormone secretion (circadian or pulsatile), which may lead to downstream adverse effects.

Ten key characteristics (KCs) of EDC have been described based on their mechanism of disruption of hormone axes or functions [23].

KC1 states that an EDC can interact with and activate hormone receptors, leading to the activation of downstream cascades and causing an increase in activity. Examples include a specific hydroxylated congener of a PCB that can activate human thyroid hormone receptor-β-mediated transcription, as well as DDT that binds to the transmembrane domain of the follicle-stimulating hormone receptor, a G protein-coupled receptor, to allosterically enhance its stimulation of cyclic adenosine monophosphate (cAMP) production.

KC2 states that an EDC can antagonize hormone receptors, inhibiting downstream pathways and decreasing the effect of hormones. The class of organochlorine (OC) pesticides which includes DDT, lindane, and dieldrin has been known to inhibit the binding of androgens to the androgen receptor (AR). In utero exposure to these compounds in male fetuses can lead to demasculinization and malformations of the male genital tract.

KC3 states that an EDC can alter hormone receptor expression. DEHP decreases the expression of the mineralocorticoid (aldosterone) receptor in the testes of adult mice, where under normal conditions it acts as a positive modulator of testosterone biosynthesis. This action decreases testosterone synthesis.

KC4 states that an EDC can alter signal transduction involving transmembrane, intracellular, or nuclear receptors in hormone-responsive cells. For example, BPA inhibits glucose-induced calcium signaling in pancreatic glucagon-secreting α-cells, which affects gluconeogenesis and glycogenolysis. In addition, EDC can act at any step in the signal transduction chain: the fungicide tolylfluanid impairs insulin action by reducing the amount of insulin receptor substrate 1 (IRS-1), potentially leading to insulin resistance. The EDC may interact with nuclear receptors through effects on coregulatory factors and gene expression. Xenoestrogens (e.g., DES, PCB, PBDDEs, octylphenol, and BPA) induce the recruitment of the coregulatory factor steroid receptor coactivator 1 by estrogen receptor α (ERα) and estrogen receptor β (ERβ) in a dose-dependent manner.

KC5 states that an EDC can induce epigenetic modifications in hormone-producing or hormone-responsive cells during development and differentiation. An EDC can do so either by interfering with the ability of a hormone to induce these epigenetic changes or inducing epigenetic changes that then interfere with hormone action by altering the transcription of hormone-responsive genes or the expression or action of a hormone receptor. For example, the pesticide methoxychlor increases the expression of DNA methyltransferase to hypermethylate DNA, including ER2 (which encodes ERβ) in the ovary of rats upon in utero exposure. This suppresses transcription. Histone modification and microRNA alteration are other epigenetic processes that modify gene transcription and translation. Epigenetic changes could have variable latencies and can manifest more severe, long-lasting, and transgenerational effects.

KC6 states that an EDC can alter hormone synthesis. For example, perchlorates are known to inhibit the sodium-iodide cotransporter, preventing iodine uptake into thyroid cells and inhibiting thyroid hormone synthesis. Phthalates reduce testosterone synthesis in fetal rat testes.

KC7 states that an EDC can alter hormone transport across cell membranes. Low-dose BPA reduces calcium entry into mouse pancreatic β-cells to reduce insulin secretion from vesicles. Imidazoline, an anti-corrosive and fungicidal agent, modulates ionic flow across membranes to enhance insulin secretion.

KC8 states that an EDC can alter hormone distribution by altering the level of binding and transport proteins. Intravenous DES administration in men results in reductions in total testosterone (by six-fold), free testosterone (to four-fifths the value), and estrogen (by five-fold), which are concurrent with an over seven-fold increase in the serum concentration of sex hormone-binding globulin.

KC9 states that an EDC can alter hormone metabolism and clearance. Many classes of compounds activate glucuronidases that increase thyroid hormone clearance from the blood. Estrogen sulfotransferase, which reduces the rate of estrogen clearance from the bloodstream, is inhibited by metabolites of the fungicide hexachlorobenzene and several chlorophenolic wood preservatives.

KC10 states that an EDC can alter the number, position, and fate of hormone-producing or hormone-responsive cells by altering cell proliferation, differentiation, migration, or cell death. The antibacterial agent triclosan results in increased decidualization of human endometrial stromal cells.

Often, a single EDC can cause hormonal disruptions through more than one KC mechanistic pathway. Over a hundred epidemiological studies show associations between BPA and adverse outcomes such as obesity and diabetes mellitus among other reproductive and homeostatic effects. Substantial evidence exists to show that BPA works through nine of the ten KCs described above [23].

4.6 EFFECT OF EDC ON CARDIOMETABOLIC DRIVERS

Recently, there has been considerable interest in exploring the association between EDC and non-communicable diseases (NCDs), such as obesity, diabetes mellitus, atherosclerotic cardiovascular disease, and cancer. Obesity and type 2 diabetes (T2D) are widely prevalent metabolic disorders that contribute significantly to morbidity and mortality among adults. Furthermore, they pose significant burdens on the healthcare system as well as the economy. The prevalence of these disorders has increased over the years, with the WHO providing estimates that obesity has almost doubled since 1980 and the CDC estimating that diabetes mellitus has increased in prevalence from 9.5% in 1999–2002 to 12.0% in 2013–2016 [5,6]. These NCDs are complex disorders that have multifactorial origins and are influenced by a range of genetic and environmental factors. Genetic determinants are also thought to influence the metabolic response of the organism to chemicals.

Much of the research to establish links between EDC and metabolic disorders was done in the last two decades. In 2002, Baillie-Hamilton hypothesized an "obesogenic" action of toxic chemicals after an extensive literature review prompted by the parallel increase in environmental pollutants and the prevalence of obesity [24]. In 2006, Grun and Blumberg defined obesogens as xenobiotic chemicals that disrupt the homeostatic controls over adipogenesis and/or energy balance [25].

Molecular models confirm that EDC promote adipogenesis and obesity in animals as well as in humans. These and other related studies resulted in the "obesogen hypothesis," which suggested that perinatal and early-life exposure to EDC predisposed individuals to develop obesity in adolescence or adulthood [25,26]. Along similar lines, any agent contributing to the derangement of glucose homeostasis leading to hyperglycemia has been referred to as a "diabetogen" [6,26]. The Parma statement issued in 2015 proposed to modify both of the above to be broadly referred to as the "metabolic-disrupting hypothesis," which pertained to obesity, insulin resistance, hyperlipidemia, as well as likely consequent hepatic steatosis – all components of the metabolic syndrome [26].

4.7   THE ASSOCIATION BETWEEN EDC AND OBESOGENESIS

4.7.1   Bisphenol A

There exist a number of studies that associate BPA with obesity in humans. Most studies are analyses of the U.S. National Health and Nutrition Examination Survey (NHANES) data in adults and children and show that BPA concentrations were strongly linked to obesity and greater waist circumference with odds ratios of 1.6–1.85 for the highest quartile of urinary BPA concentrations [27]. A study in China reported an association between urinary BPA concentrations and overweight, obesity, insulin resistance, and T2D [28]. However, a prospective study showed that girls exposed to higher concentrations of BPA in utero had a lower body weight than those exposed to nil or lower concentrations of the same, contradicting the above evidence or possibly elucidating differing dose-response characteristics [29].

4.7.2   Phthalates

The NHANES data indicate that various phthalates are associated with a significant increase in waist circumference and body mass index (BMI) in adolescent and adult males and females [30]. A Swedish study involving elderly cohorts found similar results in females, but not in males. Baseline body weight, race, ethnicity, and gender were factors found to affect outcomes post-exposure in other studies [31].

4.7.3   Persistent Organic Pollutants

These EDC have been identified in some studies as obesogens independent of gender. A comprehensive review published in 2014 examining the associations among POP with obesity and diabetes concluded that the clinical evidence for association with diabetes was strong, but that with obesity remains insufficient [28]. Nevertheless, a prospective cohort study discovered a significant association ($p < 0.01$) between low-dose developmental exposure to perfluorooctanoic acid (PFOA) and overweight in female offspring at 20 years of age. Female offspring whose mothers were in the highest quartile of serum PFOA concentration had BMI elevation of 1.6 kg/m^2

[95% confidence interval (CI): 0.6, 2.6] and waist circumference increase of 4.3 cm (95% CI: 1.4, 7.3) compared with offspring with mothers was in the lowest quartile (p <0.05) [29].

4.7.4 POLYCHLORINATED BIPHENYLS

Population studies have demonstrated a correlation between cord blood PCB levels with BMI and fat mass index in children and adolescents [32, 33, 34]. However, other longitudinal studies have reported dichotomous results with outcomes varying depending on the intensity of exposure, age and sex of children followed [34].

4.8 MECHANISMS OF EDC ACTION IN OBESOGENESIS

4.8.1 RECEPTOR-MEDIATED INCREASE IN ADIPOGENESIS

Endocrine-disrupting chemicals are known to act on receptors such as peroxisome proliferator-activated receptors (PPAR) -α and -γ and estrogen receptors (ER) to increase adipogenesis, affect adipocyte maturation, and contribute to fat metabolism and storage [5,6,35]. Examples of EDC acting through this pathway include BPA, phthalates, tributyltin (TBT), triphenyltin, parabens, and DES. Some EDC may act after mesenchymal stem cells differentiate into adipocytes (DEHP and TBT) or on preadipocytes and mesenchymal stromal cells prior to differentiation (BPA, phthalates, and the fungicide triflumizole) [6,36]. Some EDC, such as tolylfluanid, a pesticide widely used in Europe, have been shown to bind to the glucocorticoid receptor, leading to weight gain [37]. The aryl hydrocarbon receptor (AhR) was also shown to mediate adipogenesis induced by PCBs [38].

4.8.2 EFFECT ON TRANSPORT PROTEINS

Studies have shown an increase in the number of membrane receptors that are involved in glucose transport, including SGLT-1, SGLT-2, and GLUT-2 receptors, after exposure to EDC, such as dioxins [39]. This may result in an increase in the cellular uptake of glucose and conversion to lipid intermediates in the setting of a caloric surplus.

4.8.3 EFFECT ON HORMONE AXES

Tetrabromobisphenol A (TBBPA; a flame retardant) and TBT affected the expression of thyrotropin-releasing hormone (TRH) and type-4 melanocortin receptors in the paraventricular nucleus of the hypothalamus [40]. Exposure to TBBPA in animal models decreased thyroid hormone–independent TRH production and the expression of type-4 melanocortin receptors, which decrease catabolism, thermogenesis, and hypothalamic sensitivity to melanocortin, in turn stimulating orexigenic pathways [41]. These factors all decrease resting metabolic rate and stimulate appetite.

4.8.4 EFFECT ON ENZYMES

BPA increases the activity of 11ß-hydroxysteroid dehydrogenase type 1, catalyzing the conversion of cortisone to cortisol in human adipose tissues and promoting adipogenesis [42].

4.8.5 EFFECT ON ADIPOKINES AND NEUROPEPTIDES

Endocrine-disrupting chemicals, such as BPA, can modify adipokine levels, such as leptin, adiponectin, and insulin [5,6,43]. The levels of adipokines like leptin and adiponectin, which decrease appetite, are lowered. In addition, the level of neuropeptide Y, which is orexigenic, and pro-opiomelanocortin, which promotes satiety, may be altered by certain classes of EDC, including BPA, DES, and TBT [43].

4.8.6 EFFECT ON EPIGENETICS

EDC produce changes in non-coding regions of genetic material resulting in obesity. This has been observed in studies on animal models where a mix of commonly used plastic derivatives (containing BPA and phthalates) was noted to promote the transgenerational epigenetic inheritance of adult-onset obesity in rats [44]. Fetal and somatic rat cells were directly exposed to EDC in the F1 generation and epigenetic transgenerational inheritance was studied through the germline in the F3 generation. Interestingly, the F1 female rats were noted to have a normal body weight, while 1-year-old F3 female rats were noted to have increased weight, fat deposition, and visceral adiposity. In addition, these F3 obese female rats were seen to develop polycystic ovary syndrome. The disparity of phenotypes between F1 and F3 rats points to a strong indication that the mechanisms involved in the F1 generations and F3 generations are different. The doses of exposure were high compared to typical ranges of human exposure, so it is not known whether this takes place with environmentally relevant doses of these plastics.

The same study also identified methylation of sperm DNA regions in the regions of a number of genes involved in obesity and polycystic ovary syndrome, suggesting additional modification of outcomes at the levels of transcription and translation.

4.9 PHYSIOLOGICAL MODELS OF INCREASED ADIPOGENESIS

A net positive energy balance mediated through an increase in energy intake, a decrease in energy expenditure, or both leads to weight gain.

4.9.1 INCREASE IN CALORIC INTAKE

Taste-responsive neurons in the oral cavity are activated by chemicals contained in some artificial sweeteners, potentially resulting in an increase in food consumption [46]. In addition, neurons that are a part of the autonomic nervous system in the gut could be stimulated by artificial sweeteners and result in the release of insulin, which is known to increase adiposity. However, in vivo animal studies have failed to demonstrate a significant increase in insulin secretion in response to these agents. Stevia was observed to cause the opposite effect, i.e., improve insulin sensitivity and decrease adiposity [46,47].

4.9.2 Decrease in Locomotor Activity

In animal models, BPA has been shown to decrease locomotor activity after about a week of exposure, suggesting alteration of central energy regulatory pathways in the thalamus and hypothalamus [48]. However, the exact mechanisms responsible were not elucidated.

4.9.3 Alterations in Gut Microbiota

Artificial sweeteners remain unabsorbed in the colon, thus possessing the ability to modify the composition of the flora in the gastrointestinal tract. This can exert important effects on metabolism and homeostasis. Clinical studies demonstrate an alteration in the bacterial genome after as little as 1 week of EDC consumption at doses permitted by the U.S. Food and Drug Administration [49]. Interestingly, the same results were replicated after the transplantation of feces from humans given artificial sweeteners to mice. The effects of saccharin and sucralose were more pronounced than those of aspartame, which seemed relatively less harmful [49]. The effect of these sweeteners on microflora induces increased calorie consumption and weight gain among rodents [46]. Similar associations between artificial sweetener consumption and obesity are noted in human studies [46]. Stevia may cause the opposite effect and lead to decreased adiposity. Similar results that decrease adiposity have also been observed with emulsifiers in foods [46,47,49].

4.10 FACTORS AFFECTING METABOLIC RESPONSES TO EDC

4.10.1 Sex

Studies have reported sex-dependent alterations in parameters of energy homeostasis, with varied responses being observed in male and female mice exposed to BPA. It was found that exposure to similar levels of BPA in utero led to no change or decreased body weight in female offspring while causing increased weight and associated glucose intolerance in male counterparts [50].

4.10.2 Dose of EDC

Some EDC exhibit non-monotonic relationships and dose-response curves. Studies in animals show that only one BPA concentration (500 μg/kg/d) increased weight at 18 weeks of age, although lower doses promoted glucose intolerance and insulin resistance despite producing no change in weight [51,52]. Therefore, negative results obtained in studies conducted using only one dose must be interpreted with caution.

4.10.3 TIME OF EXPOSURE

Perinatal exposure seems to have a greater effect on metabolic outcomes than exposures in adult life. Study results conducted on male and female mice contradict each other with regard to the period of perinatal development during which exposure produces the greatest metabolic effects [50,52].

4.11 THE ASSOCIATION BETWEEN EDC AND DIABETES MELLITUS

Endocrine-disrupting chemicals are known to cause diabetes, both through their propensity to increase adiposity, as well as independent of changes in body fat, as proposed by the diabetogen hypothesis [45, 53]. In the former case, a combination of changes in both body fat and glucose homeostasis results in "diabesity," a form of diabetes that typically develops in later life and is associated with obesity.

An interesting example can be seen in India, which witnessed an approximate doubling in its diabetic population between the years 1980 and 2014 but without a significant increase in the levels of common risk factors, such as obesity, hypertension, hypercholesterolemia, or smoking [49]. Similar trends are observed in many other developing nations [49]. Of note, an increased prevalence of prediabetes and diabetes was observed among populations involved in farming with high persistent exposures to chemical pesticides and herbicides. Regression analysis of this data showed no association between the levels of hemoglobin A1c and common risk factors, such as BMI, blood pressure, low-density lipoprotein (LDL)-cholesterol levels, or physical inactivity, indicating that other factors may be responsible for the upsurge in T2D prevalence. A meta-analysis of 72 different epidemiological studies published by the Endocrine Society and National Toxicology Workshop concluded that there is a positive association between T2D and exposure to POP [54].

4.11.1 INDIVIDUAL COMPOUNDS AND THE RISK OF DIABETES

Early clinical evidence arose from populations exposed, accidentally or incidentally, to the rodenticide pyrinuron who then developed type 1 diabetes (T1D) [55]. While more recent data exists to support the association between EDC exposure and impaired insulin sensitivity, the quality of evidence is still lacking due to poorly designed studies (especially prospective studies), the use of self-reported diabetes, and conflicting data from existent retrospective studies. This necessitates the need for better-designed prospective studies in order to explore and elucidate this association relationship. In addition, the source of most of these organic and inorganic compounds is the lining of cans and tins containing fast foods and beverages. This confounds interpretations since the populations exposed to EDC in this manner are also more likely to develop insulin resistance and metabolic syndrome due to caloric surplus through non-EDC-mediated pathways.

4.11.1.1 Persistent Organic Pollutants

POP, especially chlorinated pesticides, are the class of compounds with the highest degree of evidence to support an association with insulin resistance and T2D. A large number of occupational and non-occupational studies demonstrate unequivocal evidence to this end [56,57]. Exposure to various POP including dioxins, DDE, and halogenated aromatics was shown, in human studies, to increase the risk of development of T2D [58].

4.11.1.2 Bisphenol A

Results drawn from the NHANES data in the years 2003–2008 demonstrate an increased risk of developing T2D with an increase in the urinary concentration of BPA, with an odds ratio of 1.68 in the quartile with the highest concentration, in comparison to the reference population [59,60]. A prospective study established an association between BPA and phthalate exposures with the risk of T2D in middle-aged women [61]. However, a similar study from China found conflicting evidence regarding the above association [62].

4.11.1.3 Phthalates

Published cross-sectional studies in Mexico, United States, and Sweden consistently demonstrate a borderline statistically significant association between phthalates and T2D, with the relative risk of T2D ranging between 1.02 and 1.64 for different compounds [60]. Greater concentrations of these POP were found in women, possibly due to higher exposure through household products [60].

4.11.1.4 Perfluoroalkyl Substances

The first evidence that perfluoroalkyl substances (PFAs) had diabetogenic potential arose from occupational studies of a population exposed to the compound in the workplace [63]. In another study of a population exposed to the chemical through drinking water in West Virginia, no association with diabetes was found at measured levels of exposure. In other studies, serum concentrations of total PFAs have been associated with diabetes in Sweden and the United States [63].

4.11.1.5 Metals

While some studies point to an association between the concentrations of metals like aluminum, cadmium, and mercury and the likelihood of T2D [60], the lack of large prospective studies and well-established criteria for the diagnosis of diabetes limits interpretation.

4.12 MECHANISMS IMPLICATED IN DIABETES

4.12.1 Insulin Resistance and Prediabetes

4.12.1.1 Altered Insulin and Glucagon Secretion

4.12.1.1.1 Decreased Insulin Secretion

Tetrachlorodibenzodioxin (TCDD; a POP-like compound) was shown to alter the glucose entry into pancreatic ß-cells, thereby decreasing insulin secretion. BPA has been shown, among other EDC, to result in blockage of K and Ca channels involved in β-cell depolarization and insulin release [23,60,64]. Compounds like BPA and

DES were also shown to affect glucagon secretion by altering calcium levels in pancreatic α-cells [23,64].

4.12.1.1.2 Increased Insulin Secretion

Interestingly, compounds like PCBs and dioxins may lead to an increase in insulin secretion, which is hypothesized to deplete cellular insulin, leading to β-cell exhaustion [61]. Imidazoline has also been shown to decrease insulin secretion by altering transmembrane ionic flow across the membranes to enhance insulin secretion [23].

4.12.1.1.3 Altered Insulin Signaling

Polychlorinated biphenyl mixtures, OC pesticide mixtures, and DDT among the POP were found to decrease the insulin-mediated uptake of glucose into the skeletal muscle and adipose tissues [60,65]. Park et al. demonstrated that mitochondrial dysfunction induced by EDC suppressed IRS-1 expression, a downstream mediator of insulin signaling [66]. Tolylfluanid has also been shown to decrease the amount of IRS-1 [23].

4.12.1.1.4 Promotion of Inflammation

POP, through the activation of steroid receptors including the AhR, pregnane X receptor (PXR), and constitutive androstane receptor, alter the expression of genes. These include TLR5, ROCK2, and YWHAZ and proteins such as CD14 involved in the inflammatory pathway, lipid oxidation, and lipogenesis, thereby contributing to the development of insulin resistance [65]. In addition, POP have been shown to increase the levels of pro-inflammatory cytokines, such as interleukin (IL)-1, IL-6, and tumor necrosis factor-α which contribute to insulin resistance [64,65].

4.12.1.1.5 Advanced Glycation End Products

Advanced glycation end products (AGE) are harmful compounds contained in cigarette smoke, plastics, and linings of packaged food and beverages. They bind to a specific receptor – receptor of advanced glycation end products – and lead to the generation of reactive oxygen species (ROS), causing oxidative stress and tissue injury. This alters insulin signaling and glucose homeostasis. Animal and human studies indicate worsened glycemic control in those exposed to AGE [5].

4.12.1.1.6 Alterations of Gut Microbiota

EDC alter the number, structure, and functioning of the diverse microorganisms in the gastrointestinal tract [49]. These bacteria, upon fermentation of undigested carbohydrates, fiber, and other dietary and xenobiotic compounds, produce short-chain fatty acids, choline, and bile metabolites, among other by-products. These by-products may act as hormones or signal molecules that influence different host metabolic processes. Microbial genes, proteins, and metabolites alter key metabolic pathways including gluconeogenesis, glycogenolysis, and lipogenesis [49]. The effects of this alteration have been noted in animal studies involving heavy metals, such as arsenic, cadmium, and lead, as well as with POP-like OC pesticides, PCBDEs, and organophosphates. Artificial sweeteners have also been shown to alter gut microbiota and decrease insulin sensitivity, increase hepatic gluconeogenesis, and potentially increase the risk of T2D. Studies show that these effects are reproducible through fecal transplantation in rodents and are nullified by the use of antibiotics, suggesting that these metabolic changes are mediated through gut bacteria [49].

4.12.1.1.7 Genetic Changes

When POP accumulate in fatty fish, the functioning of various genes (*Insig-1* and *Lpin1*) that regulate lipogenesis is inhibited [65]. There is an increase in the expression of sterol regulatory element-binding protein 1C (SREBP1C) that stimulates the lipogenic pathway, and fatty acid synthase, a well-known target gene of SREBP1C. The increase in adiposity that results from these effects on gene expression contributes to the development of insulin resistance [65].

4.12.2 β-CELL DEPLETION AND TYPE 1 DIABETES

The most prominent effects on β-cell structure and insulin secretion have been noted during gestational exposure to EDC, especially phthalates and BPA [67].

4.13 THE ASSOCIATION BETWEEN EDC AND ATHEROSCLEROSIS

4.13.1 PATHOGENESIS OF ATHEROSCLEROSIS

Atherosclerosis is thought to result as a part of the "response to injury hypothesis" based on a chronic inflammatory process that recruits mononuclear cells in the subendothelial space and causes their differentiation into macrophages [68–71]. A vicious cycle results when these macrophages produce more cytokines that drive the process, eventually forming atherosclerotic lesions in the form of fatty streaks and then plaques. A key inflammatory mediator in this process is IL-8, known to be produced by macrophages and expressed at high levels in atheromas, specifically in foamy macrophages [70].

4.13.2 DATA ON EDC AND ATHEROSCLEROSIS

Animal studies show that exposure to EDC including polycyclic aromatic hydrocarbons (PAH) found in cigarette smoke and generated through fuel combustion as well as dioxins can lead to the formation of complex atheromas, even in mice not fed a high-fat diet [70]. This is mediated through an increased expression of inflammatory genes, inflammatory mediators, and lipoproteins including LDL cholesterol [70].

Data obtained from the NHANES registry between the years 1999 and 2004 demonstrate a positive correlation between serum levels of organochlorine (OC) pesticides and the presence of peripheral arterial disease (PAD) using the ankle–brachial pressure index but only in individuals with obesity [71]. Although obesity may alter PAD risk in those exposed to POP, these results must be interpreted with caution since higher-circulating OCs are found in obese individuals, compared to leaner sedentary or athletic individuals. Since OCs are lipid soluble, increased body fat can lead to increased total body OC content with consequent increases in OC free fractions and activities [71].

Population studies among workers exposed to dioxins reveal a higher incidence of hyperlipidemia, atherosclerotic plaques, increased carotid artery intima-media thickness, and a higher risk of ischemic heart disease [70]. A mixture of various organic compounds derived from combustion was shown to increase the risk of atherosclerosis and downstream effects including coronary artery disease and peripheral arterial disease [72]. BPA has been associated with CVD in several large and well-controlled cross-sectional and longitudinal studies, independent of traditional CVD risk factors [73,74].

4.13.3 MECHANISMS OF EDC-MEDIATED ATHEROSCLEROSIS

4.13.3.1 Hyperlipidemia

Various EDC, including OCs and organophosphate pesticides, phthalates, PCBDEs, BPA and their analogs, and citrate esters have been shown to activate the PXR, a nuclear receptor in a potent manner [75]. PXR functions as a xenobiotic sensor to regulate the metabolism of toxic compounds [70,71]. PXR ligands have been demonstrated to cause hyperlipidemia in humans. In addition, genome-wide association studies show that common genetic variants of PXR are associated with alterations in the levels of LDL cholesterol. In mouse models, chronic activation of PXR increases the size of atherosclerotic lesions, while loss of PXR decreases atherosclerosis [65,71]. OC pesticides can exacerbate hyperlipidemia by decreasing the hepatic binding and elimination of LDL particles, raising the risk of the formation of fatty streaks and atherosclerotic plaques [71]. Lastly, OC decreases the activity of lipoprotein lipase, leading to hypertriglyceridemia and furthering the risk of atherosclerosis [71].

4.13.3.2 Chronic Inflammation

EDC including dioxins have been shown to increase the expression of IL-8 and monocyte chemoattractive protein-1. Dioxin exposure is also shown to increase the expression of VEGF, produced by the activation of CXC chemokine receptor 2, as well as that of the cytokine CXCL5, which is co-regulated with IL-8 [66,72,75]. This series of pro-inflammatory cytokine signaling is associated with an increase in oxidative stress, endothelial cell dysfunction, and thrombosis and initiates the cascade causing atherosclerosis and associated macrovascular complications. AGE compounds too have been shown to alter endothelial function, cause chronic inflammation, and lead to vascular diseases, even after a single exposure [5,76]. Exposure to chemicals contained in smoke, through combustion of fuels as well as through suspended particulate matter in air, has been shown to increase vasoconstriction, thrombogenicity, atherosclerotic plaque size, and endothelial inflammation in animal and human studies [77–80]. In addition, a prospective study in Iran notes increased cardiovascular mortality in those with exposure to fine particulate matter ($<2.5\ \mu$) [79].

4.13.3.3 Mitochondrial Dysfunction

Mitochondrial damage causes endothelial damage and dysfunction in more ways than one. There is an increase in the number of ROS that cause oxidative stress and damage to the endothelium [66,72]. It has been shown that mitochondrial dysfunction may also decrease the production of nitric oxide, accentuating endothelial dysfunction [66]. Mitochondrial dysfunction also results in alteration in heat and energy production and lowered body temperature causing an increased body mass in an attempt to maintain optimal core temperature. Many prospective studies show that individuals with decreased rates of energy expenditure are predisposed to weight gain [81–85]. Weyer et al. conducted a longitudinal study over 3.6 years that found an association between 24-hour energy expenditure and weight changes in Pima Indians [86]. In addition, mitochondrial damage decreases metabolic demand and causes a consequent decrease in blood flow to tissues, measured by decreased vessel lumen diameters as an adaptation to the decreased need for oxygen delivery [66].

Exposure to POP can induce mitochondrial dysfunction through mitochondrial DNA depletion and damage [66]. For instance, the triazine herbicide, atrazine, can result in structural alterations in mitochondria, including ring- and cup-shaped mitochondria, and the loss of cristae, although the structure of protein complexes involved in oxidative phosphorylation may not be directly affected [66]. Mitochondrial damage, caused by EDC, causes endothelial cells to release damage-associated molecular pattern molecules (e.g., high-mobility group protein B1, heat shock proteins, and S100 proteins), which recruit inflammatory cells, such as macrophages that are a key component of fatty streaks and atheromatous plaques [66,70]. Other mitochondrial proteins can activate formyl peptide receptor-1 on neutrophils, thus activating the inflammatory cascade through another route [66].

4.13.3.4 Epigenetic Changes

EDC cause epigenetic changes through alterations in DNA methylation, histone acetylation, and non-coding RNA (e.g., micro-RNA), affecting gene expression. An increase in inflammation and alterations in lipid metabolism and vascular smooth muscle activity result as a consequence of altered genetic activity, transcription, and translation [75]. EDC can also epigenetically affect PXR gene expression [75].

4.14 METHODS FOR EDC DETECTION AND EXPOSURE MITIGATION

Over 1800 chemicals that disrupt at least one of three hypothalamic-pituitary endocrine pathways have been identified in an examination by the FDA. Of the 575 chemicals screened by the European Commission, 320 showed potential evidence for EDC classification [63]. Crucial steps in alleviating exposure include:

1. establishing the specific toxicities of each compound
2. delineating the individual EDC posing risk among an individual's exposome (an aggregate measure of all environmental exposures over a lifetime) and the interaction among them
3. assessing exposure most precisely
4. taking into account exposure variability, distribution, and timing

To address these questions, well-designed prospective studies are needed. Based on the evidence gathered, implementation tactics, with logistical and ethical considerations, must aim to optimize the manufacturing, use, and disposal of EDC. Presently, intervention studies have been successful at resulting in rapid decreases in exposure to EDC, such as organophosphate pesticides, bisphenols, and phthalates, but have not examined changes in disease or intermediate markers of adverse health outcomes [63].

4.14.1   SCREENING FOR EDC EXPOSURE

The Endocrine Disruptor Screening Program (EDSP) has been developed by the EPA and uses a two-tiered approach to screen chemicals and environmental contaminants for their potential effect on various hormone systems [3]. The EDSP is outlined in two Federal Register Notices published in 1998.

It is mandated to use validated methods to screen and test chemicals and identify potential endocrine disruptors, determine adverse effects and dose responses, assess the risk, and ultimately alleviate the risk under current laws. The EDSP has developed a set of animal- and cell-based assays to test the endocrine toxicities of multiple EDC at a time [3]. However, currently, the vast majority of the focus is on the thyroid, estrogen, and androgen hormones among the various endocrine pathways because most mechanistic assays that screen compounds detect chemicals that alter steroid hormone synthesis or interact with steroid or other nuclear receptors. The U.S. EPA Toxicity Forecaster (ToxCast) and the Toxicity Testing in the 21st century (Tox21) are two federally funded tools to screen chemicals for adverse human health effects [87,88]. These tools compare endocrine-disrupting activities across a number of structurally related compounds. However, neither of these tools examines all potential routes of endocrine disruption. High-throughput mechanistic assays which screen thousands of chemicals for a variety of toxicities, including endocrine disruption, are widely available. Tiered Protocol for Endocrine Disruption is a strategy that offers five levels of testing during chemical development, to screen for potential endocrine disruption [3].

At present, these assays have not undergone international validation, limiting their use to only certain contexts.

4.14.2   ORGANIZED EFFORTS TO DECREASE EDC EXPOSURE

At the 2001 Stockholm Convention, it was agreed that there will be attempts to reduce or eliminate the production, use, and release of major persistent organic pollutants, primarily due to their endocrine-disrupting potential [89]. The Endocrine Society released two position statements on the role of EDC in human health and disease [5,6]. A number of dangerous EDC, such as DDT, have been banned as a result of these ongoing efforts.

In order to protect consumer health, the levels of potential contaminants in food are internationally regulated. For example, tolerable levels of certain POP, including dioxins and dioxin-like PCBs, in food are regulated in accordance with the European Union legislation in 2006 [90,91]. However, it must be noted that the estimation of the tolerable upper levels of intake of individual compounds is based on their potential biologic toxicities and therefore may not be reliable. This is because many studies that estimate safe levels of exposure oversimplify mechanistic processes, eliminating interactions among different EDC, as well as preexistent genetic or metabolic conditions in susceptible populations. In 2006, the EPA issued a cumulative risk assessment of triazine herbicides (including AZT), while concluding that they posed "no harm that would result to the general U.S. population, infants, children, or other consumers" [92]. This conclusion was made despite evidence that these agents may damage mitochondrial function, affect insulin signaling, and induce insulin resistance and obesity, especially when associated with a high-fat diet. No doubt, there is a potential conflict of interest between industries that profit from the use of cheaper, potentially hazardous chemicals, and organizations that try to eliminate or reduce the widespread use of these same chemicals. This potential conflict requires concentrated efforts, lobbying, and involvement by citizens' groups to ensure that health is prioritized for present and future generations.

Policy makers and manufacturers must also ensure accurate product labeling with appropriate ingredient lists and concentrations. This is necessary to allow consumers to make informed decisions regarding the use of commercial products. While cosmetic companies are required by the FDA to display intentionally added ingredients [93] and pesticides and disinfectants must be labeled per EPA guidelines [94], other products such as cleaners, fabrics, and durable goods have few regulations in place. This creates a systemic practice gap, necessitating effective regulatory intervention.

4.14.3 INDIVIDUAL EFFORTS TO DECREASE EDC EXPOSURE

While more studies are needed to reveal clear relationships between EDC and toxic metabolic consequences, the "Precautionary Principle" may be put into effect, wherein anticipatory avoidance of products with high concentrations of EDC is practiced to prevent potential harm, even in the absence of ratifying evidence [5,6]. Governments and large industries and organizations have the ability to draft and execute policies to reduce the generation, use, and exposure to EDC. But individuals and groups of individuals can also take steps to reduce EDC exposures. Those in the highest quartiles of personal care product use have significantly higher exposure to a range of EDC (e.g., parabens, triclosan, and phenol congeners), compared to the lower quartiles. Also, consumers who reported scrutinizing ingredient labels had lower levels of exposure in comparison to those who did not. Thus, reduced use of products containing EDC is likely to translate into lower circulating levels and the likelihood of associated adverse health outcomes [95].

Specifically, individuals can lower EDC exposures by avoiding or reducing their use of certain products as follows:

1. By increasing awareness regarding the widespread use of these compounds, sources of exposure, and approximate daily levels of exposure within safe limits. Increased knowledge regarding the potential adverse effects of EDC on metabolic processes in not just subjects directly exposed to EDC but also successive generations of progeny is likely to shift the decision-making process to avoid chemically laced products
2. By exploring resources, such as the Breast Cancer and the Environment Research Program [96], PROTECT Superfund Research Program [97], Silent Spring Institute's Digital Exposure Report-Back Interface [98], and

Detox Me smartphone application, which provide guidance in general decision-making. These may prompt users to avoid selected ingredients on labels, reduce the use of products containing EDC unless absolutely necessary, and/or substitute certain products with less harmful, more sustainably produced alternatives with lower impacts on the environment

3. By avoiding the use of plastic containers for food and beverage preparation/consumption and minimizing consumption of processed, tinned, or canned foods

4. By avoiding the handling of carbonless copy paper when possible as it may contain BPA and its congeners

5. By avoiding the use of personal care or domestic products that contain parabens, sulfates, and triclosan (the latter commonly found in personal and home care products labeled as "antibacterial")

6. Using clean-burning stoves and fuel, improved household ventilation devices, and air-filtration devices which help improve air quality and decrease cardiovascular risk, among other health benefits [80].

4.15 CONCLUSION

It is recommended that regulatory authorities, including the FDA, EPA, and WHO, focus attention on evidence-based regulation of EDC production and use. Better-designed clinical studies on EDC are needed to institute corrective measures. In general, all EDC should be replaced by safer chemicals that are thoroughly tested prior to widespread use. Successful implementation of these regulatory stipulations on both population and individual scales can decrease the social and biological burden of chronic disease and promote cardiometabolic health.

Disclosures:
Jeffrey I. Mechanick received honoraria from Abbott Nutrition for lectures and serves on the Advisory Boards for Aveta.Life and Twin Health.

REFERENCES

1. Mechanick JI. Molecular nutrition: the good, the bad, and the uncertain. *Lancet Diabetes Endocrinol.* 2013 Oct;1(2):86–87. Doi:10.1016/S2213-8587(13)70110-4
2. Hall JM, Korach KS. Endocrine disrupting chemicals (EDCs) and sex steroid receptors. *Adv Pharmacol.* 2021;92:191–235. Doi:10.1016/bs.apha.2021.04.001
3. Schug TT, Johnson AF, Birnbaum LS, et al. Minireview: endocrine disruptors: past lessons and future directions. Mol Endocrinol. 2016;30(8):833–847. Doi:10.1210/me.2016-1096
4. Carson RL. *Silent Spring*, Anniversary Edition. New York: Houghton Miffin Co; 1962.
5. Diamanti-Kandarakis E, Bourguignon JP, Giudice LC, et al. Endocrine-disrupting chemicals: an Endocrine Society scientific statement. *Endocr Rev.* 2009;30(4):293–342. Doi:10.1210/er.2009-002
6. Gore AC, Chappell VA, Fenton SE, Flaws JA, Nadal A, Prins GS, Toppari J, Zoeller RT. EDC-2: the Endocrine Society's second scientific statement on endocrine-disrupting chemicals. *Endocr Rev.* 2015;36(6):E1–E150. Doi:10.1210/er.2015-1010
7. Dodds EC, Lawson W. Synthetic oestrogenic agents without the phenanthrene nucleus. *Nature.* 1936;137:996.

8. Calafat AM, Ye X, Wong LY, Reidy JA, Needham LL. Exposure of the U.S. population to bisphenol A and 4-tertiary-octylphenol: 2003–2004. *Environ Health Perspect.* 2008;116:39–44.

9. Hannon PR, Flaws JA. The effects of phthalates on the ovary. *Front Endocrinol.* 2015;6:8.

10. Agency for Toxic Substances and Disease Registry. *Toxicological Profile for Atrazine.* Atlanta, GA: U.S. Department of Health and Human Services, Public Health Service; 2003.

11. Agency for Toxic Substances and Disease Registry. *Toxicological Profile for Polybrominated Biphenyls and Polybrominated Diphenyl Ethers (PBBs and PBDEs).* Atlanta, GA: U.S. Department of Health and Human Services, Public Health Service; 2004.

12. Lauby-Secretan B, Loomis D, Grosse Y, et al. Carcinogenicity of polychlorinated biphenyls and polybrominated biphenyls. *Lancet Oncol.* 2013;14:287–288.

13. National Toxicology Program. *Report on Carcinogens*, 12th Edition. Washington, DC: U.S. Department of Health and Human Services, Public Health Service; 2011;12:iii–499.

14. Guo W, Pan B, Sakkiah S, et al. Persistent organic pollutants in food: contamination sources, health effects and detection methods. *Int J Environ Res Public Health.* 2019;16(22):4361. Doi:10.3390/ijerph16224361

15. Calafat AM, Needham LL. Human exposures and body burdens of endocrine-disrupting chemicals. In *Endocrine-Disrupting Chemicals.* Edited by Gore AC. Totowa, NJ: Humana Press; 2007:253–268.

16. Hales CN, Barker DJ. The thrifty phenotype hypothesis. *Br Med Bull.* 2001;60:5–20.

17. Anway MD, Skinner MK Epigenetic transgenerational actions of endocrine disruptors. *Endocrinology.* 2006;147:S43–S49.

18. Anway MD, Skinner MK. Transgenerational effects of the endocrine disruptor vinclozolin on the prostate transcriptome and adult onset disease. *Prostate.* 2008;68:517–529.

19. Anway MD, Cupp AS, Uzumcu M, Skinner MK. Epigenetic transgenerational actions of endocrine disruptors and male fertility. *Science.* 2005;308:1466–1469.

20. Li S, Hursting SD, Davis BJ, McLachlan JA, Barrett JC. Environmental exposure, DNA methylation and gene regulation. Lessons from diethylstilbestrol-induced cancers. *Ann NY Acad Sci.* 2003;983:161–169.

21. Skinner MK. What is an epigenetic transgenerational phenotype? F3 or F2. *Reprod Toxicol.* 2008;25(1):2–6. Doi:10.1016/j.reprotox.2007.09.001

22. Fan AM, Chou WC, Lin P. Toxicity and risk assessment of bisphenol A. In *Reproductive and Developmental Toxicology*, 2nd Edition. Edited by Gupta R. Cambridge, MA: Academic Press; 2017:765–795.

23. La Merrill, M.A., Vandenberg, L.N., Smith, M.T. et al. Consensus on the key characteristics of endocrine-disrupting chemicals as a basis for hazard identification. *Nat Rev Endocrinol.* 2020;16:45–57. Doi:10.1038/s41574-019-0273-8

24. Baillie-Hamilton PF. Chemical toxins: a hypothesis to explain the global obesity epidemic. *J Altern Complement Med.* 2002;8:185–192.

25. Grün F, Blumberg B 2006 Environmental obesogens: organotins and endocrine disruption via nuclear receptor signaling. *Endocrinology* 147:S50–S55.

26. Heindel JJ, Blumberg B, Cave M, et al. Metabolism disrupting chemicals and metabolic disorders. *Reprod Toxicol.* 2017;68:3–33. Doi:10.1016/j.reprotox.2016.10.001

27. Carwile JL, Michels KB. Urinary bisphenol A and obesity: NHANES 2003–2006. *Environ Res.* 2011;111:825–830.

28. Wang T, Li M, Chen B, et al. Urinary bisphenol A (BPA) concentration associates with obesity and insulin resistance. *J Clin Endocrinol Metab.* 2012;97:E223–E227.

29. Harley KG, Aguilar Schall R, Chevrier J, et al. Prenatal and postnatal bisphenol A exposure and body mass index in childhood in the CHAMACOS cohort. *Environ Health Perspect.* 2013;121:514–520.

30. Stahlhut RW, van Wijngaarden E, Dye TD, Cook S, Swan SH. Concentrations of urinary phthalate metabolites are associated with increased waist circumference and insulin resistance in adult U.S. males. *Environ Health Perspect.* 2007;115:876–882.
31. Lind PM, Roos V, Rönn M, et al. Serum concentrations of phthalate metabolites are related to abdominal fat distribution two years later in elderly women. *Environ Health.* 2012;11:21.
32. Lee DH, Porta M, Jacobs DR, Jr, Vandenberg LN. Chlorinated persistent organic pollutants, obesity, and type 2 diabetes. *Endocr Rev.* 2014;35:557–601.
33. Halldorsson TI, Rytter D, Haug LS, et al. Prenatal exposure to perfluorooctanoate and risk of overweight at 20 years of age: a prospective cohort study. *Environ Health Perspect.* 2012;120:668–673.
34. Tahir E, Cordier S, Courtemanche Y, et al. Effects of polychlorinated biphenyls exposure on physical growth from birth to childhood and adolescence: a prospective cohort study. *Environ Res.* 2020;189:109924. Doi:10.1016/j.envres.2020.109924
35. Tontonoz P, Spiegelman BM. Fat and beyond: the diverse biology of PPARγ. *Annu Rev Biochem.* 2008;77:289–312.
36. Biemann R, Santos AN, Santos AN, et al. Endocrine disrupting chemicals affect the adipogenic differentiation of mesenchymal stem cells in distinct ontogenetic windows. *Biochem Biophys Res Commun.* 2012;417:747–752.
37. Neel BA, Brady MJ, Sargis RM. The endocrine disrupting chemical tolylfluanid alters adipocyte metabolism via glucocorticoid receptor activation. *Mol Endocrinol.* 2013;27:394–406.
38. Arsenescu V, Arsenescu RI, King V, Swanson H, Cassis LA. Polychlorinated biphenyl-77 induces adipocyte differentiation and proinflammatory adipokines and promotes obesity and atherosclerosis. *Environ Health Perspect.* 2008;116:761–768.
39. Tonack S, Kind K, Thompson JG, Wobus AM, Fischer B, Santos AN. Dioxin affects glucose transport via the arylhydrocarbon receptor signal cascade in pluripotent embryonic carcinoma cells. *Endocrinology.* 2007;148(12):5902–5912. Doi:10.1210/en.2007-0254
40. Decherf S, Seugnet I, Fini JB, Clerget-Froidevaux MS, Demeneix BA. Disruption of thyroid hormone-dependent hypothalamic set-points by environmental contaminants. *Mol Cell Endocrinol.* 2010;323:172–182.
41. Decherf S, Demeneix BA. The obesogen hypothesis: a shift of focus from the periphery to the hypothalamus. *J Toxicol Environ Health B Crit Rev.* 2011;14:423–448.
42. Wang J, Sun B, Hou M, Pan X, Li X. The environmental obesogen bisphenol A promotes adipogenesis by increasing the amount of 11β-hydroxysteroid dehydrogenase type 1 in the adipose tissue of children. *Int J Obes.* 2013;37:999–1005.
43. Angle BM, Do RP, Ponzi D, et al. Metabolic disruption in male mice due to fetal exposure to low but not high doses of bisphenol A (BPA): evidence for effects on body weight, food intake, adipocytes, leptin, adiponectin, insulin and glucose regulation. *Reprod Toxicol.* 2013;42:256–268.
44. Marraudino M, Bo E, Carlini E, et al. Hypothalamic expression of neuropeptide Y (NPY) and pro-opiomelanocortin (POMC) in adult male mice is affected by chronic exposure to endocrine disruptors. *Metabolites.* 2021;11(6):368. Doi:10.3390/metabo11060368
45. Manikkam M, Tracey R, Guerrero-Bosagna C, Skinner MK. Plastics derived endocrine disruptors (BPA, DEHP and DBP) induce epigenetic transgenerational inheritance of obesity, reproductive disease and sperm epimutations. *PLoS One.* 2013;8(1):e55387. Doi:10.1371/journal.pone.0055387
46. Pearlman M, Obert J, Casey L. The association between artificial sweeteners and obesity. *Curr Gastroenterol Rep.* 2017;19(12):64. Doi:10.1007/s11894-017-0602-9
47. Pang MD, Goossens GH, Blaak EE. The impact of artificial sweeteners on body weight control and glucose homeostasis. *Front Nutr.* 2021;7:598340. Doi:10.3389/fnut.2020.598340

48. Batista TM, Alonso-Magdalena P, Vieira E, et al. Short-term treatment with bisphenol-A leads to metabolic abnormalities in adult male mice. *PLoS One.* 2012;7:e33814.

49. Velmurugan G, Ramprasath T, Gilles M, Swaminathan K, Ramasamy S. Gut microbiota, endocrine-disrupting chemicals, and the diabetes epidemic. *Trends Endocrinol Metab.* 2017;28(8):612–625. Doi:10.1016/j.tem.2017.05.001

50. Alonso-Magdalena P, Vieira E, Soriano S, et al. Bisphenol A exposure during pregnancy disrupts glucose homeostasis in mothers and adult male offspring. *Environ Health Perspect.* 2010;118(9):1243–1250. Doi:10.1289/ehp.1001993

51. Vandenberg LN, Colborn T, Hayes TB, et al. Hormones and endocrine-disrupting chemicals: low-dose effects and nonmonotonic dose responses. *Endocr Rev.* 2012;33:378–455.

52. Angle BM, Do RP, Ponzi D, et al. Metabolic disruption in male mice due to fetal exposure to low but not high doses of bisphenol A (BPA): evidence for effects on body weight, food intake, adipocytes, leptin, adiponectin, insulin and glucose regulation. *Reprod Toxicol.* 2013;42:256–268.

53. Alonso-Magdalena P, Quesada I, Nadal A. Endocrine disruptors in the etiology of type 2 diabetes mellitus. *Nat Rev Endocrinol.* 2011;7:346–353.

54. Taylor KW, Novak RF, Anderson HA, et al. Evaluation of the association between persistent organic pollutants (POPs) and diabetes in epidemiological studies: a national toxicology program workshop review. *Environ Health Perspect.* 2013;121(7):774–783. Doi:10.1289/ehp.1205502

55. Heindel JJ, Blumberg B, Cave M, et al. Metabolism disrupting chemicals and metabolic disorders. *Reprod Toxicol.* 2017;68:3–33. Doi:10.1016/j.reprotox.2016.10.001

56. Lee DH, Porta M, Jacobs DR, Jr, Vandenberg LN. Chlorinated persistent organic pollutants, obesity, and type 2 diabetes. *Endocr Rev.* 2014;35:557–601.

57. Magliano DJ, Loh VH, Harding JL, Botton J, Shaw JE. Persistent organic pollutants and diabetes: a review of the epidemiological evidence. *Diabetes Metab.* 2014;40:1–1448.

58. Wu H, Bertrand KA, Choi AL, et al. Persistent organic pollutants and type 2 diabetes: a prospective analysis in the Nurses' Health Study and meta-analysis. *Environ Health Perspect.* 2013;121:153–161.

59. Silver MK, O'Neill MS, Sowers MR, Park SK. Urinary bisphenol A and type-2 diabetes in U.S. adults: data from NHANES 2003–2008. *PLoS One.* 2011;6(10):e26868. Doi:10.1371/journal.pone.0026868

60. Kuo CC, Moon K, Thayer KA, Navas-Acien A. Environmental chemicals and type 2 diabetes: an updated systematic review of the epidemiologic evidence. *Curr Diab Rep.* 2013;13:831–849.

61. Sun Q, Cornelis MC, Townsend MK, et al. Association of urinary concentrations of bisphenol A and phthalate metabolites with risk of type 2 diabetes: a prospective investigation in the Nurses' Health Study (NHS) and NHSII cohorts. *Environ Health Perspect.* 2014;122:616–623.

62. Duan Y, Yao Y, Wang B, et al. Association of urinary concentrations of bisphenols with type 2 diabetes mellitus: a case-control study. *Environ Pollut.* 2018;243(Pt B):1719–1726. Doi:10.1016/j.envpol.2018.09.093

63. Kahn LG, Philippat C, Nakayama SF, Slama R, Trasande L. Endocrine-disrupting chemicals: implications for human health. *Lancet Diabetes Endocrinol.* 2020;8(8):703–718. Doi:10.1016/S2213-8587(20)30129-7

64 Mimoto MS, Nadal A, Sargis RM. Polluted pathways: mechanisms of metabolic disruption by endocrine disrupting chemicals. *Curr Environ Health Rep.* 2017;4(2):208–222. Doi:10.1007/s40572-017-0137-0

65. Ruzzin J, Petersen R, Meugnier E, et al. Persistent organic pollutant exposure leads to insulin resistance syndrome. *Environ Health Perspect.* 2010;118(4):465–471. Doi:10.1289/ehp.0901321

66. Park SY, Choi GH, Choi HI, Ryu J, Jung CY, Lee W. Depletion of mitochondrial DNA causes impaired glucose utilization and insulin resistance in L6 GLUT4myc myocytes. *J Biol Chem.* 2005 Mar 18;280(11):9855–9864.

67. Bodin J, Bølling AK, Becher R, Kuper F, Løvik M, Nygaard UC. Transmaternal bisphenol A exposure accelerates diabetes type 1 development in NOD mice. *Toxicol Sci.* 2014;137:311–323.

68. Ross R. Rous-Whipple award lecture. atherosclerosis: a defense mechanism gone awry. *Am J Pathol.* 1993;143:987–1002.

69. Helsley RN, Zhou C. Epigenetic impact of endocrine disrupting chemicals on lipid homeostasis and atherosclerosis: a pregnane X receptor-centric view. *Environ Epigenet.* 2017;3(4):dvx017. Doi:10.1093/eep/dvx017

70. Wu D, Nishimura N, Kuo V, et al. Activation of aryl hydrocarbon receptor induces vascular inflammation and promotes atherosclerosis in apolipoprotein E-/- mice. *Arterioscler Thromb Vasc Biol.* 2011;31(6):1260–1267. Doi:10.1161/ATVBAHA.110.220202

71. Min JY, Cho JS, Lee KJ, Park JB, Park SG, Kim JY, Min KB. Potential role for organochlorine pesticides in the prevalence of peripheral arterial diseases in obese persons: results from the National Health and Nutrition Examination Survey 1999–2004. *Atherosclerosis.* 2011 Sep;218(1):200–206. Doi:10.1016/j.atherosclerosis.2011.04.044

72. Hoffmann B, Moebus S, Kröger K, et al. Residential exposure to urban air pollution, ankle-brachial index, and peripheral arterial disease. *Epidemiology.* 2009;20:280–208.

73. Lang IA, Galloway TS, Scarlett A, Henley WE, Depledge M, Wallace RB, Melzer D. Association of urinary bisphenol a concentration with medical disorders and laboratory abnormalities in adults. *JAMA* 2008;300:1303–1310.

74. Melzer D, Rice NE, Lewis C, Henley WE, Galloway TS. Association of urinary bisphenol a concentration with heart disease: evidence from NHANES 2003/06. *PLoS One.* 2010;5:e8673.

75. Helsley RN, Zhou C. Epigenetic impact of endocrine disrupting chemicals on lipid homeostasis and atherosclerosis: a pregnane X receptor-centric view. *Environ Epigenet.* 2017;3(4):dvx017. Doi:10.1093/eep/dvx017

76. Uribarri J, Stirban A, Sander D, Cai W, Negrean M, Buenting CE, Koschinsky T, Vlassara H. Single oral challenge by advanced glycation end products acutely impairs endothelial function in diabetic and nondiabetic subjects. *Diabetes Care.* 2007 Oct;30(10): 2579–2582.

77. Sun Q, Wang A, Jin X, et al. Long-term air pollution exposure and acceleration of atherosclerosis and vascular inflammation in an animal model. *JAMA.* 2005;294(23): 3003–3010. Doi:10.1001/jama.294.23.3003

78. Niemann B, Rohrbach S, Miller MR, Newby DE, Fuster V, Kovacic JC. Oxidative stress and cardiovascular risk: obesity, diabetes, smoking, and pollution: part 3 of a 3-part series. *J Am Coll Cardiol.* 2017;70(2):230–251. Doi:10.1016/j.jacc.2017.05.043

79. Mitter SS, Vedanthan R, Islami F, et al. Household fuel use and cardiovascular disease mortality: golestan cohort study. *Circulation.* 2016;133(24):2360–2369. Doi:10.1161 /CIRCULATIONAHA.115.020288

80. Hadley MB, Vedanthan R, Fuster V. Air pollution and cardiovascular disease: a window of opportunity. *Nat Rev Cardiol.* 2018;15(4):193–194. Doi:10.1038/nrcardio.2017.207

81. Ravussin E, Lillioja S, Knowler WC, et al. 1988 Reduced rate of energy expenditure as a risk factor for body weight gain. *N Engl J Med.* 318:467–482.

82. Buscemi S, Di Maggio O, Blunda G, Maneri R, Verga S, Bompiani GD. A low resting metabolic rate is associated to body weight gain in adult Caucasian subjects: preliminary results of a 8–10 year longitudinal study. *Int J Obes.* 1998;22(Suppl 1):S75.

83. Griffiths M, Payne PR, Stunkard AJ, Rivers JPW, Cox M. Metabolic rate and physical development in children at risk for obesity. *Lancet.* 1990;336:76–77.

84. Roberts SB, Savage J, Coward WA, Chew B, Lucas A. Energy expenditure and intake in infants born to lean and overweight mothers. *Lancet*. 1990;318:461–466.

85. Zurlo F, Lillioja S, Puente A, et al. Low ratio of fat to carbohydrate oxidation as a predictor of weight gain: study of 24-RQ. *Am J Physiol*. 1991;259:E650–E657.

86. Weyer C, Pratley RE, Salbe AD, Bogardus C, Ravussin E, Tataranni PA. Energy expenditure, fat oxidation, and body weight regulation: a study of metabolic adaptation to long-term weight change. *J Clin Endocrinol Metab*. 2000;85(3):1087–1094. Doi:10.1210/jcem.85.3.6447

87. Tice RR, Austin CP, Kavlock RJ, Bucher JR. Improving the human hazard characterization of chemicals: a Tox21 update. *Environ Health Perspect*. 2013;121:756–765.

88. Kavlock R, Chandler K, Houck K, et al. Update on EPA's ToxCast program: providing high throughput decision support tools for chemical risk management. *Chem Res Toxicol*. 2012;25:1287–1302.

89. Takagi K. Study on the biodegradation of persistent organic pollutants (POPs). *J Pestic Sci*. 2020;45(2):119–123. Doi:10.1584/jpestics.J19-06

90. Heindel JJ, Blumberg B. Environmental obesogens: mechanisms and controversies. *Annu Rev Pharmacol Toxicol*. 2019;59:89–106. Doi:10.1146/annurev-pharmtox-010818-021304

91. https://ec.europa.eu/environment/chemicals/endocrine/documents/index_en.htm\

92. https://archive.epa.gov/pesticides/reregistration/web/pdf/atrazine_ired_finalization

93. https://www.epa.gov/laws-regulations/summary-federal-food-drug-and-cosmetic-act

94. https://www.epa.gov/pesticide-labels

95. James-Todd TM, Chiu YH, Zota AR. Racial/ethnic disparities in environmental endocrine disrupting chemicals and women's reproductive health outcomes: epidemiological examples across the life course. *Curr Epidemiol Rep*. 2016;3(2):161–180. Doi:10.1007/s40471-016-0073-9

96. https://bcerp.org/

97. https://www.niehs.nih.gov/research/supported/centers/srp/index.cfm

98. https://silentspring.org/project/digital-exposure-report-back-interface-derbi

5 Primordial Prevention of Cardiometabolic Risk Factors Using Lifestyle Medicine – Implementing Early Childhood Health Promotion

Ana Devesa and Valentin Fuster
Centro Nacional de Investigaciones Cardiovasculares (CNIC)
Icahn School of Medicine at Mount Sinai

Alexandra Turco
Icahn School of Medicine at Mount Sinai

Gloria Santos-Beneit
Icahn School of Medicine at Mount Sinai
Foundation for Science, Health and Education (SHE)

Rodrigo Fernandez-Jimenez
Centro Nacional de Investigaciones Cardiovasculares (CNIC)
Hospital Universitario Clínico San Carlos
Centro de Investigación Biomédica En Red en
enfermedades CardioVasculares (CIBERCV)

CONTENTS

DOI: 10.1201/9781003206637-5

5.1 INTRODUCTION: WHAT IS PRIMORDIAL PREVENTION, ITS BIOLOGICAL BASIS, AND THE OBSTACLES TO EFFECTIVE IMPLEMENTATION?

5.1.1 DEFINITION

Cumulative exposure to cardiovascular risk factors from young ages is an important contributor to adverse outcomes in adulthood.[1] Primordial prevention strategies aim to halt the development of cardiovascular risk factors. As opposed to primary prevention, which is focused on the treatment of the risk factors to avoid the development of cardiovascular disease, primordial prevention is focused on the prevention of these factors from appearing in the first place.[2]

In order to combat growing risk factors for and the burden of cardiovascular disease, the American Heart Association (AHA) defined ideal cardiovascular health (ICH) in children as the simultaneous presence of four favorable health behaviors (related to non-smoking, body mass index [BMI], healthy diet, and physical activity) and three favorable health factors (total cholesterol, blood pressure, and fasting glucose levels).[2] Starting at a very young age, most children experience a decline in ICH as they reach adolescence, correlating with an increased risk for future disease. Particularly, data for the population of U.S. children (12–19 years of age) showed that from 2015 to 2016, <1% of children met the ideal status for the healthy diet component of the ICH score. For most components of the ICH score, the prevalence of ideal levels is higher in U.S. children (12–19 years) than in adults (≥20 years) with the exception of healthy diet and physical activity scores, for which the prevalence of ideal levels is lower in children than adults.[3]

Previous studies have suggested that the process of subclinical atherosclerosis begins in youth.[4] The number of ICH metrics has been inversely correlated with aortic intima-media thickness and directly associated with elasticity.[5] Moreover, the ICH score has a long-lasting effect on cardiac structure and function, and the association is already evident in childhood.[6] The different factors and behaviors included in the ICH are associated with vascular health from a young age, supporting the relevance of targeting these metrics as part of primordial prevention.[5]

5.1.2 BIOLOGICAL BASIS: LINK BETWEEN CARDIOVASCULAR RISK FACTORS IN CHILDREN AND DISEASE IN ADULTHOOD

The link between the presence of modifiable cardiovascular risk factors in children and the development of disease in adulthood is becoming more evident. A recent study in a prospective cohort of more than 38,000 participants evaluated the relationship between childhood risk factors and cardiovascular events in adulthood after a 35-year follow-up. In the analysis of fatal cardiovascular events that occurred, the hazard ratios for a fatal cardiovascular event in adulthood ranged from a 1.3 per unit increase in the z-score for total cholesterol to 1.61 for youth smoking (as designated by a binary-smoking versus non-smoking status).[7] The seven components of the ICH score as they relate to children's cardiovascular health are described below.

5.1.2.1 Unhealthy Weight

Higher BMI during childhood is associated with an increased risk of coronary heart disease in adulthood;[8] this association increases as the age of the child increases. Childhood obesity by 7 years of age, if continued, has been associated with an increased risk of adult diabetes.[9] However, children who normalized their weights before the age of 13 showed a risk of adult diabetes similar to those who were never overweight, which supports the potential to reverse adverse outcomes with childhood interventions.[9] Higher BMI has also resulted in increased blood pressure in early midlife.[10]

The increase in risk factors associated with obesity as well as the reversibility supports the fact that interventions should start in childhood. Further, some studies suggest that obesity prevention should start as early as in the prenatal period since excessive weight gain during pregnancy along with other risk factors can alter fetal growth and metabolism and lead to higher adiposity in the newborn.[11]

5.1.2.2 Unhealthy Diet

Healthy dietary behaviors directly influence multiple cardiovascular risk factors such as obesity, dyslipidemia, hypertension, and hyperglycemia.[12] Diet quality and energy balance are two of the primary features of healthy eating. The AHA provided a definition of a healthy diet based on different components, including intakes of fruits and vegetables, fish, fiber, sodium, and sugar-sweetened beverages.[2] Strong evidence supports the association of added sugars with increased cardiovascular disease risk in children through increased energy intake, adiposity, and dyslipidemia.[13] Moreover, poorer food choices at preschool age have been associated with reduced scores in verbal and cognitive abilities. Interventions at this level are crucial since 91% of U.S. children are classified as having a poor diet score, according to the AHA definition.[12]

5.1.2.3   Insufficient Physical Activity

Physical activity is crucial to the physical and cognitive health of school-aged children; U.S. guidelines recommend that children spend a minimum of 60 minutes each day in moderate-to-vigorous physical activity.[14] Different studies have reported benefits on children's health factors that were associated with physical activity, including decreased adiposity, lower odds of becoming overweight or obese, and larger reductions in cardiometabolic biomarkers, including blood pressure, triglycerides, total cholesterol, insulin resistance, fasting insulin, fasting glucose, and carotid–femoral pulse wave velocities.[15] Additionally, interventions in youth are necessary to increase positive attitudes toward physical activity, which could lead to lifelong preventive behaviors. There is evidence linking the development of fundamental movement skills during preschool with a greater willingness to participate in physical activity of all types during early childhood and beyond.[16]

5.1.2.4   Smoking/Smoking Exposure

In the United States, 13.8% of high school students report current smoking;[17] smoking in teenage years is a strong predictor of adult smoking. Those who start early and continue to smoke may be more susceptible to diseases in adulthood than smokers who start later in life. With regard to its effect on cardiovascular health, cigarette smoking has been associated with increased blood pressure in adulthood.[10] Moreover, it has been shown that the detrimental effect of exposure to parental smoking is independent of other cardiovascular risk factors.[12] Childhood secondhand tobacco smoke exposure is associated with cardiometabolic risk factors such as obesity, dyslipidemia, and insulin resistance. Health interventions in childhood can target smoking in a multilevel manner through the encouragement of protective behavioral mechanisms in childhood, which might reduce future substance dependence, as well as through paired education to parents on the dangers of secondhand smoke.

5.1.2.5   Blood Pressure, Blood Cholesterol, and Blood Glucose

Increased arterial stiffness in adulthood is connected to metabolic syndrome in childhood, which manifests as a cluster of risk factors for cardiovascular diseases including high blood pressure, dyslipidemia, and insulin resistance. However, evidence shows that recovery from childhood metabolic syndrome can lead to favorable outcomes in adulthood, including decreased arterial pulse wave velocity.[18] The Bogalusa Heart study[4] showed a correlation of LDL cholesterol and blood pressure with aortic and coronary fatty streaks in autopsy results in teens, indicating that the number of cardiovascular risk factors increases, so does the severity of asymptomatic coronary and aortic atherosclerosis in young people. This evidence supports the need for comprehensive early childhood intervention, including both primordial and primary prevention strategies that could halt or slow the development and progression of risk factors, respectively.

Data from a large number of studies show that there is evidence for blood pressure tracking from childhood into adulthood: childhood blood pressure is associated with blood pressure in later life, with the strength of tracking increasing with the baseline age of measurement.[19] The main tool for reducing the deleterious effects of high blood pressure focuses on the reduction of salt in the diet beginning in infancy. In a randomized, double-blind trial among 476 newborn Dutch infants conducted in 1980, sodium intake was positively related to blood pressure during the first 6 months of life after an intervention with a normal sodium diet group and low-sodium diet group.[20] Because parental diet preferences largely govern food intake, especially at this early age, it is vitally important that primordial prevention strategies for the long-term reduction of children's blood pressure include outreach and education of parents beginning at birth or even pregnancy.

Furthermore, studies have revealed significant tracking of total cholesterol and LDL cholesterol levels from childhood to adulthood. Abnormal lipid levels in childhood are associated with increased evidence of atherosclerosis. However, puberty has a strong influence, with total and LDL cholesterol levels falling 10%–20% or more.[12,21] Therefore, it is important to note that the higher the childhood results and the older the post-pubertal age of assessment, the better the correlation with results in adulthood.[22]

Currently, pediatric guidelines suggest lipid screening for children 9–11 years, particularly non-HDL cholesterol, and in children 2–8 years only in populations with especially high risk of cardiovascular diseases.[22] However, in a major systematic review on screening and treatment for lipid disorders in children by the U.S. Preventive Services Task Force, due to a lack of standardization of family history questions, reliance on family history as a primary factor for screening would miss between 30% and 60% of children with high total cholesterol levels.[22] In accordance with studies showing no consistent harm, lipid screenings could pose an interesting avenue for the early detection of cardiovascular risk factors.

Measurements of fasting blood glucose levels give an important insight into the risk for future cardiovascular diseases and comorbidities such as type 2 diabetes. The burden of diabetes is predicted to worsen and parallel increasing obesity and sedentary lifestyle in children.[23] Children with diabetes are at a 40% greater risk of heart failure compared to non-diabetic counterparts and carry significant heterogeneity in risk for cardiovascular diseases.[24]

5.1.3 SCHOOLS AS THE MAIN FOCUS FOR PRIMORDIAL PREVENTION STRATEGIES

Further support for the necessity of early intervention is that knowledge acquired during childhood will have an influence on adulthood behaviors. Children spend so much of their time in school so this environment has great potential as a setting for intervention.[25] Additionally, schools are considered key sites for the implementation of health promotion programs due to their potential to reach the whole population in particular age-groups.[26] The implementation of primordial prevention strategies in childhood is a way to increase children's health literacy, which is defined as the ability to find, understand, and use information and services to inform health-related decisions and actions.[27] Prior studies have used health literacy-related scores[28–30] and have shown an improvement in children's health literacy after interventions. Additionally, interventions in schools that contain family components might encourage parental participation in healthy lifestyle changes.

Limitations to primordial prevention through school-based interventions largely revolve around the need for buy-in from relevant stakeholders, as well as the lack of a strong evidence base to draw on when creating structured randomized control trials (RCTs) in this setting. First, for an educational intervention to be successful in youth, the parents must adapt to the health needs of their children. Regardless of children's knowledge acquisition, substantial changes in health behaviors, such as diet, center on parental participation in feeding their children healthy foods. Furthermore, public policy and the school administration need to be in line with educational strategies, including improved nutrition of school lunches and greater time for physical activity throughout the school day. So far, public policy lags behind a growing evidence base calling for these changes. While parental and institutional participation may be limited at first, primordial prevention through education can still be successful in improving the health literacy of children so that they can be informed actors when making their own future decisions. The second limitation of school-based interventions is the need for growing evidence to inform the implementation of primordial prevention strategies. While large-scale RCTs are increasing in prevalence, there is a strong need for the rigorous scientific evaluation of proposed educational strategies in order to adequately inform proper delivery and ensure cost-effective solutions.

5.2 EVIDENCE: DESIGN OF STUDIES, CLINICAL EVIDENCE, AND CONCLUSIONS FROM LARGE-SCALE STUDIES ON PRESCHOOL-BASED INTERVENTIONS ON CARDIOVASCULAR HEALTH PROMOTION

5.2.1 SCHOOL-BASED INTERVENTIONS FOR PRIMORDIAL PREVENTION

Interventions for primordial prevention in the school environment are gaining traction as the primary avenue for health promotion. While numerous factors affect the cardiovascular disease risk of a child, most preschool interventions have targeted only physical activity and/or dietary components.[31] In large part, this is because children's weight during the preschool years is a key determinant of obesity later in life. A recent study of 51,505 children found that almost 90% of those who were obese at 3 years of age were overweight or obese in adolescence.[32] However, a systematic review of childhood obesity prevention programs showed significant effects on BMI with interventions that involve multiple components of the ICH score, demonstrating the need for multidimensional interventions.[33] Since lifestyle practices later in life can also be influenced by psychosocial factors in childhood,[34] emotional learning is an essential piece in primordial prevention.[35,36] The regulation of thoughts, emotions, and responses involves executive action, which mainly develops during preschool years[37]. Programs such as the SI! Program (Salud Integral – Comprehensive Health) implemented in large-scale trials across Spain, Colombia, and the United States involved an emotional management component, seeking to instill protective behavioral mechanisms against substance abuse, mainly smoking, later in life by working on self-awareness, self-esteem, decision-making, listening, and communication skills.[30] However, more research is needed to define which specific intervention characteristics and strategies contribute to the effectiveness of school-based interventions for health promotion and obesity prevention.[31]

5.2.2　Scientific Evaluation of School-Based Interventions on Health Promotion

Published RCT results on preschool-based interventions could help ensure the replicability of interventions in diverse settings.[31] Nevertheless, there are several scientific challenges to measuring the efficacy of an intervention in the school setting. For instance, at all study phases (from design to statistical analysis), a cluster effect can occur (e.g., when individuals from the same classroom or school show some correlation with each other in terms of their habits and routines). The implementation of the intervention itself is a complex procedure that needs to involve the whole educational community and the role of teaching staff is fundamental to ensuring that the program is carried out effectively. Developing awareness of implementation issues is becoming an increasingly prominent concern in educational contexts, offering an interesting perspective on its scientific dimensions. Before expanding a health promotion program, it is appropriate to evaluate the effectiveness of the intervention, as well as possible limitations, while adhering to evidence-based practice. There is now consensus that RCTs are the gold standard for assessing relationships between interventions and outcomes.[31]

5.2.3　Assessment Tools within RCTs

One of the main challenges with intervention evaluation is the nature of the assessment tools, particularly for research on preschoolers. The use of age-appropriate questionnaires is especially important. Preschool-age children cannot yet read well, so questionnaires need to include simple pictures to support both questions and answers and be administered individually by a trained team of early childhood education professionals. Questions should also be adapted to the sociocultural context, for example, by using names and pictures of local foods, pictures of local playgrounds, and pictures reflecting local ethnic diversity. In addition, the duration of the intervention will determine the need to adjust the methodology (individual vs. group administration) or questionnaire items (number and complexity) according to the stages of maturation in children.[28,38,39]

Questionnaires can carry a subjective component that may impact the results; however, individual administration by trained staff helps standardize the process and minimize this problem. An example of a response bias is social desirability, which has been widely studied in relation to reported eating habits.[40,41] On the other hand, direct measurements are an accurate and reliable source of information, and a combination of questionnaires and direct measurements can allow cross-validation. Data collection should be standardized and carried out by trained technical personnel such as nutritionists or nurses. The chosen measurement tools should pose zero or minimal risk to the children and be associated with health indicators such as BMI, waist circumference, or blood pressure. Given the lack of consensus regarding BMI cut-offs, large-scale comparisons might be aided by using both local percentiles and growth charts from the World Health Organization or the U.S. Centers for Disease Control and Prevention.[42] Some indicators of fat amount and distribution, such as skinfolds or circumferences, may add additional information widely used in the pediatric setting.[43] Also, the waist-to-height ratio is an accurate indicator of the presence of metabolic syndrome components, especially hypertension, in childhood and adolescence.[44] The use of other indicators, such as a blood glucose or lipid profile, or accelerometers to assess physical activity, may be more suitable for older children.[45,46]

5.2.4 IMPLEMENTATION OF RCTS ON HEALTH PROMOTION IN EARLY CHILDHOOD

The SI! Program is a large-scale heart health intervention, which is a school-based program for the promotion of cardiovascular health aimed at achieving lasting lifestyle changes in children from preschool ages.[30] The four components of the SI! Program curriculum are diet, physical activity, emotional management, and body and heart; the four levels of intervention are classroom, family, teachers, and the school environment (Figure 5.1).

SI! Program RCTs included a questionnaire assessing children's Knowledge, Attitude, and Habits (KAH) in relation to a healthy lifestyle, demonstrating the workability of early childhood assessments through questionnaires. The KAH metric is based on the progressive acquisition and retention of healthy habits in children according to the "Transtheoretical Model of Change," which includes five stages of behavior modification.[47] The KAH score aggregates the "pre-contemplative" and "contemplative" stages as the acquisition of knowledge (K), the "preparation" phase as setting this knowledge into attitudes (A), and the final "action" and "maintenance" stages as the acquisition of the desired habit (H). The KAH system has been shown to serve as a surrogate of improved lifestyle and therefore as a successful measure of the ability of the intervention to instill these concepts and provide children with tools for self-promotion of health.[31]

The SI! Program has been assessed in a cluster RCT in three countries: Colombia, Spain, and the United States. The first intervention took place in Colombia in 2009, in the Usaquén neighborhood of Bogotá.[28] The effect of the SI! Program for preschoolers was assessed in an RCT in 14 preschool facilities, involving 1,216 children aged 3–5 years, their parents, and their teachers. A structured survey was conducted at baseline and at the end of the intervention to assess changes in KAH toward a healthy lifestyle. Children in the interventional group showed a significantly larger increase in KAH scores than those in the control group.[28]

From 2011 to 2014, the program was assessed in Madrid (Spain) using a similar cluster randomized controlled strategy. This study enrolled 2,062 children aged 3–5 years, their parents/caregivers, and teachers, who all participated in a 3-year intervention.[48] The results after 1 year of the intervention indicated that the SI! Program significantly increased children's KAH scores. At the end of the 3-year intervention period, the overall KAH score change was significantly higher in children in the interventional group than in the control group.[29]

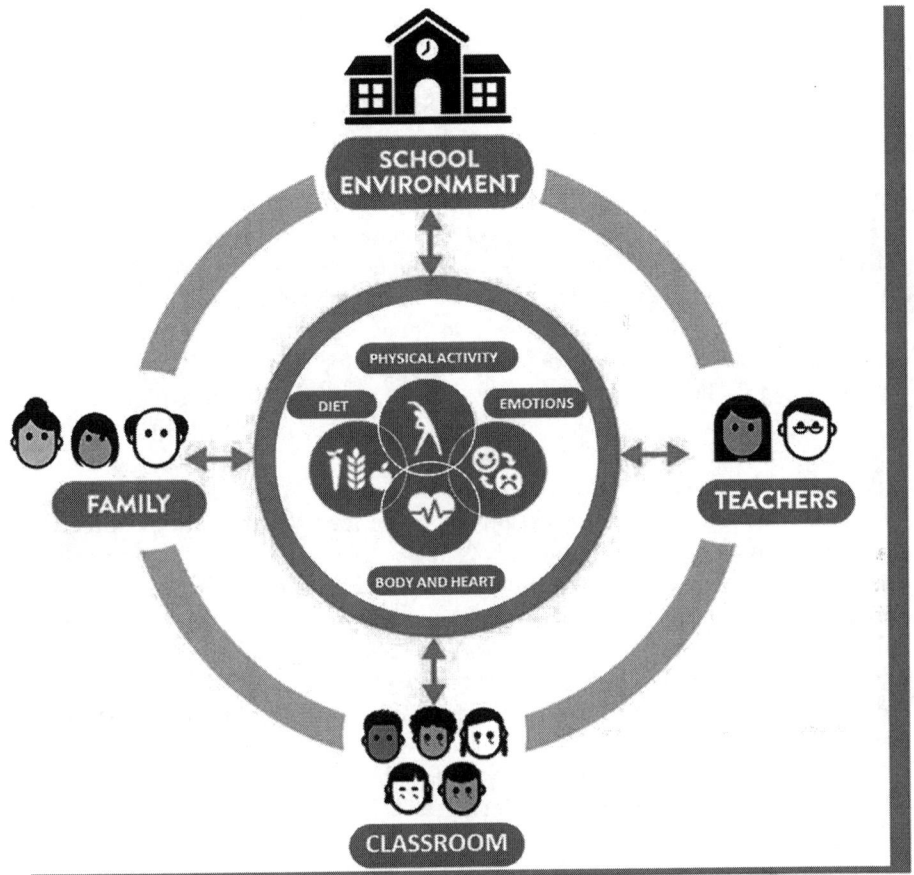

FIGURE 5.1 The SI!-Program components. (Reproduced with permission from the authors.[31])

Most recently, the impact of the SI! Program was assessed in a vulnerable multiracial urban community in Harlem, New York (USA). A total of 562 children aged 3–5 years from 15 preschools were randomized in the FAMILIA trial to receive the SI! Program for 4 months or to the control group.[49] Consistent with the results obtained in Colombia and Spain, the change from baseline in overall KAH score was significantly higher among intervened children than children in the control group.[50] The impact of intervention adherence or fidelity on intervention effects was explored in the SI! Program study in Harlem. The project analyzed a potential dose-response effect of the intervention through the differences in KAH scores between children receiving <50% of the program modules (low adherence) vs. those receiving 50%–75% (intermediate adherence) or >75% (high adherence). Compared with the low-adherence group, the high-adherence group showed a significantly larger change from baseline in overall KAH score (mean difference of 3.10 points [95% CI, 0.32–5.89]). The significant impact of intervention adherence on outcomes highlights the importance of strategies to promote high adherence and therefore achieve the highest benefits for the targeted population.[50]

In accordance with the emphasis on the bioecological contributions to health in the SI! Program, the Healthy Start-Depart Santé (HSDS) intervention was a 2-arm cluster randomized controlled childhood obesity prevention trial, aiming to improve motor skills, physical activity, and fruit and vegetable consumption among 897 children (ages 3–5 years) enrolled in 61 early childhood care centers in Chicago, Illinois (USA).[16] The HSDS involved a direct educational intervention in childcare facilities delivered by preschool teachers, who were trained and supported by research staff. Of the 12 main outcome variables analyzed (including physical activity, fundamental motor skills, and healthy eating), only two showed a statistically significant difference: locomotor skills and fruit/vegetable consumption. The significant difference in locomotor skills shows promise in its long-term ability to increase participation in physical activity and therefore its preventive capacities against obesity and cardiovascular diseases.

While early intervention is necessary to improve long-term cardiovascular health outcomes, the RCT of the Child Health Initiative for Lifelong Eating and Exercise (CHILE) Study[51] displayed limitations of shorter-term assessment measures. CHILE was a 5-year evidence-based intervention that used a socioecological approach to improve dietary intake and increase physical activity of 1,898 Hispanic and American Indian preschoolers in New Mexico, USA.[51] At the end of the intervention, no significant group differences existed in the primary outcome variable of BMI. Despite successful implementation, the CHILE study showed that significant changes in BMI may take longer than 2 years to achieve.

The sustainability of effects is a question needing more attention within school-based interventions, yet strategies exist to overcome these barriers. The SI! Program for children aged 9–13 years in Bogotá, Colombia, tested the possibility of sustained results over a 7-year period. The effects of a 4-month intervention in preschool, as measured by a change in KAH score, dissipated at the 7-year post-intervention follow-up among the 596 children in the interventional cohort.[52] Additionally, after a successive re-intervention, there were no differences found between the re-interventional group and those receiving an intervention for the first time. This is likely because multiple factors in a child's life, including socioeconomic status, school environment, age, and engagement with the curriculum, affect their ability and likelihood to practice healthy habits. However, a dose-response effect was observed after delivering the curriculum, with the largest effect observed in the high-adherence group (i.e., those receiving >75% of the educational program modules). Compared with the low-adherence group, the high-adherence group showed a significantly greater change from baseline in the overall KAH score (mean difference of 3.72 points [95% CI: 1.71–5.73; $p < 0.001$]). For everyday participation in the intervention, the change from baseline in the overall KAH score increased by 0.64 points (95% CI: 0.34–0.94; $p < 0.001$).[52] The results of this study show a need for integrated approaches to combat the development of risk factors in children, including but not limited to multilevel educational intervention, rigorous implementation monitoring, and policy change such as healthier school lunches and physical activity programs.

5.3 SYNTHESIS: CORE ELEMENTS (THEORY, DATA, CHALLENGES, UPDATED STRATEGIES, AND IMPLEMENTATION TACTICS)

5.3.1 BUILDING A TEAM AND STAKEHOLDER RELATIONSHIPS

Achieving sustainable lifestyle changes in preschool children through health promotion programs is likely to require the integration of several factors such as multidisciplinary teams, multidimensional educational program targeting several levels of intervention, and a strong local program coordination for subsequent community engagement. The multifaceted nature of cardiovascular diseases requires complex interventions targeting several behaviors and/or levels of influence.[25] The interventional materials should be designed by a multidisciplinary team of experts, facilitating the integration of methodologies from different fields proven to be the most effective at generating significant learning.[31] Combining the scientific evidence with optimal teaching strategies requires synergy among experts in each domain to ensure that the message reaches the target population in the most effective way. It is essential to include local health and educational professionals to adjust the educational strategies to the socioeconomic and cultural context of each setting. Moreover, establishing a close relationship with stakeholders and building trust in the community is essential for generating support for school-based health promotion interventions.[53] This requires working partners and leaders from the community who have a longstanding relationship with and deep commitment to their local community.

5.3.2 NEED FOR INTERVENTION ADAPTABILITY

Interventions can be tailored to the study population and the local environment to increase the likelihood of behavioral change. Focus groups conducted in a pilot phase of the study, before trial initiation, are a very effective qualitative analysis tool for this purpose.[54] This strategy can help the research team to adapt the whole approach of the intervention.[55]

According to the cognitive social theory, the environment has a fundamental influence on the learning process and behavior change,[56] and children are engaged more effectively if the intervention includes their immediate surrondings.[57] In particular, the cognitive social theory highlights the role of social modeling, motivational factors, and self-efficacy to support the adoption of desirable behaviors. Thus, a family-based approach is also desirable and surely complementary to school-based programs, given that parents normally manage most access to food at home or lead physical activity routines.[31] Family members are young children's primary social context, providing experiences and access to food and physical activity through which children begin to acquire healthy or unhealthy lifestyles.[58] In the Cardiovascular Risk in Young Finns Study, childhood parental smoking exposure was associated with increased risk for life-course overweight/obesity.[59] The Identification and Prevention of Dietary and Lifestyle-Induced Health Effects in Children and Infants study (IDEFICS) analyzed characteristics and intervention involvement in 4,180 parents of 2- to 9-year-old children in seven European countries (Belgium, Cyprus, Estonia, Germany, Italy, Spain, and Sweden).[60] The authors found that parental exposure and involvement in the

IDEFICS intervention in all countries were much less than aimed for. The reasons for this shortfall could include an overly diverse focus (six key messages) and the high intensity and duration of the intervention. In an IDEFICS qualitative interview substudy of 20 children and 36 parental focus groups in southwest Sweden, parents described lack of time, financial constraints, availability, and food marketing techniques as barriers to promoting healthy eating.[61] Providing information and guidance to families based on their children's results is also a great incentive for participation, especially in communities with low access to medical care, as shown by the FAMILIA study conducted in Harlem. The objectives within each component of the intervention must be addressed in a very direct and simple way so they can be easily adapted to different socioeconomic settings or coexist with health promotion strategies at the local level.

5.3.3 ROLE OF TEACHERS ON SCHOOL-BASED INTERVENTION SUCCESS

Teachers have a fundamental role in transmitting knowledge and shaping children's behavior during learning[62]. Teachers are also crucial for the success of school-based interventions, especially those involving preschool-age children. The trusting relationship developed between children and teachers allows the message to be received with greater attention and credibility than if it came from external personnel. In a meta-analysis of 213 school-based social and emotional learning programs involving 270,034 students from kindergarten through high school,[35] programs delivered by non-school personnel (e.g., university researchers or outside consultants) were less likely than teacher-led programs to meet recommended practices related to skill development (65% vs. 90%) and were more likely to encounter problems during program implementation (31% vs. 22%). Teacher-delivery models have been used in several recent interventions in preschoolers.[31]

A school-based program to encourage behavior change goes beyond standard preservice teacher education, and specific training is therefore fundamental to supporting the needed transformation of teacher practices with consistency across classrooms and schools in order to promote the fidelity of the intervention.[63] Teachers' roles in school-based interventions are crucial because they can determine how the curriculum is implemented.

5.3.4 ROLE OF FAMILIES IN INTERVENTION SUCCESS

Parental participation in primordial prevention strategies is crucial for the success of health interventions. Sustained lifestyle changes must be supported in the home environment through the provision of healthy foods at mealtimes, encouragement to participate in physical activity, and the avoidance of negative lifestyle habits, such as smoking. At such a young age, children have little control over the home sphere, so it is vital that parents and other family members acknowledge the importance of healthy living and that they are given the tools, such as knowledge or community support, to achieve those health goals. Considering the importance of familial participation, a new RCT – "Vive la Salud en Familia" or Live Healthy as a Family – is being developed in Spain by the SI! Program Team. This project is an educational program applicable to the entire family in order to inspire a culture of health. The home environment and family lifestyles are crucial in forming habits; therefore, the concept of collective health is a facilitating factor when modifying and maintaining healthy routines.

5.3.5 Sustained Efficacy of School-Based Interventions

The evidence suggests that the peak effect is seen immediately after school-based interventions and reinforcement is required to achieve a sustained effect.[25,31] Transferring and sustaining effective programs in real-world settings are complex, long-term processes that require effective strategies for dealing with subsequent phases of program scale-up. Achieving the commitment of teaching staff, school leaders, and other stakeholders is critical for the success of a health promotion program. A recent study of school-based interventions in adolescents found that a passionate, well-trained layperson can effectively change students' and teachers' practices.[57,64] The inclusion of a local program coordinator (i.e., a non-school staff layperson) is a recommended strategy to support the school community, school team coordinator (school staff), and teachers. The local program coordinator ensures effective coordination with school-level interventions in terms of teacher training, meetings, curriculum presentation, and frequent motivational communication. The effectiveness of a health promotion program depends not only on the quality of the materials and curriculum offered to teachers and families but also on the follow-up and support provided by the program developers.[38] To promote the commitment of the educational community, program developers can create a feeling of belonging by providing feedback on the results through meetings and social and/or mass media.[31] Successful engagement in the educational community will mostly depend on whether people believe the issue is directly relevant to them, see evidence of progress, and have a sense that their actions can make a difference. Beyond the school, the sustainability of the effect of school interventions may be promoted by interventions at different strata such as workplace health promotion programs, active aging programs, or more intense parallel health promotion programs specifically targeting parents/caregivers. Although the maximum possibly sustained public health benefit would come from implementing multiple interventions at all levels of the ecological model, the single interventions with the greatest impact on population health are those focusing on the physical and social environmental context and socioeconomic and policy factors.

It is very important to engage all potential partners as strategic collaborators to ensure that interventions address the full spectrum of cardiovascular diseases, from prevention and risk factor reduction to diagnosis and treatment (Figure 5.2). Moreover, the collaboration of community health and government agencies is necessary to give the public a coherent message on health matters, for example through advertising, food labeling, adaptation of local infrastructures to promote physical activity as healthy leisure, price regulation of healthy foods, etc.[65] All of these strategies, added to school programs and legislative actions, can contribute to the comprehensive approach needed to curb the burden of cardiovascular diseases.[66]

A core challenge in global health is translating scientific evidence into educational and community practices. This challenge becomes more complex when it requires

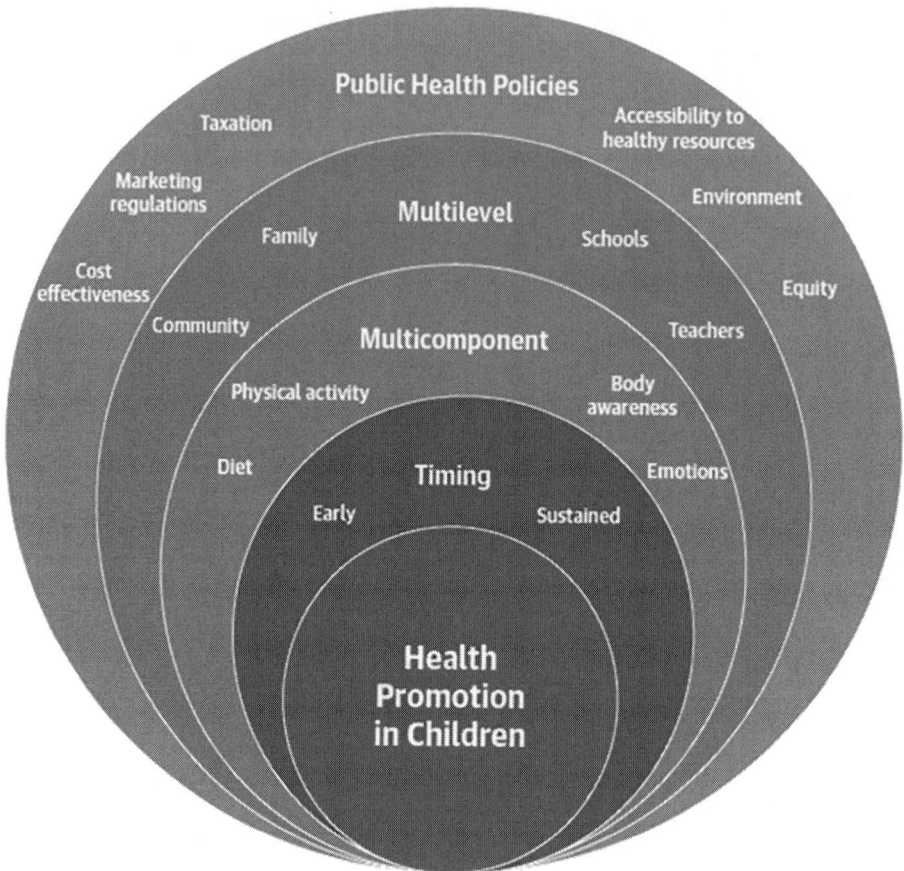

FIGURE 5.2 Factors of health promotion in children. (Reproduced with permission from the authors.[25])

individual, organizational, and systemic behavior change. By matching rigorous scientific impact studies with implementation studies, the divide between science and educational practice can be bridged.[31]

5.4 CONCLUSIONS

Cardiovascular disease is the leading cause of death and disability in the world. The development of protective health behaviors and the acquisition of health knowledge must begin as early as possible to prevent an increased risk of cardiovascular diseases. Primordial prevention strategies that aim to prevent risk factors for cardiovascular diseases before they develop are vitally necessary to fight against future cardiovascular diseases. This is in light of the growing obesity epidemic and increased sedentary lifestyle but requires coordination among the school, family, and community, as well as wide support across multiple sectors through the implementation of public policy.

Lifestyle interventions in childhood may provide an opportunity to implement primordial prevention strategies and increase health literacy in children. However, more RCTs are needed to determine the most effective and cost-efficient interventions.

The time is now to focus our efforts on the long-term prevention of cardiovascular diseases by encouraging healthy lifestyle changes, improving health literacy, and increasing access to preventive care.

Disclosures:
None.

REFERENCES

1. O'Connor EA, Evans CV, Burda BU, Walsh ES, Eder M, Lozano P. Screening for obesity and intervention for weight management in children and adolescents evidence report and systematic review for the us preventive services task force. *JAMA - J Am Med Assoc.* 2017;317(23):2427–2444. doi:10.1001/jama.2017.0332

2. Lloyd-Jones DM, Hong Y, Labarthe D, et al. Defining and setting national goals for cardiovascular health promotion and disease reduction: The American Heart Association strategic impact goal through 2020 and beyond. *Circulation.* 2010;121(4):586–613. doi: 10.1161/CIRCULATIONAHA.109.192703

3. Virani SS, Alonso A, Aparicio HJ, et al. Heart disease and stroke statistics-2021 update a report from the American Heart Association. *Circulation.* 2021;143:E254–E743. doi: 10.1161/CIR.0000000000000950

4. Berenson GS, Srinivasan SR, Bao W, Newman WP, Tracy RE, Wattigney WA. Association between multiple cardiovascular risk factors and atherosclerosis in children and young adults. *N Engl J Med.* 1998 Jun 4;338(23):1650–1656. doi:10.1056/nejm199806043382302

5. Pahkala K, Hietalampi H, Laitinen TT, et al. Ideal cardiovascular health in adolescence effect of lifestyle intervention and association with vascular intima-media thickness and elasticity (the Special Turku Coronary Risk Factor Intervention Project for Children [STRIP] Study). *Circulation.* 2013;127(21):2088–2096. doi:10.1161/CIRCULATIONAHA.112.000761

6. Laitinen TT, Ruohonen S, Juonala M, et al. Ideal cardiovascular health in childhood—Longitudinal associations with cardiac structure and function: The Special Turku Coronary Risk Factor Intervention Project (STRIP) and the Cardiovascular Risk in Young Finns Study (YFS). *Int J Cardiol.* 2017;230:304–309. doi:10.1016/j.ijcard.2016.12.117

7. Jacobs DR, Woo JG, Sinaiko AR, et al. Childhood cardiovascular risk factors and adult cardiovascular events. *N Engl J Med.* 2022;386(20):1877–1888. doi:10.1056/NEJMoa2109191

8. Baker JL, Olsen LW, Sørensen TIA. Childhood Body-mass index and the risk of coronary heart disease in adulthood. *N Engl J Med.* 2007;357(23):2329–2337. doi:10.1056/nejmoa072515

9. Bjerregaard LG, Jensen BW, Ängquist L, Osler M, Sørensen TIA, Baker JL. Change in overweight from childhood to early adulthood and risk of type 2 diabetes. *N Engl J Med.* 2018;378(14):1302–1312. doi:10.1056/nejmoa1713231

10. Zhang T, Li S, Bazzano L, He J, Whelton P, Chen W. Trajectories of childhood blood pressure and adult left ventricular hypertrophy: The bogalusa heart study. *Hypertension.* 2018;72(1):93–101. doi:10.1161/HYPERTENSIONAHA.118.10975

11. Gillman MW, Ludwig DS. How early should obesity prevention start? *N Engl J Med.* 2013;369(23):2173–2175. doi:10.1056/nejmp1310577

12. Steinberger J, Daniels SR, Hagberg N, et al. Cardiovascular health promotion in children: Challenges and opportunities for 2020 and beyond: A scientific statement from the American Heart Association. *Circulation.* 2016;134(12):e236–e255. doi:10.1161/CIR.0000000000000441

13. Vos MB, Kaar JL, Welsh JA, et al. Added sugars and cardiovascular disease risk in children: A scientific statement from the American Heart Association. *Circulation.* 2017;135(19):e1017–e1034. doi:10.1161/CIR.0000000000000439

14. Poitras VJ, Gray CE, Borghese MM, et al. Systematic review of the relationships between objectively measured physical activity and health indicators in school-aged children and youth. *Appl Physiol Nutr Metab.* 2016;41(6):S197–S239. doi:10.1139/apnm-2015-0663

15. Aatola H, Koivistoinen T, Hutri-Kähönen N, et al. Lifetime fruit and vegetable consumption and arterial pulse wave velocity in adulthood: The cardiovascular risk in young finns study. *Circulation.* 2010;122(24):2521–2528. doi:10.1161/CIRCULATIONAHA.110.969279

16. Leis A, Ward S, Vatanparast H, et al. Effectiveness of the Healthy Start-Départ Santé approach on physical activity, healthy eating and fundamental movement skills of preschoolers attending childcare centres: A randomized controlled trial. *BMC Public Health.* 2020;20(1):1–12. doi:10.1186/s12889-020-08621-9

17. Fanshawe TR, Halliwell W, Lindson N, Aveyard P, Livingstone-Banks J, Hartmann-Boyce J. Tobacco cessation interventions for young people. *Cochrane Database Syst Rev.* 2017;2017(11). doi:10.1002/14651858.CD003289.pub6

18. Koivistoinen T, Hutri-Kähönen N, Juonala M, et al. Metabolic syndrome in childhood and increased arterial stiffness in adulthood - The Cardiovascular Risk in Young Finns Study. *Ann Med.* 2011;43(4):312–319. doi:10.3109/07853890.2010.549145

19. Chen X, Wang Y. Tracking of blood pressure from childhood to adulthood: A systematic review and meta-regression analysis. *Circulation.* 2008;117(25):3171–3180. doi:10.1161/CIRCULATIONAHA.107.730366

20. Hofman A, Hazebroek A, Valkenburg HA. A randomized trial of sodium intake and blood pressure in newborn infants. *JAMA J Am Med Assoc.* 1983;250(3):370–373. doi:10.1001/jama.1983.03340030030023

21. De Jesus JM. Expert panel on integrated guidelines for cardiovascular health and risk reduction in children and adolescents: Summary report. *Pediatrics.* 2011;128(SUPPL. 5). doi:10.1542/peds.2009-2107C

22. NHLBI. Integrated Guidelines for Cardiovascular Health and Risk Reduction in Children and Adolescents - NHLBI, NIH. Report. http://www.nhlbi.nih.gov/health-pro/guidelines/current/cardiovascular-health-pediatric-guidelines. Published 2012. Accessed April 8, 2022.

23. Truong UT, Maahs DM, Daniels SR. Cardiovascular disease in children and adolescents with diabetes: Where are we, and where are we going? *Diabetes Technol Ther.* 2012;14(SUPPL. 1). doi:10.1089/dia.2012.0018

24. Glovaci D, Fan W, Wong ND. Epidemiology of diabetes mellitus and cardiovascular disease. *Curr Cardiol Rep.* 2019;21(4):1–8. doi:10.1007/s11886-019-1107-y

25. Fernandez-Jimenez R, Al-Kazaz M, Jaslow R, Carvajal I, Fuster V. Children present a window of opportunity for promoting health: JACC review topic of the week. *J Am Coll Cardiol.* 2018;72(25):3310–3319. doi:10.1016/j.jacc.2018.10.031

26. Pearson M, Chilton R, Wyatt K, et al. Implementing health promotion programmes in schools: A realist systematic review of research and experience in the United Kingdom. *Implement Sci.* 2015;10(1):1–20. doi:10.1186/s13012-015-0338-6

27. US Department of Health and Human Services. Health Literacy in Healthy People 2030. https://health.gov/our-work/national-health-initiatives/healthy-people/healthy-people-2030/health-literacy-healthy-people-2030. Published 2021. Accessed April 8, 2022.

28. Céspedes J, Briceño G, Farkouh ME, et al. Targeting preschool children to promote cardiovascular health: Cluster randomized trial. *Am J Med.* 2013;126(1):27–35.e3. doi:10.1016/j.amjmed.2012.04.045

29. Peñalvo JL, Santos-Beneit G, Sotos-Prieto M, et al. The SI! program for cardiovascular health promotion in early childhood a cluster-randomized trial. *J Am Coll Cardiol.* 2015;66(14):1525–1534. doi:10.1016/j.jacc.2015.08.014

30. Fernandez-Jimenez R, Jaslow R, Bansilal S, et al. Different lifestyle interventions in adults from underserved communities: The FAMILIA trial. *J Am Coll Cardiol.* 2020;75(1):42–56. doi:10.1016/j.jacc.2019.10.021

31. Santos-Beneit G, Fernández-Jiménez R, de Cos-Gandoy A, et al. Lessons learned from 10 years of preschool intervention for health promotion: JACC state-of-the-art review. *J Am Coll Cardiol.* 2022;79(3):283–298. doi:10.1016/j.jacc.2021.10.046

32. Geserick M, Vogel M, Gausche R, et al. Acceleration of BMI in early childhood and risk of sustained obesity. *N Engl J Med.* 2018;379(14):1303–1312. doi:10.1056/nejmoa 1803527

33. Wang Y, Cai L, Wu Y, et al. What childhood obesity prevention programmes work? A systematic review and meta-analysis. *Obes Rev.* 2015;16(7):547–565. doi:10.1111/obr.12277

34. Bermejo-Martins E, Mujika A, Iriarte A, et al. Social and emotional competence as key element to improve healthy lifestyles in children: A randomized controlled trial. *J Adv Nurs.* 2019;75(8):1764–1781. doi:10.1111/jan.14024

35. Durlak JA, Weissberg RP, Dymnicki AB, Taylor RD, Schellinger KB. The impact of enhancing students' social and emotional learning: A meta-analysis of school-based universal interventions. *Child Dev.* 2011;82(1):405–432. doi:10.1111/j.1467-8624.2010. 01564.x

36. Rueda MR, Checa P, Cómbita LM. Enhanced efficiency of the executive attention network after training in preschool children: Immediate changes and effects after two months. *Dev Cogn Neurosci.* 2012;2(SUPPL. 1). doi:10.1016/j.dcn.2011.09.004

37. Jones LB, Rothbart MK, Posner MI. Development of executive attention in preschool children. *Dev Sci.* 2003;6(5):498–504. doi:10.1111/1467-7687.00307

38. Chiang M, Torres M, Maldonado M, González U. Proposal for a program to promote a healthy lifestyle in preschool children through a multidisciplinary intervention. *Cuba J Biomed Res.* 2003;22(4):245–252.

39. Santos-Beneit G, Sotos-Prieto M, Bodega P, et al. Development and validation of a questionnaire to evaluate lifestyle-related behaviors in elementary school children. *BMC Public Health.* 2015;15(1):1–7. doi:10.1186/s12889-015-2248-6

40. Guinn CH, Baxter SD, Royer JA, Hardin JW, MacKelprang AJ, Smith AF. Fourth-grade childrens dietary recall accuracy for energy intake at school meals differs by social desirability and body mass index percentile in a study concerning retention interval. *J Health Psychol.* 2010;15(4):505–514. doi:10.1177/1359105309353814

41. Baxter SD, Smith AF, Litaker MS, Baglio ML, Guinn CH, Shaffer NM. Children's social desirability and dietary reports. *J Nutr Educ Behav.* 2004;36(2):84–89. doi:10.1016/ S1499-4046(06)60138-3

42. Grossman DC, Bibbins-Domingo K, Curry SJ, et al. Screening for obesity in children and adolescents us preventive services task force recommendation statement. *JAMA - J Am Med Assoc.* 2017;317(23):2417–2426. doi:10.1001/jama.2017.6803

43. Santos-Beneit G, Sotos-Prieto M, Pocock S, Redondo J, Fuster V, Peñalvo JL. Association between anthropometry and high blood pressure in a representative sample of preschoolers in Madrid. *Rev Española Cardiol.* 2015;68(6):477–484. doi:10.1016/j. rec.2014.09.002

44. Martínez Álvarez JR, Villarino Marín A, García Alcón RM, López Ejeda N, Marrodán Serrano MD. El Índice Cintura-Talla Es Un Eficaz Indicador Antropométrico De La Hipertensión En Escolares. *Nutr Hosp.* 2016;33(2). doi:10.20960/nh.140

45. Fernandez-Jimenez R, Santos-Beneit G, Tresserra-Rimbau A, et al. Rationale and design of the school-based SI! Program to face obesity and promote health among Spanish adolescents: A cluster-randomized controlled trial. *Am Heart J.* 2019;215:27–40. doi:10.1016/j.ahj.2019.03.014

46. Steene-Johannessen J, Hansen BH, Dalene KE, et al. Variations in accelerometry measured physical activity and sedentary time across Europe-harmonized analyses of 47,497 children and adolescents. *Int J Behav Nutr Phys Act.* 2020;17(1):1–14. doi:10.1186/s12966-020-00930-x

47. Zask A, Barnett LM, Rose L, et al. Three year follow-up of an early childhood intervention: Is movement skill sustained? *Int J Behav Nutr Phys Act.* 2012;9(1):1–9. doi:10.1186/1479-5868-9-127

48. Peñalvo JL, Sotos-Prieto M, Santos-Beneit G, Pocock S, Redondo J, Fuster V. The Program SI! intervention for enhancing a healthy lifestyle in preschoolers: First results from a cluster randomized trial. *BMC Public Health.* 2013;13(1). doi:10.1186/1471-2458-13-1208

49. Bansilal S, Vedanthan R, Kovacic JC, et al. Rationale and design of family-based approach in a minority community integrating systems–biology for promotion of health (FAMILIA). *Am Heart J.* 2017;187:170–181. doi:10.1016/j.ahj.2017.02.020

50. Fernandez-Jimenez R, Jaslow R, Bansilal S, et al. Child health promotion in underserved communities: The FAMILIA trial. *J Am Coll Cardiol.* 2019;73(16):2011–2021. doi:10.1016/j.jacc.2019.01.057

51. Davis SM, Myers OB, Cruz TH, et al. CHILE: Outcomes of a group randomized controlled trial of an intervention to prevent obesity in preschool Hispanic and American Indian children. *Prev Med.* 2016;89:162–168. doi:10.1016/j.ypmed.2016.05.018

52. Fernández-Jiménez R, Briceño G, Céspedes J, et al. Sustainability of and adherence to preschool health promotion among children 9 to 13 years old. *J Am Coll Cardiol.* 2020;75(13):1565–1578. doi:10.1016/j.jacc.2020.01.051

53. Dabravolskaj J, Montemurro G, Ekwaru JP, et al. Effectiveness of school-based health promotion interventions prioritized by stakeholders from health and education sectors: A systematic review and meta-analysis. *Prev Med Rep.* 2020;19. doi:10.1016/j.pmedr.2020.101138

54. Haerens L, De Bourdeaudhuij I, Barba G, et al. Developing the IDEFICS community-based intervention program to enhance eating behaviors in 2- to 8-year-old children: Findings from focus groups with children and parents. *Health Educ Res.* 2009;24(3):381–393. doi:10.1093/her/cyn033

55. Carral Bielsa V, Rodríguez C, Orrit X, et al. the Si! program for promoting heart-healthy habits in children aged 3 to 5 years: Pedagogical strategies. *EDULEARN20 Proc.* 2020;1:3490–3499. doi:10.21125/edulearn.2020.0985

56. Bandura A. Health promotion by social cognitive means. *Heal Educ Behav.* 2004;31(2):143–164. doi:10.1177/1090198104263660

57. Shinde S, Weiss HA, Varghese B, et al. Promoting school climate and health outcomes with the SEHER multi-component secondary school intervention in Bihar, India: A cluster-randomised controlled trial. *Lancet.* 2018;392(10163):2465–2477. doi:10.1016/S0140-6736(18)31615-5

58. Bogl LH, Mehlig K, Ahrens W, et al. Like me, like you-relative importance of peers and siblings on children's fast food consumption and screen time but not sports club participation depends on age. *Int J Behav Nutr Phys Act.* 2020;17(1):1–11. doi:10.1186/s12966-020-00953-4

59. Jaakkola JM, Rovio SP, Pahkala K, et al. Childhood exposure to parental smoking and life-course overweight and central obesity. *Ann Med.* 2021;53(1):208–216. doi:10.1080/07853890.2020.1853215

60. de Bourdeaudhuij I, Verbestel V, de Henauw S, et al. Implementation of the IDEFICS intervention across European countries: Perceptions of parents and relationship with BMI. *Obes Rev.* 2015;16:78–88. doi:10.1111/obr.12330

61. Regber S. Barriers and facilitators of health promotion and obesity prevention in early childhood : A focus on parents results from the IDEFICS study by. 2014:91. http://hdl.handle.net/2077/34815. Accessed April 8, 2022.

62. Cheung P. Teachers as role models for physical activity: Are preschool children more active when their teachers are active? *Eur Phys Educ Rev.* 2020;26(1):101–110. doi:10.1177/1356336X19835240

63. Renko E, Knittle K, Palsola M, Lintunen T, Hankonen N. Acceptability, reach and implementation of a training to enhance teachers' skills in physical activity promotion. *BMC Public Health.* 2020;20(1):1–13. doi:10.1186/s12889-020-09653-x

64. Ameratunga S, Clark T, Banati P. Changing school climates to promote adolescent wellbeing: Two trials with one goal. *Lancet.* 2018;392(10163):2416–2418. doi:10.1016/S0140-6736(18)32280-3

65. Mozaffarian D. Dietary and policy priorities for cardiovascular disease, diabetes, and obesity. *Circulation.* 2016;133(2):187–225. doi:10.1161/CIRCULATIONAHA.115.018585

66. Fuster V. Stratified approach to health integration of science and education at the right time for each individual. *J Am Coll Cardiol.* 2015;66(14):1627–1629. doi:10.1016/j.jacc.2015.08.039

6 Primary Prevention of Type 2 Diabetes and Cardiometabolic-Based Chronic Disease Using Lifestyle Medicine

Hajira Amir and Michael A. Via
Icahn School of Medicine at Mount Sinai

Jeffrey I. Mechanick
Kravis Center for Cardiovascular Health at Mount Sinai Heart
Icahn School of Medicine at Mount Sinai

CONTENTS

DOI: 10.1201/9781003206637-6

119

6.1   INTRODUCTION

Cardiometabolic-based chronic disease (CMBCD) (1,2) is a pathophysiological state consisting of three dimensions that lead to cardiovascular disease (CVD):

1. Progression by stage over time (stage 1 = risk; stage 2 = predisease; stage 3 = disease; and stage 4 = complications);
2. Causation by primary drivers (genetics, environment, and behavior culminating in a personalized lifestyle) and secondary metabolic drivers (adiposity-based chronic disease [ABCD] (3), dysglycemia-based chronic disease [DBCD] (4), hypertension-based chronic disease, lipid-based chronic disease, and other metabolic syndromes [MetS] traits) (1,2); and
3. Social determinants of health and transcultural factors (1,2).

In DBCD, stage 1 refers to the impact of primary drivers and abnormal adiposity on insulin resistance, stage 2 refers to the early impact of a β-cell defect resulting in mild hyperglycemia, stage 3 refers to the persistence/worsening of the β-cell defect and more severe hyperglycemia, and stage 4 refers to vascular complications (micro- and macro-, especially CVD) (4). This driver-based chronic disease modeling approach is specifically designed to expose opportunities for early and sustainable preventive care. Accordingly, primordial prevention is situated between stages 1 and 2, primary stages 2 and 3, secondary stages 3 and 4, and tertiary at stage 4. Regarding the dysglycemia driver, primary prevention of T2D is situated between DBCD stages 2 and 3, and though judicious pharmacotherapy is indicated in certain conditions, this chapter will focus on the role of lifestyle medicine.

Diabetes is a major health epidemic with the International Diabetes Federation reporting that a staggering 537 million adults between 20 and 79 years of age are living with this chronic disease globally in 2021, and this number is projected to rise to 634 million by 2030 and then 783 million by 2045 (4)! As reported for the years 1980–2004, the incidence and prevalence of type 2 diabetes (T2D) have quadrupled, believed to be due to risk of obesity, an aging population, and changes in environmental factors, including those promoting physical inactivity and energy-dense diets (5). T2D accounts for over 90% of all diabetes cases (6). Type 1 diabetes (T1D) is a hyperglycemic condition, arising from the primary destruction of pancreatic β-cells (typically due to autoimmune processes), leading to a state of near-absolute insulin deficiency. Diabetes poses a major economic burden – about $760 billion spent on related health expenditures in 2019, projected to approach $845 billion by 2045 (7). Complications from diabetes are a major contributor to morbidity and mortality and are often present at the time of T2D diagnosis (5). Therefore, preventing or postponing the development of T2D in patients with prediabetes would logically prevent or postpone the development of these complications.

6.2   PROGRESSION OF IMPAIRED GLUCOSE TOLERANCE AND IMPAIRED FASTING GLUCOSE TO T2D

The biochemical descriptors of prediabetes include impaired glucose tolerance (IGT) and impaired fasting glucose (IFG), as well as a fasting plasma glucose of 100–125 mg/dL and hemoglobin A1c (A1C) of 5.7%–6.4%. Prediabetes represents a pathophysiological state in which patients do not meet the diagnostic criteria of diabetes but still have abnormal glycemic markers. The American Diabetes Association (ADA) defines IGT as 2-hour 75-gram oral glucose tolerance test (OGTT) with values of 140–199 mg/dL and IFG as fasting plasma glucose levels of 100–125 mg/dL (8). Risk factors for glucose intolerance are represented as DBCD stage 1 and include a family history of T2D, body mass index (BMI) >25 kg/m², physical inactivity, dyslipidemia, history of gestational diabetes, history of polycystic ovary syndrome or other conditions with insulin resistance, and certain ethnocultural populations (e.g., African American, Latino/Hispanics, and Native Americans and Asian-Pacific Islanders) (9). Individuals with IGT or IFG have a high risk of developing T2D in the future – approximately 3.6%–8.5%/year in patients with IGT as defined by World Health Organization criteria (10). Moreover, elevated fasting glucose, 2-hour postchallenge glucose, and BMI (>27 kg/m²) were each associated with an increased risk for T2D (10). In 2021, it was reported that 541 million adults are at risk of developing T2D (4), emphasizing the need for lifestyle interventions to prevent or at least postpone this chronic disease progression.

6.3   DIETARY MODIFICATION AND PRIMARY PREVENTION OF T2D

The rising epidemic of T2D and obesity can be partly attributed to a change in dietary trends given more accessibility to unhealthy foods. There has been an expansion of fast-food restaurants and supermarkets leading to easy access of high-caloric diets with processed meats and unhealthy fats as well as sugar-sweetened beverages. An increase in the refinement of grains leading to decreased nutritional content has also been seen (11). Dietary composition can play a vital role in improving insulin sensitivity (Table 6.1).

TABLE 6.1
Dietary Macronutrient Components and Cardiometabolic Risks

Dietary Components	Effect on Risk
	Fats
PUFA (15,16)	Reduction in insulin resistance proportional to PUFA intake
MUFA (19)	Reduction in LDL-C, lipoprotein(a), and insulin resistance
	Improvement in pancreatic β-cell function
	Carbohydrates
Glycemic index (25)	High GI intake associated with a 1.37 relative risk for T2D
Glycemic load (25)	High GL intake associated with a 1.47 relative risk for T2D
Fiber (25)	High dietary fiber associated with a 28% risk reduction for T2D

Abbreviations: GI, glycemic index; LDL-C, low-density lipoprotein cholesterol; MUFA, monounsaturated fatty acid; PUFA, polyunsaturated fatty acid; T2D, type 2 diabetes.

6.3.1 MACRONUTRIENTS – FAT

Historically, diets containing a higher amount of total fat were believed to lead to the development of T2D through weight gain and induction of insulin resistance, though human studies have not supported this contention (11). In fact, numerous observational studies have shown that total fat intake was not associated with an increased risk for T2D. The Women's Health Initiative was a randomized controlled trial (RCT) that, among other studies, investigated the effect of a low-fat diet on the incidence of T2D in healthy postmenopausal women (12). Women were randomly assigned to a usual diet in the control group or a 20% low-fat diet in the interventional group. Despite high levels of protocol adherence, results showed no difference in the annual incidence of T2D after 8.1 years, which was observed as 7.1% in the interventional group and 7.4% in the control group (12). Therefore, it was believed that the quality of fat is more important than the quantity of fat (11). This includes the fatty acid composition of ingested foods, which in turn affects cell membrane function (e.g., membrane and ion permeability), as well as binding and affinity of the insulin receptor and consequently insulin sensitivity. Recent experimental data also suggest that fatty acids have a direct regulatory effect on gene expression and enzyme activity (13).

Numerous studies on the effect of dietary fat on insulin sensitivity have shown that replacing saturated fatty acids (SFA) with unsaturated fats has a beneficial effect. For instance, Borkman et al. (14) investigated the association of the fatty acid composition of skeletal muscle phospholipids with insulin sensitivity in two groups. In the first group, a sample was obtained from the rectus abdominis muscle from 27 patients undergoing coronary artery surgery and fasting serum insulin levels were checked as a marker of insulin sensitivity. Results showed that fasting serum insulin levels were significantly inversely associated with the percentage of individual long-chain polyunsaturated fatty acids (PUFA), suggesting that low PUFA content is associated with insulin resistance. The second group consisting of 13 men had a biopsy of the vastus lateralis muscle and measurement of insulin sensitivity by euglycemic clamp studies. Results showed a significant positive association of insulin sensitivity with the percentage of arachidonic acid (a PUFA) in the muscle, total percentage of 20–22 carbon PUFAs, and average degree of fatty acid unsaturation. In conclusion, improved insulin sensitivity correlated with increased concentrations of PUFA in skeletal muscle phospholipids (14). Similarly, a cross-sectional study was performed on 52 adult male Pima Indians (15), a population with one of the highest prevalence rates of T2D in the world (16). The euglycemic clamp technique was used to compare insulin action with body fat and muscle phospholipid fatty acid composition, obtained by a percutaneous biopsy of vastus lateralis. Insulin action reflected by glucose uptake at supraphysiological insulin concentrations was positively correlated with the percentage of C20–22 PUFA, unsaturation index, and delta-5 desaturase activity. The percentage of body fat was inversely associated with delta-5 desaturase activity, an enzyme required for the generation of long-chain PUFA and the main determinant for serum and tissue PUFA levels (17). Delta-5 desaturase activity was independently associated with both insulin resistance and obesity (15). In another study, subjects with T2D but not obesity ($N=6$), without T2D but with obesity

($N=5$), and without T2D or obesity ($N=6$) were randomized to spend two 5-week periods on a diet rich in SFA or PUFA in a crossover study design (18). Results in all three groups showed improved insulin sensitivity (measured using the hyperinsulinemic euglycemic clamp method). In the PUFA group, there was reduced low-density lipoprotein cholesterol (LDL-C; measured via a fasting lipid panel) along with a decrease in the abdominal subcutaneous fat area (18).

Diets enriched in monounsaturated fatty acid (MUFA) have also shown a positive effect on insulin sensitivity as shown in the KANWU study (19), which included 162 healthy people who received a controlled isocaloric diet for 3 months containing either a high amount of SFA or MUFA. Results showed significantly impaired insulin sensitivity in the SFA group, while no change was seen in the MUFA group. The MUFA group had both lower LDL-C and lipoprotein(a) levels (19), which are independent risk factors for CVD (20). Given that family history is a significant risk factor for the development of T2D (9), Paniagua et al. (21) examined 11 subjects with insulin resistance who were the offspring of patients with both obesity and T2D. Enrolled subjects were given three 28-day periods of diets enriched in SFA, MUFA, and carbohydrates in a randomized crossover design. Results showed increased accumulation of fat in the trunk with decreased fat in the legs in the carbohydrate diet group as compared to the SFA and MUFA diet groups. The MUFA group had significantly improved insulin sensitivity, decreased fasting glucose levels, and improved insulin secretion compared to the SFA-enriched diet group. These effects were observed despite a short intervention period of 28 days and high total fat content (21).

Studies have shown the negative effects of *trans*-fatty acids (TFA) on CVD (22); however, human studies on the effect of TFA on insulin sensitivity have been inconsistent, and data to assess an association between TFA intake and incidence of T2D is limited (23). Still, there may be a weak association between high TFA intake levels and the development of T2D, but the amount of TFA consumed as part of a standard Western diet is much lower (23).

6.3.2 MACRONUTRIENTS – CARBOHYDRATES

Disruption of carbohydrate metabolism is the hallmark of DBCD, particularly stage 3 (T2D), where more severe hyperglycemia can lead to clinical symptoms and vascular complications. In general, blood glucose levels after a meal are determined by the rate at which glucose appears in the bloodstream and its clearance from the circulation, which is driven by the secretion and action of insulin. Different dietary components influence this process. With carbohydrates, both the quality and quantity have significant effects on glycemic status. The glycemic index (GI) reflects the change in the blood glucose levels following ingestion of a carbohydrate-containing food, whereas the glycemic load (GL) considers the GI and the amount of carbohydrate in the serving. Additionally, the physical form of the food (e.g., juice versus whole fruit), degree of processing, type of starch, and manner of preparation play important roles in postprandial glycemic excursions. There are even other factors that influence GI/GL, such as co-ingestion of a protein which augments insulin release and fat which slows the intestinal absorption of glucose, thus delaying peak glycemic response (24).

Studies to determine whether there is an association between the intake of foods with high GI/GL and the development of T2D have mixed results. In a 1986 cohort study by Salmeron et al. (25) of 65,173 women from the Nurses' Health Study with no diabetes, CVD, or cancer at baseline, dietary questionnaires were used to calculate the intake of dietary fiber and dietary GI/GL. Results showed that during the 6 years of follow-up, dietary GI was positively associated with the risk of T2D, even after adjustment of other known risk factors, such as age, BMI, and physical activity, with a relative risk (RR) of 1.37 (95% confidence interval [CI], 1.09–1.71, p trend = 0.005) when comparing the highest and lowest quintiles of intake (25). The GL had a similar association with a RR of 1.47 (95% CI, 1.16–1.86, p trend = 0.003) when comparing the highest and lowest quintiles (25). Cereal fiber intake was inversely linked to the risk of T2D, with a RR of 0.72 (95% CI, 0.58–0.90, p trend = 0.001) when comparing the highest and lowest quintiles of intake (25). The combination of a high GL and a low cereal fiber diet further increased the risk of T2D (RR = 2.50, 95% CI, 1.14–5.51) when compared with a low GL and high cereal fiber diet (25). Similarly, another study of 42,759 men from the Health Professionals Follow-up Study with no diabetes or CVD at baseline showed a significant positive association of GI and T2D with a RR of 1.37 (95% CI, 1.02–1.83, p trend = 0.03) even after adjustment for age, BMI, smoking, physical activity, family history of diabetes, alcohol consumption, cereal fiber, and total energy intake and a significant inverse association between dietary cereal fiber intake and the risk of developing T2D (RR = 0.70; 95% CI, 0.51–0.96, p trend = 0.007) during the 6-year follow-up period (26). An increased risk of T2D was found in those who had a combination of high GL and low cereal fiber diet (RR = 2.17, 95% CI, 1.04–4.54) as compared to a low GL and high cereal fiber diet independently of other currently known risk factors (26). On the other hand, a prospective cohort study of 35,988 women with no diabetes at baseline found an inverse relationship between dietary intake of total grains – particularly whole grains and cereal fiber – and the development of T2D (27). In this study, the intake of total carbohydrates, GI, refined grains, fruits, and vegetables was unrelated to T2D risk (27). Thus, even though many studies have reported a positive association between high GI/GL and the risk of developing T2D, this association has not been observed in others.

6.3.3 Vitamins and Minerals

In a meta-analysis of 13 prospective cohort studies involving 536,318 participants, there was a significant inverse relationship between magnesium intake and the risk of developing T2D in a dose-response manner (28). A systematic review and meta-analysis showed that a higher intake of heme iron and increased levels of ferritin, which is the storage form of iron, was associated with a higher risk of T2D (29). A meta-analysis of 21 prospective cohort studies showed a significant inverse relationship between serum levels of 25-hydroxyvitamin D and the risk of T2D (30). However, the ADA recommends against the routine use of minerals and vitamins for people with prediabetes or T2D unless there is a demonstrable underlying deficiency (31). Moreover, a large study investigating the prevention of T2D development showed no benefit to supplementation with 4,000 units daily of vitamin D_3 in patients with prediabetes (32).

6.3.4 INDIVIDUAL FOODS

There are numerous studies evaluating the effects of different individual foods on the risk of T2D. A systematic review and meta-analysis of prospective studies showed a positive association between whole grain intake and reduced risk of T2D even after adjustment of BMI (33). Conversely, higher consumption of white rice, which is a processed grain, is associated with a significantly increased risk of T2D, especially in Chinese and Japanese populations (34). Similarly, red meat is associated with an increased risk of T2D as shown in a meta-analysis of 37,083 men in the Health Professionals Follow-Up Study (1986–2006), 79,570 women in the Nurses' Health Study I (1980–2008), and 87,504 women in the Nurses' Health Study II (1991–2005) (35). After adjustment for age, BMI, and other lifestyle and dietary risk factors, red meat consumption, particularly processed red meat, was associated with an increased risk of T2D (35). Seafood consumption and the association with the risk of T2D were evaluated in a meta-analysis that revealed no significant association (36). Opposite associations depending on geographical locations were observed, with a lower risk seen in studies from Asia and a higher risk seen in studies from North America and Europe (36). A greater intake of green leafy vegetables was associated with a 14% risk reduction of developing T2D (37). Sugar-sweetened beverages have been linked with high risk for T2D development (38). A meta-analysis of 11 prospective cohort studies showed that individuals in the highest quintile of sugar-sweetened beverage intake (more than 1–2 servings per day) had a 26% greater risk of developing T2D as compared to those in the lowest quintile (0–1 serving/month) (38). This study also showed that the increased intake of sugar-sweetened beverages was associated with a higher risk of MetS, with a 20% greater risk in the highest quintile compared to the lowest quintile (38). Based on these studies, patients with IGT should be advised to decrease their dietary intake of red meat, processed meat, processed grains, and sugar-sweetened beverages, with an increased intake of whole grains and green leafy vegetables to reduce the risk of progressing to T2D.

6.3.5 DIETARY PATTERNS

Various individual macronutrients, micronutrients, and foods are associated with a reduction in the risk of developing T2D. However, the assessment of dietary patterns to assess the cumulative effects of an overall meal is being increasingly recognized as useful. Different studies have been performed to evaluate the effect of healthy dietary patterns on the risk of developing T2D, though no specific dietary pattern has been recommended for prevention (39).

The Dietary Approaches to Stop Hypertension (DASH) dietary pattern emphasizes the intake of fruits, vegetables, fat-free/low-fat dairy, whole grains, nuts, and legumes, while limiting the intakes of sodium and salt, as well as saturated fat, red and processed meats, sweets, added sugars, and sugar-sweetened beverages (40). There are many different Mediterranean diets depending on the specific geographical region and culture examined. In general, a Mediterranean diet emphasizes a high consumption of polyphenols, as well as certain fats (ranging between 30% and 40% of daily energy intake) primarily from foods rich in MUFA, encouraging increased consumption of fruits, vegetables, tree nuts, legumes, whole grains, and fish, with only moderate consumption of alcohol. In other words, a Mediterranean diet includes a large amount of plant foods with olive oil being the principal source of fat, low-to-moderate amounts of fish and poultry, relatively low amounts of red meat, and moderate amounts of wine as the source of alcohol normally with meals (41).

There is mounting evidence that adherence to these healthy dietary patterns is associated with a decrease in the risk of developing T2D and has favorable effects on cardiovascular health. A meta-analysis of 18 prospective studies with 20 cohorts in four world regions to discern the effect of healthy dietary patterns on the risk of developing T2D showed that participants with the highest adherence to healthy dietary patterns had a lower risk of developing T2D with a 20% risk reduction compared to those with the lowest adherence (42). There was no change in the result depending on the different geographical regions of cohort studies (Europe, United States, or Asia), duration of follow-up (≤10 or >10 years), or the type of dietary pattern used (Mediterranean versus DASH diet) (42).

It is also paramount to examine the effect of these dietary patterns on cardiovascular health given that CVD is the most common cause of morbidity and mortality in patients with T2D (40). A review of systematic reviews and meta-analysis was done to assess the association between the DASH dietary pattern and the development of CVD, as well as other cardiometabolic outcomes (37). Results showed that the DASH dietary pattern was associated with a decrease in the incidence of T2D, CVD, coronary heart disease (macrovascular [coronary artery disease] + microvascular [structural and electrical remodeling in heart muscle]) (43), and stroke, in prospective cohort studies, and decreased systolic and diastolic blood pressure, total cholesterol, LDL-C, A1C, fasting blood insulin levels, and body weight in controlled trials (40).

Similarly, another meta-analysis of prospective cohort studies showed that greater adherence to a Mediterranean diet was associated with a significant reduction in overall mortality, mortality from CVD, incidence of mortality from cancer, and incidence of Parkinson's and Alzheimer's disease (44). Comparable results were also obtained in the PREDIMED trial, which was a large randomized multi-center trial in Spain that evaluated the effects of a Mediterranean diet on primary cardiovascular prevention (45,46) (Note that the originally published study was retracted due to errors in randomization and allocation, but results and implications were essentially unchanged after re-analysis in the republished paper). Inclusion criteria included men (55–80 years of age) or women (60–80 years of age) at high risk for CVD, which included a diagnosis of T2D, or having at least three major risk factors, including smoking, hypertension, elevated LDL-C levels, low high-density lipoprotein cholesterol (HDL-C) levels, elevated BMI in the overweight or obese category, or a family history of premature CVD. Study participants were randomly assigned in a 1:1:1 ratio to three dietary intervention groups – Mediterranean diet supplemented with extra-virgin olive oil (encouraged to take at least ≥4 tablespoons/day), Mediterranean diet supplemented with nuts (recommended consumption was one daily serving of 30 grams, consisting of 15 grams of walnuts, 7.5 grams of almonds, and 7.5 grams of hazelnuts), or a control diet with advice to reduce dietary fat. Drug treatment regimens at baseline were similar in the three groups and remained so during the follow-up period. The study participants were followed for a median of 4.8 years. Results showed that the primary end point, which was defined as a composite of myocardial infarction, stroke, and death from any cardiovascular cause, was 96 (3.8%) in the group assigned to a Mediterranean diet with extra-virgin oil, compared to 83 (3.4%) in the group assigned to a Mediterranean diet with nuts, and 109 (4.4%) in the control group, with incidence rates of 8.1, 8.0, and 11.2 per 1,000 person-years, respectively (42). Thus, the results of this study supported a beneficial effect of a Mediterranean diet for the primary prevention of CVD (46).

Mediterranean diets have been shown to have favorable impacts on body weight and are associated with a lower prevalence of MetS, which is closely linked to insulin resistance, prediabetes, and T2D development. A longitudinal analysis of 6,319 participants in a Spanish prospective study demonstrated that participants in the group with the lowest baseline adherence to the Mediterranean dietary pattern had more weight gain compared to those in the highest baseline adherence group (47). Similarly, data from the Spanish cohort of the European Prospective Investigation into Cancer and Nutrition, in which 17,238 women and 10,589 men who were not obese at baseline were followed, found that high Mediterranean diet adherence was significantly associated with a lower chance of becoming obese in overweight subjects (48). In a randomized prospective trial, 101 overweight men and women were randomized to receive a moderate-fat Mediterranean-style energy-restricted diet (35% energy from fat) or a low-fat, energy-restricted diet (20% energy from fat), with the main outcome being a change in body weight (49). Results showed that after 18 months, in the moderate-fat diet group, there were mean decreases in body weight of 4.1 kg, BMI of 1.6 kg/m², and waist circumference of 6.9 cm, compared to the low-fat diet group, which had increases in body weight of 2.9 kg, BMI of 1.4 kg/m², and waist circumference of 2.6 cm (49). The ATTICA study, in which 1,128 men and 1,154 women with no baseline evidence of CVD or T2D were followed to determine the effect of leisure time physical activity and a Mediterranean diet on the prevalence of MetS, showed that this intervention was associated with a 20% lower risk of developing MetS, irrespective of confounding variables that included age, sex, physical activity, lipids, and blood pressure (50).

In conclusion, there are various dietary patterns that have been associated with a decrease in the risk of developing T2D as well as a reduction in adverse cardiometabolic outcomes. Although exact compositions vary somewhat, similarities among the DASH and Mediterranean diets include features such as emphasis on the intake of whole grains, fruits, vegetables, nuts, legumes with reduced intake of red and processed meats, processed grains, sugar, and sweetened beverages. Also, there are many dietary patterns, programs, and approaches espoused and lauded by the community, such as intermittent fasting, time-restricted eating, paleo, and ketogenic, to name a few, but there are currently insufficient compelling and valid clinical trial data in people with DBCD stage 2, to prevent DBCD stage 3, to include commentary here.

6.4   ROLE OF PHYSICAL ACTIVITY IN THE PREVENTION OF T2D

Insulin resistance is the inability of an exogenous or endogenous amount of insulin to exert predictable effects on glucose metabolism compared to someone without insulin resistance. Mechanisms include genetic abnormalities in the insulin receptor, proteins involved in insulin receptor signal transduction, and other downstream metabolic pathways; body composition changes such as high visceral adiposity and ectopic fat; detrimental effects of comorbidities such as sepsis; and various pharmacological agents (51). Insulin resistance is commonly seen with MetS and these individuals have a higher risk of developing T2D (51) along with other cardiovascular risk factors such as elevated blood pressure and cholesterol. Acute exercise and chronic training lead to improvements in insulin sensitivity and glucose disposal which could improve insulin resistance in patients with prediabetes. Both processes may prevent or postpone the development of T2D.

6.4.1 ACUTE EFFECTS OF EXERCISE

Physical activity causes a shift from the use of free fatty acids (FFA) at rest for myocyte energy substrate to a combination of fat, glucose, and muscle glycogen. Glycogen is the main source of energy for muscles during the earlier part of the exercise. As glycogen stores are utilized, glucose uptake from the circulation is increased by the active contracting muscles. With a continued duration of the activity, hepatic gluconeogenesis is increased to balance the increase in peripheral glucose uptake and maintain circulating blood glucose levels. Myocyte glucose uptake occurs via two pathways: insulin dependent and insulin independent. The insulin-independent pathway occurs during exercise whereby muscular contractions lead to increased glucose uptake to supplement glycogen breakdown in the muscle to provide energy. Peripheral glucose is transported into the muscles via the glucose transporter (GLUT) proteins with GLUT4 being the main isoform in the muscles that is influenced by both insulin action and muscle contractions, however, through different mechanisms. Insulin activates GLUT4 translocation via a signaling cascade whereas muscular contractions activate GLUT4 translocation in part through the activation of 5' adenosine monophosphate-activated protein kinase. Exercise, both aerobic and resistance forms, also increase the abundance of GLUT4 separate from insulin activity, leading to an increase in blood glucose uptake by skeletal muscles. This uptake remains elevated postexercise, with the contraction-mediated mechanism lasting for several hours and the insulin-mediated pathway for even longer. This means that even though in patients with T2D or insulin resistance insulin-mediated glucose uptake is impaired, exercise can still stimulate glucose uptake via a separate mechanism and control hyperglycemia (52).

6.4.2 POSTEXERCISE EFFECTS

For people with normal glucose tolerance, physical activity stimulates increased glucose uptake by the active muscles, which is balanced by an increase in hepatic glucose production (52). This leads to stable blood glucose levels, except if the duration of exercise is so prolonged that glycogen stores are depleted (52). For people who have IGT or T2D, the rise in glucose uptake by the muscles is greater than the hepatic glucose production, which causes a drop in peripheral blood glucose levels. A single bout of aerobic exercise improves insulin action and glucose metabolism for more than 24 hours but less than 72 hours (52).

6.4.3   Resistance Exercise Effects

Resistance training results in lower fasting blood glucose levels in people with IFG up to 24 hours after the exercise, with increased volume and intensity leading to a greater drop in levels. This can be explained by increased muscle mass, which could increase glucose uptake (52). A trial included 248 adults from ages 50 to 75 with prediabetes who were randomized to resistance training three times weekly, aerobic training three times weekly, or control (no formal exercise regimen given) for 2 years (53). In both the resistance training and aerobic training groups, A1c reduced by 0.2%, whereas A1c increased by 0.2% in the control group ($p < 0.001$). Homeostasis modeling of insulin resistance (HOMA-IR) decreased by 15% in the aerobic group and 36% in the resistance group, compared to no change in the control group ($p = 0.045$ for both compared to control, no significant difference, $p = 0.506$ when comparing aerobic training with resistance training) (53). Another 2-year randomized trial that included adults with prediabetes demonstrates similar improvement in HOMA-IR with resistance training compared to aerobic training and both with 12% reductions in HOMA-IR compared to control ($p < 0.01$) (54).

6.4.4   Effects of Chronic Training

Chronic training can increase insulin sensitivity and glucose metabolism as shown in studies comparing trained subjects with matched untrained subjects (55). Björntorp et al. (56) observed lower insulin levels and glucose values with OGTT in middle-aged, physically well-trained men in comparison to randomly selected men of the same age. Cholesterol and triglyceride levels were also lower in the well-trained group compared to the controls (56). Similarly, Houmard et al. (57) demonstrated that 14 weeks of exercise training in previously sedentary middle-aged men led to changes in insulin action using the insulin sensitivity index, which increased by two-fold ($p < 0.05$), changes in the percentage of GLUT4-rich type IIa muscle fibers, which increased by 10% ($p < 0.01$), and changes in GLUT4 protein concentration, which increased by 1.8-fold ($p < 0.001$).

The effect of training intensity was demonstrated by DiPietro et al. (58) in a 9-month randomized study of healthy older women. High-intensity training improved insulin sensitivity more than moderate-intensity training independent of changes in body composition or training volume (58). Physical training also counteracts the decrease in insulin sensitivity found with aging where lean older athletes had a similar glucose and insulin response to an OGTT compared to young athletes (59).

Moderate-to-vigorous aerobic training leads to improvement of whole-body insulin sensitivity for hours to days. Mechanisms include improving the skeletal muscle response to insulin via increased expression and activity of proteins involved in glucose metabolism and insulin signaling (52). Endurance training in rats has been shown to enhance gene expression of the insulin receptor and insulin receptor substrate-1 (IRS-1) in skeletal muscle (55). Defects in the insulin signal transduction pathway, specifically IRS-1 phosphorylation, have been shown in the skeletal muscle of patients with obesity and/or T2D. In addition, capillary density has been shown to be increased with endurance training in both patients with and without T2D. Insulin stimulates muscle blood flow, which is increased with endurance training (55). These changes are important since changes in muscle blood flow are necessary to ensure an adequate supply of glucose (55). Glucose uptake in the muscle depends on the amount of glucose transporters in the plasma membrane, transverse (or T)-tubules, and GLUT4 translocation in response to insulin stimulation (55). Moderate training increases glycogen synthase activity and GLUT4 protein expression (52). Hughes et al. (60) demonstrated that 12 weeks of training in 18 sedentary participants with impaired or non-diagnostic OGTT led to an improvement in oral glucose tolerance by 11%, increased GLUT4 concentration in skeletal muscle by 60%, and increased skeletal muscle glycogen by 24%, despite no changes in body composition.

Patients with T2D have been found to have an elevated number of glycolytic fibers and glycolytic enzymes, as compared to oxidative fibers and oxidative enzymes, which correlates negatively with insulin sensitivity. Physical training increases enzyme capacity for glucose transport and metabolism in patients with/without T2D, leading to an increase in insulin sensitivity (55).

An increase in visceral adiposity is associated with insulin resistance (51). Moreover, women with a BMI of ≥ 30 kg/m^2 had a 28 times greater risk of developing T2D than women of normal weight (61). Plasma-free FFA are increased in patients with T2D, which can impair the uptake and metabolism of glucose in skeletal muscle and also cause an increase in hepatic glucose output. Of note, visceral adipocytes have a decrease in their response to the antilipolytic effect of insulin (55). Physical training reduces visceral body fat which could potentially lead to a decrease in plasma FFA levels, and this may improve glucose metabolism (55). In a study by Goodpaster et al. (62), volunteers with obesity but without T2D underwent 16 weeks of daily moderate-intensity physical activity combined with caloric reduction. Results demonstrated improved insulin sensitivity with enhanced fasting rates of lipid oxidation accounting for 52% of the variance (62). Similarly, a study of ten adult children of parents with T2D and eight normal subjects who underwent 6 weeks of an aerobic exercise training program showed a 40% improvement in whole-body insulin sensitivity and an improvement in whole-body non-oxidative glucose metabolism by 60%–70% in both groups (63).

Resistance exercise training also has beneficial impacts as shown in an RCT where twice weekly resistance training for 16 weeks by older men that had a new diagnosis of T2D led to a 46.3% increase in insulin action, a 7.1% reduction in fasting blood glucose levels, and loss of visceral fat (52).

6.5 PHYSICAL ACTIVITY AND EFFECT ON OXIDATIVE STRESS AND INFLAMMATION

Another key factor in the pathogenesis of DM is inflammation. Cross-sectional studies have demonstrated increased levels of interleukin (IL)-6 and C-reactive protein (CRP), which are sensitive markers of subclinical inflammation, in individuals with insulin resistance and T2D (51). A prospective study done with 1,047 individuals without diabetes found that over 5 years, there was an increase in levels of inflammatory markers, including fibrinogen and CRP, and the incidence of new-onset T2D (64). Increased IL-1 levels have been found in pancreatic secretions obtained in individuals with T2D and are associated with the failure of the pancreatic β-cells to secrete sufficient insulin (51). IL-1 signaling is thought to also be involved in the autoimmune destruction of β-cells leading to T1D. IL-1 activates nuclear factor kappa B and leads to the inhibition of β-cell function and an increase in β-cell apoptosis (51). A study done by Claus et al. (65) demonstrated that the antagonism of IL-1 leads to an improvement in glucose control in individuals with T2D.

With regular exercise and physical activity, there is increased production of anti-inflammatory cytokines as compared to pro-inflammatory cytokines (51). A study done in women with obesity to reduce body weight via a low-calorie diet and increased physical activity showed decreased levels of pro-inflammatory cytokines including IL-6, IL-18, and CRP and increased adiponectin, which has both anti-inflammatory and insulin-sensitizing properties (3). Physical activity also leads to reduced inflammation with improvement of endothelial function and reduction in oxidative stress, both of which are expected to reduce the development of T2D and CMBCD (1,2,51).

6.6 OVERVIEW OF KEY LIFESTYLE MEDICINE CLINICAL TRIALS

Recently, numerous clinical trials have demonstrated a favorable impact of lifestyle medicine on the prevention of T2D, primarily through changes in diet and physical activity (Table 6.2). The Diabetes Prevention Program (DPP) was an RCT that compared the effects of three different interventions on the development of T2D in high-risk individuals: intensive lifestyle, standard lifestyle, and metformin 850 mg twice a day with standard lifestyle and placebo medication (66). Inclusion criterion was IGT based on a single 75-g OGTT with no prior diagnosis of T2D as these individuals are at increased risk of developing T2D in the future. The primary end point measured was significant prevention or delay of diabetes development of any type, as defined by the 1997 ADA criteria based on fasting plasma glucose or 2-hour postchallenge glucose on the OGTT. Participants in all three groups received general information regarding healthy lifestyles to prevent diabetes, including diet and weight loss counseling, but the

TABLE 6.2
Prevention Trials in Patients with Prediabetes

Trial	T2D Risk Reduction	Cardiometabolic Risk Reduction
Diabetes Prevention Program (68–70)	34% at 10 years 27% at 15 years	14% reduction in the need for lipid-lowering medications 8% reduction in the need for blood pressure–lowering medications
Diabetes Prevention Study (71)	58% at 3 years	Reduced total cholesterol to HDL-C ratio by 0.4 Reduced triglycerides by 18 mg/dL 4.5 kg weight loss
Da Qing Trial (73)	Delay in the onset of T2D by 3.96 years	26% risk reduction in cardiovascular diseases over 30 years

Abbreviations: HDL-C, high-density lipoprotein cholesterol; T2D, type 2 diabetes.

intensive lifestyle intervention group received more comprehensive, personalized, and regular education in order to achieve their goals. The intensive lifestyle participants were given a weight loss goal of losing 7% of their initial body weight in the first 6 months at a recommended loss of 1–2 pounds/week and maintaining this weight loss throughout the trial. This goal was chosen because prior clinical trials have reported that weight loss of this magnitude is attainable and appears to improve insulin sensitivity in patients with T2D. A physical activity goal of 700 kcal (kilocalories)/week expenditure via at least 150 minutes of moderate physical activity, which was described to be of similar intensity such as brisk walking, was given to all participants; this is in agreement with the national activity recommendations of the Centers for Disease Control and Prevention and the American College of Sports Medicine (66). The mean BMI of the participants was 34.0 and the mean age was 51 years (67).

Results showed that during the average follow-up period of 2.8 years, the incidence rate of diabetes was 4.8, 7.8, and 11.0 cases per 100 person-years in the lifestyle, metformin, and placebo groups, respectively (67). The incidence of developing diabetes was reduced by 58% (95% CI, 48%–66%) and 31% (95% CI, 17%–43%) as compared to the placebo group in the intensive lifestyle intervention group and standard lifestyle intervention with metformin group respectively; of which all cases were T2D. The incidence of developing T2D was 39% lower (95% CI, 24%–51%) in the lifestyle intervention group than in the metformin group (67).

The participants in the DPP are being followed by the Diabetes Prevention Program Outcomes Study, which examined the long-term effects in each of these groups. The lifestyle intervention group participants had a delay in the development of T2D by 34% and 27% as compared to the placebo group at the 10- and 15-year follow-up respectively, whereas the metformin group had a delay by 18% as compared to the placebo group at the 10- and 15-year follow-up (68,69). No significant difference in the prevalence of aggregate microvascular end points, which included nephropathy, retinopathy, and neuropathy, was seen among treatment groups. However, results showed a 28% lower prevalence of microvascular complications in those who did not progress to diabetes, compared to those who did progress to diabetes (69). There was a reduction in systolic blood pressure, diastolic blood pressure, LDL-C, and triglycerides, as well as an elevation in HDL-C in all three groups with no significant differences among the groups after the 10-year follow-up; however, the lifestyle intervention group achieved these results with a smaller requirement of lipid-lowering medications (32% vs 37%; $p = 0.012$) and a trend for less requirement of blood pressure–lowering medications (47% vs 51%; $p = 0.09$) (70).

Similarly, the Finnish Diabetes Prevention Study was a multicenter RCT that demonstrated a 58% reduction in the incidence of T2D within the lifestyle intervention group as compared to the control group (71). Subjects with ages of 40–64 years, BMI >25 kg/m^2, and IGT test based on WHO criteria were included in this study. Baseline characteristics were similar, reflecting an increased risk of T2D in both groups. The lifestyle intervention group goals included weight reduction ≥5%, moderate-intensity physical activity ≥30 minute/day, limited dietary and saturated fat consumption, and fiber intake of ≥15 g/1,000 kcal. The control group received general information regarding diet and lifestyle changes; however, the difference was that the lifestyle intervention group received their counseling through more frequent face-to-face consultations throughout the study and their guidance was more individualized and personalized as implemented in the DPP. Results included a statistically significant mean weight reduction of 4.5 kg in the intervention group, compared to 1.0 kg in the control group at 1 year. Improvements were observed after 1 year in fasting plasma glucose, 2-hour plasma glucose with OGTT, A1C, serum total cholesterol to HDL ratio, and serum triglycerides in the intervention group as compared to the control group. The proportion of sedentary individuals also decreased in the intervention group as compared to the control group, with 14% at year 1 and 17% at year 3, compared to 30% and 29% in the control group, respectively. Over the first 3 years of the study, 9% of the subjects in the intervention group developed T2D, compared to 20% of the subjects in the control group (71).

Another landmark trial highlighting the importance of lifestyle modifications for the primary prevention of T2D was the Da Qing study (72). This RCT began in 1986, in which participants with IGT based on WHO criteria were followed over a 6-year period to compare the effects of diet alone, exercise alone, and diet plus exercise on the incidence of T2D, compared to the control group in Da Qing, China (72). The interventions were carried out by 33 local health clinics. Participants were randomized by the particular clinic to carry out the interventions rather than randomization of the participants themselves. In each clinic, participants were stratified according to BMI: <25 kg/m^2 as lean and ≥25 kg/m^2 as overweight. In the diet-alone intervention group, participants with BMI <25 kg/m^2 were prescribed a diet containing 25–30 kcal/kg body weight (55%–65% carbohydrate, 10%–15% protein, and 25%–30% fat), compared to those with BMI ≥25 kg/m^2, who were advised to reduce the caloric intake to lose weight at a rate of 0.5–1.0 kg per month until they reached a BMI of 23 kg/m^2. The exercise-alone intervention group participants were advised to increase their physical activity, which was predefined depending on the intensity and timing of the activity. In the diet-plus-exercise group, participants received counseling for dietary and exercise interventions similar to the diet- and exercise-only groups. All three intervention groups received counseling on an individual basis regarding daily food intake and exercise, followed by sessions in small groups weekly for 1 month, monthly for 3 months, and then every 3 months for the rest of the study duration. The control group received general information about diabetes, diet, and physical activity, but there were no individual instructions or formal counseling sessions provided. No statistically significant difference was found in baseline characteristics in all groups. Results showed that the mean for a 6-year incidence of T2D was statistically significantly higher in the control group, 15.7/100 person-years, as compared to the three active treatment intervention groups (10, 8.3, and 9.6 per 100 person-years in the diet-alone, exercise-alone, and diet-plus-exercise groups, respectively). No statistically significant difference was found in the incidence of T2D among the groups providing active treatment (72).

These study participants were followed for up to 30 years after randomization in the Da Qing Diabetes Prevention Outcomes Study. After 30 years of follow-up, the combined intervention groups had a median delay in the development of T2D onset by 3.96 years (95% CI 1.25–6.67; $p = 0.0042$), decrease in the incidence of CVD (hazard ratio [HR] 0.74, 95% CI 0.59–0.92; $p = 0.0060$), decrease in deaths due to CVD (HR 0.67, 95% CI 0.48–0.94; $p = 0.022$), decrease in microvascular complications (HR

0.65, 95% CI 0.45–0.95; $p = 0.025$), and lower all-cause mortality (0.74, 95% CI 0.61–0.89; $p = 0.0015$) as compared to the control group (73).

In summary, these trials showed that lifestyle interventions can significantly postpone the development of T2D in high-risk individuals (abnormal adiposity and/or prediabetes), as well as a reduction in the incidence of CVD and metabolic risk factors, including blood pressure and cholesterol. The observed difference in T2D incidence, cardiometabolic risk, and development of both microvascular and macrovascular complications indicates that these interventions should be individualized with frequent follow-ups and interval checkups performed by skilled healthcare professionals.

6.7   CONCLUSION

Type 2 diabetes is a major health epidemic and the recent rise in its prevalence could be attributed to a change in lifestyle with increases in unhealthy dietary choices, lack of physical activity, and causative association with abnormal adiposity. These phenomena have been interpreted in the ABCD, DBCD, and CMBCD models. Evidence shows that a structured lifestyle intervention that involves dietary changes and increased physical activity can significantly impact insulin sensitivity through a variety of mechanisms. Landmark primary prevention clinical trials, such as the Diabetes Prevention Program, the Finnish Diabetes Prevention Study, and Da Qing Study, have shown that changes in lifestyle with more individualized care by skilled healthcare professionals can lead to a significant postponement in the development of T2D, as well as cardiometabolic complications.

Disclosures:
Jeffrey I. Mechanick received honoraria from Abbott Nutrition for lectures and serves on the Advisory Boards for Aveta.Life and Twin Health.

REFERENCES

1. Mechanick JI, Farkouh ME, Newman JD, Garvey WT. Cardiometabolic-based chronic disease, adiposity and dysglycemia drivers: JACC state-of-the-art review. *J Am Coll Cardiol.* 2020;75(5):525–38.
2. Mechanick JI, Farkouh ME, Newman JD, Garvey WT. Cardiometabolic-based chronic disease, addressing knowledge and clinical practice gaps: JACC state-of-the-art review. *J Am Coll Cardiol.* 2020;75(5):539–55.
3. Mechanick JI, Hurley DL, Garvey WT. Adiposity-based chronic disease as a new diagnostic term: the American Association of Clinical Endocrinologists and American College of Endocrinology position statement. *Endocr Pract.* 2017;23(3):372–8.
4. Mechanick JI, Garber AJ, Grunberger G, Handelsman Y, Garvey WT. Dysglycemia-based chronic disease: an American Association of Clinical Endocrinologists position statement. *Endocr Pract.* 2018;24(11):995–1011.
5. Chatterjee S, Khunti K, Davies MJ. Type 2 diabetes. *Lancet.* 2017;389(10085):2239–51.
6. Carlsson LMS, Sjoholm K, Jacobson P, Andersson-Assarsson JC, Svensson PA, Taube M, et al. Life expectancy after bariatric surgery in the Swedish obese subjects study. *N Engl J Med.* 2020;383(16):1535–43.
7. Williams R, Karuranga S, Malanda B, Saeedi P, Basit A, Besancon S, et al. Global and regional estimates and projections of diabetes-related health expenditure: results from

the International Diabetes Federation Diabetes Atlas, 9th edition. *Diabetes Res Clin Pract.* 2020;162:108072.

8. Expert Committee on the Diagnosis and Classification of Diabetes Mellitus. Report of the expert committee on the diagnosis and classification of diabetes mellitus. *Diabetes Care.* 2003;26(Suppl 1):S5–20.

9. Rao SS, Disraeli P, McGregor T. Impaired glucose tolerance and impaired fasting glucose. *Am Fam Physician.* 2004;69(8):1961–8.

10. Edelstein SL, Knowler WC, Bain RP, Andres R, Barrett-Connor EL, Dowse GK, et al. Predictors of progression from impaired glucose tolerance to NIDDM: an analysis of six prospective studies. *Diabetes.* 1997;46(4):701–10.

11. Ley SH, Hamdy O, Mohan V, Hu FB. Prevention and management of type 2 diabetes: dietary components and nutritional strategies. *Lancet.* 2014;383(9933):1999–2007.

12. Tinker LF, Bonds DE, Margolis KL, Manson JE, Howard BV, Larson J, et al. Low-fat dietary pattern and risk of treated diabetes mellitus in postmenopausal women: the Women's Health Initiative randomized controlled dietary modification trial. *Arch Intern Med.* 2008;168(14):1500–11.

13. Riserus U, Willett WC, Hu FB. Dietary fats and prevention of type 2 diabetes. *Prog Lipid Res.* 2009;48(1):44–51.

14. Borkman M, Storlien LH, Pan DA, Jenkins AB, Chisholm DJ, Campbell LV. The relation between insulin sensitivity and the fatty-acid composition of skeletal-muscle phospholipids. *N Engl J Med.* 1993;328(4):238–44.

15. Pan DA, Lillioja S, Milner MR, Kriketos AD, Baur LA, Bogardus C, et al. Skeletal muscle membrane lipid composition is related to adiposity and insulin action. *J Clin Invest.* 1995;96(6):2802–8.

16. Pearson ER. Dissecting the etiology of type 2 diabetes in the Pima Indian population. *Diabetes.* 2015;64(12):3993–5.

17. Tosi F, Sartori F, Guarini P, Olivieri O, Martinelli N. Delta-5 and delta-6 desaturases: crucial enzymes in polyunsaturated fatty acid-related pathways with pleiotropic influences in health and disease. *Adv Exp Med Biol.* 2014;824:61–81.

18. Summers LK, Fielding BA, Bradshaw HA, Ilic V, Beysen C, Clark ML, et al. Substituting dietary saturated fat with polyunsaturated fat changes abdominal fat distribution and improves insulin sensitivity. *Diabetologia.* 2002;45(3):369–77.

19. Vessby B, Uusitupa M, Hermansen K, Riccardi G, Rivellese AA, Tapsell LC, et al. Substituting dietary saturated for monounsaturated fat impairs insulin sensitivity in healthy men and women: the KANWU Study. *Diabetologia.* 2001;44(3):312–9.

20. Saeedi R, Frohlich J. Lipoprotein (a), an independent cardiovascular risk marker. *Clin Diabetes Endocrinol.* 2016;2:7.

21. Paniagua JA, Gallego de la Sacristana A, Romero I, Vidal-Puig A, Latre JM, Sanchez E, et al. Monounsaturated fat-rich diet prevents central body fat distribution and decreases postprandial adiponectin expression induced by a carbohydrate-rich diet in insulin-resistant subjects. *Diabetes Care.* 2007;30(7):1717–23.

22. Erkkila A, de Mello VD, Riserus U, Laaksonen DE. Dietary fatty acids and cardiovascular disease: an epidemiological approach. *Prog Lipid Res.* 2008;47(3):172–87.

23. Thompson AK, Minihane AM, Williams CM. Trans fatty acids, insulin resistance and diabetes. *Eur J Clin Nutr.* 2011;65(5):553–64.

24. Sheard NF, Clark NG, Brand-Miller JC, Franz MJ, Pi-Sunyer FX, Mayer-Davis E, et al. Dietary carbohydrate (amount and type) in the prevention and management of diabetes: a statement by the American Diabetes Association. *Diabetes Care.* 2004;27(9):2266–71.

25. Salmeron J, Manson JE, Stampfer MJ, Colditz GA, Wing AL, Willett WC. Dietary fiber, glycemic load, and risk of non-insulin-dependent diabetes mellitus in women. *JAMA.* 1997;277(6):472–7.

26. Salmeron J, Ascherio A, Rimm EB, Colditz GA, Spiegelman D, Jenkins DJ, et al. Dietary fiber, glycemic load, and risk of NIDDM in men. *Diabetes Care.* 1997;20(4):545–50.

27. Meyer KA, Kushi LH, Jacobs DR, Jr., Slavin J, Sellers TA, Folsom AR. Carbohydrates, dietary fiber, and incident type 2 diabetes in older women. *Am J Clin Nutr.* 2000;71(4):921–30.

28. Dong JY, Xun P, He K, Qin LQ. Magnesium intake and risk of type 2 diabetes: meta-analysis of prospective cohort studies. *Diabetes Care.* 2011;34(9):2116–22.

29. Zhao Z, Li S, Liu G, Yan F, Ma X, Huang Z, et al. Body iron stores and heme-iron intake in relation to risk of type 2 diabetes: a systematic review and meta-analysis. *PLoS One.* 2012;7(7):e41641.

30. Song Y, Wang L, Pittas AG, Del Gobbo LC, Zhang C, Manson JE, et al. Blood 25-hydroxy vitamin D levels and incident type 2 diabetes: a meta-analysis of prospective studies. *Diabetes Care.* 2013;36(5):1422–8.

31. Evert AB, Dennison M, Gardner CD, Garvey WT, Lau KHK, MacLeod J, et al. Nutrition therapy for adults with diabetes or prediabetes: a consensus report. *Diabetes Care.* 2019;42(5):731–54.

32. Pittas AG, Dawson-Hughes B, Sheehan P, Ware JH, Knowler WC, Aroda VR, et al. Vitamin D supplementation and prevention of type 2 diabetes. *N Engl J Med.* 2019;381(6):520–30.

33. Aune D, Norat T, Romundstad P, Vatten LJ. Whole grain and refined grain consumption and the risk of type 2 diabetes: a systematic review and dose-response meta-analysis of cohort studies. *Eur J Epidemiol.* 2013;28(11):845–58.

34. Hu EA, Pan A, Malik V, Sun Q. White rice consumption and risk of type 2 diabetes: meta-analysis and systematic review. *BMJ.* 2012;344:e1454.

35. Pan A, Sun Q, Bernstein AM, Schulze MB, Manson JE, Willett WC, et al. Red meat consumption and risk of type 2 diabetes: 3 cohorts of US adults and an updated meta-analysis. *Am J Clin Nutr.* 2011;94(4):1088–96.

36. Wu JH, Micha R, Imamura F, Pan A, Biggs ML, Ajaz O, et al. Omega-3 fatty acids and incident type 2 diabetes: a systematic review and meta-analysis. *Br J Nutr.* 2012;107(Suppl 2):S214–27.

37. Carter P, Gray LJ, Troughton J, Khunti K, Davies MJ. Fruit and vegetable intake and incidence of type 2 diabetes mellitus: systematic review and meta-analysis. *BMJ.* 2010;341:c4229.

38. Malik VS, Popkin BM, Bray GA, Despres JP, Willett WC, Hu FB. Sugar-sweetened beverages and risk of metabolic syndrome and type 2 diabetes: a meta-analysis. *Diabetes Care.* 2010;33(11):2477–83.

39. American Diabetes Association. 8. Obesity management for the treatment of type 2 diabetes: standards of medical care in diabetes-2021. *Diabetes Care.* 2021;44(Suppl 1):S100–S10.

40. Chiavaroli L, Viguiliouk E, Nishi SK, Blanco Mejia S, Rahelic D, Kahleova H, et al. DASH dietary pattern and cardiometabolic outcomes: an umbrella review of systematic reviews and meta-analyses. *Nutrients.* 2019;11(2):338.

41. Giugliano D, Esposito K. Mediterranean diet and metabolic diseases. *Curr Opin Lipidol.* 2008;19(1):63–8.

42. Esposito K, Chiodini P, Maiorino MI, Bellastella G, Panagiotakos D, Giugliano D. Which diet for prevention of type 2 diabetes? A meta-analysis of prospective studies. *Endocrine.* 2014;47(1):107–16.

43. Farkouh ME, Rayfield EJ, Fuster V. Diabetes and cardiovascular disease. In: Fuster V, Narula J, Vaishnava P, Leon MB, Callans DJ, Rumsfeld J, Poppas A, editors. *Fuster and Hurst's The Heart, 15e.* New York: McGraw Hill. 2022.

44. Sofi F, Cesari F, Abbate R, Gensini GF, Casini A. Adherence to Mediterranean diet and health status: meta-analysis. *BMJ.* 2008;337:a1344.

45. Estruch R, Ros E, Salas-Salvado J, Covas MI, Corella D, Aros F, et al. Primary prevention of cardiovascular disease with a Mediterranean diet. *N Engl J Med.* 2013;368(14):1279–90.

46. Estruch R, Ros E, Salas-Salvado J, Covas MI, Corella D, Aros F, et al. Primary prevention of cardiovascular disease with a Mediterranean diet supplemented with extra-virgin olive oil or nuts. *N Engl J Med.* 2018;378(25):e34.

47. Sanchez-Villegas A, Bes-Rastrollo M, Martinez-Gonzalez MA, Serra-Majem L. Adherence to a Mediterranean dietary pattern and weight gain in a follow-up study: the SUN cohort. *Int J Obes.* 2006;30(2):350–8.

48. Mendez MA, Popkin BM, Jakszyn P, Berenguer A, Tormo MJ, Sanchez MJ, et al. Adherence to a Mediterranean diet is associated with reduced 3-year incidence of obesity. *J Nutr.* 2006;136(11):2934–8.

49. McManus K, Antinoro L, Sacks F. A randomized controlled trial of a moderate-fat, low-energy diet compared with a low fat, low-energy diet for weight loss in overweight adults. *Int J Obes Relat Metab Disord.* 2001;25(10):1503–11.

50. Panagiotakos DB, Pitsavos C, Chrysohoou C, Skoumas J, Tousoulis D, Toutouza M, et al. Impact of lifestyle habits on the prevalence of the metabolic syndrome among Greek adults from the ATTICA study. *Am Heart J.* 2004;147(1):106–12.

51. Venkatasamy VV, Pericherla S, Manthuruthil S, Mishra S, Hanno R. Effect of physical activity on insulin resistance, inflammation and oxidative stress in diabetes mellitus. *J Clin Diagn Res.* 2013;7(8):1764–6.

52. Colberg SR, Albright AL, Blissmer BJ, Braun B, Chasan-Taber L, Fernhall B, et al. Exercise and type 2 diabetes: American College of Sports Medicine and the American Diabetes Association: joint position statement. Exercise and type 2 diabetes. *Med Sci Sports Exerc.* 2010;42(12):2282–303.

53. Chen X, Zhao S, Hsue C, Dai X, Liu L, Miller JD, et al. Effects of aerobic training and resistance training in reducing cardiovascular disease risk for patients with prediabetes: a multi-center randomized controlled trial. *Prim Care Diabetes.* 2021;15(6):1063–70.

54. Liu L, Ma X, Xu H, Ruan S, Yuan X. Comparing the effects of 12 months aerobic exercise and resistance training on glucose metabolism among prediabetes phenotype: a explorative randomized controlled trial. *Prim Care Diabetes.* 2021;15(2):340–6.

55. Borghouts LB, Keizer HA. Exercise and insulin sensitivity: a review. *Int J Sports Med.* 2000;21(1):1–12.

56. Bjorntorp P, Fahlen M, Grimby G, Gustafson A, Holm J, Renstrom P, et al. Carbohydrate and lipid metabolism in middle-aged, physically well-trained men. *Metabolism.* 1972;21(11):1037–44.

57. Houmard JA, Shinebarger MH, Dolan PL, Leggett-Frazier N, Bruner RK, McCammon MR, et al. Exercise training increases GLUT-4 protein concentration in previously sedentary middle-aged men. *Am J Physiol.* 1993;264(6 Pt 1):E896–901.

58. DiPietro L, Dziura J, Yeckel CW, Neufer PD. Exercise and improved insulin sensitivity in older women: evidence of the enduring benefits of higher intensity training. *J Appl Physiol.* 2006;100(1):142–9.

59. Seals DR, Hagberg JM, Allen WK, Hurley BF, Dalsky GP, Ehsani AA, et al. Glucose tolerance in young and older athletes and sedentary men. *J Appl Physiol Respir Environ Exerc Physiol.* 1984;56(6):1521–5.

60. Hughes VA, Fiatarone MA, Fielding RA, Kahn BB, Ferrara CM, Shepherd P, et al. Exercise increases muscle GLUT-4 levels and insulin action in subjects with impaired glucose tolerance. *Am J Physiol.* 1993;264(6 Pt 1):E855–62.

61. Barnes AS. The epidemic of obesity and diabetes: trends and treatments. *Tex Heart Inst J.* 2011;38(2):142–4.

62. Goodpaster BH, Katsiaras A, Kelley DE. Enhanced fat oxidation through physical activity is associated with improvements in insulin sensitivity in obesity. *Diabetes.* 2003;52(9):2191–7.

63. Perseghin G, Price TB, Petersen KF, Roden M, Cline GW, Gerow K, et al. Increased glucose transport-phosphorylation and muscle glycogen synthesis after exercise training in insulin-resistant subjects. *N Engl J Med.* 1996;335(18):1357–62.

64. Festa A, D'Agostino R, Jr., Tracy RP, Haffner SM, Insulin Resistance Atherosclerosis Study Investigators. Elevated levels of acute-phase proteins and plasminogen activator inhibitor-1 predict the development of type 2 diabetes: the insulin resistance atherosclerosis study. *Diabetes.* 2002;51(4):1131–7.

65. Larsen CM, Faulenbach M, Vaag A, Volund A, Ehses JA, Seifert B, et al. Interleukin-1-receptor antagonist in type 2 diabetes mellitus. *N Engl J Med.* 2007;356(15):1517–26.

66. Mancusi C, Izzo R, di Gioia G, Losi MA, Barbato E, Morisco C. Insulin resistance the hinge between hypertension and type 2 diabetes. *High Blood Press Cardiovasc Prev.* 2020;27(6):515–26.

67. Esposito K, Pontillo A, Di Palo C, Giugliano G, Masella M, Marfella R, et al. Effect of weight loss and lifestyle changes on vascular inflammatory markers in obese women: a randomized trial. *JAMA.* 2003;289(14):1799–804.

68. The Diabetes Prevention Program. Design and methods for a clinical trial in the prevention of type 2 diabetes. *Diabetes Care.* 1999;22(4):623–34.

69. Knowler WC, Barrett-Connor E, Fowler SE, Hamman RF, Lachin JM, Walker EA, et al. Reduction in the incidence of type 2 diabetes with lifestyle intervention or metformin. *N Engl J Med.* 2002;346(6):393–403.

70. Diabetes Prevention Program Research Group, Knowler WC, Fowler SE, Hamman RF, Christophi CA, Hoffman HJ, et al. 10-year follow-up of diabetes incidence and weight loss in the Diabetes Prevention Program Outcomes Study. *Lancet.* 2009;374(9702):1677–86.

71. Lindstrom J, Louheranta A, Mannelin M, Rastas M, Salminen V, Eriksson J, et al. The Finnish Diabetes Prevention Study (DPS): lifestyle intervention and 3-year results on diet and physical activity. *Diabetes Care.* 2003;26(12):3230–6.

72. Pan XR, Li GW, Hu YH, Wang JX, Yang WY, An ZX, et al. Effects of diet and exercise in preventing NIDDM in people with impaired glucose tolerance. The Da Qing IGT and Diabetes Study. *Diabetes Care.* 1997;20(4):537–44.

73. Gong Q, Zhang P, Wang J, Ma J, An Y, Chen Y, et al. Morbidity and mortality after lifestyle intervention for people with impaired glucose tolerance: 30-year results of the Da Qing Diabetes Prevention Outcome Study. *Lancet Diabetes Endocrinol.* 2019; 7(6):452–61.

7 Secondary Prevention Example

Using Lifestyle Medicine in Patients with Type 2 Diabetes

Kaveeta Marwaha and
Stephanie Behringer-Massera
Icahn School of Medicine at Mount Sinai

CONTENTS

7.1   INTRODUCTION

Insulin resistance underlies prediabetes, type 2 diabetes (T2D), and cardiovascular disease (CVD) development and is extremely prevalent in both the U.S. population and the world (1,2). Unhealthy dietary patterns, poor sleep hygiene, lack of regular exercise, and high levels of stress, all in the setting of an aging population, contribute to these cardiometabolic risks. Cardiometabolic-based chronic disease (CMBCD) is a new model that configures chronic diseases with three dimensions: I - stage (1-risk; 2-predisease; 3-disease; and 4-complications); II - drivers (primary [genetics, environment, and behavior] and secondary/metabolic [abnormal adiposity, dysglycemia, hypertension, and dyslipidemia]); and III - social determinants of disease and transcultural factors, which populate each cell in this 2×2 stage $\times$ driver matrix (3,4). Insulin resistance is a key pathophysiological step, mediating the effects of lifestyle and adiposity on dysglycemia, other metabolic syndrome traits, and CVD. This driver-based chronic disease approach exposes early pathophysiological targets for preventive care: primordial, or the prevention of risk in stage 1; primary, or the prevention of progression of predisease in stage 2 to disease or complications; secondary, or the

DOI: 10.1201/9781003206637-7

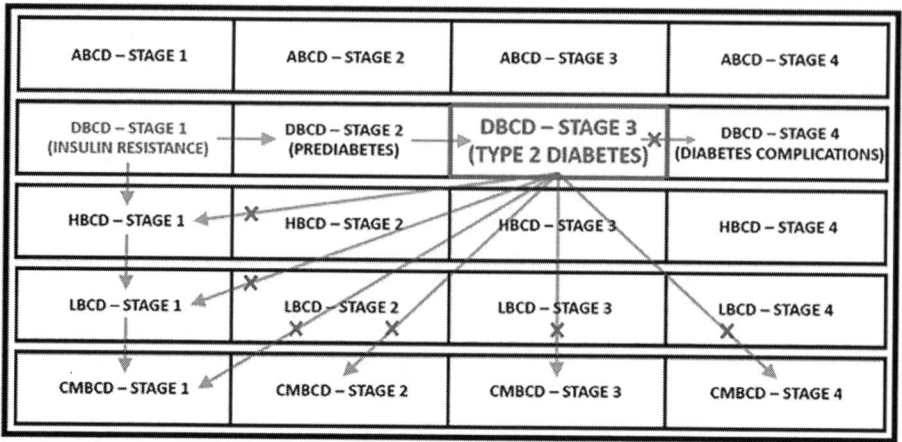

FIGURE 7.1 Secondary Prevention of Cardiovascular Disease by Focusing on Type 2 Diabetes. The cardiometabolic-based chronic disease model highlighting in blue the key role of insulin resistance and in red the impact of secondary prevention strategies in patients with type 2 diabetes to mitigate or even abrogate progression to diabetes complications, risk for hypertension, risk for dyslipidemia, and/or any cardiovascular disease (CMBCD) stage. Stage 1 is "risk;" stage 2 is "predisease;" stage 3 is "disease;" and stage 4 is "complications." Abbreviations: ABCD, adiposity-based chronic disease; CMBCD, cardiometabolic-based chronic disease; DBCD, dysglycemia-based chronic disease; HBCD, hypertension-based chronic disease; LBCD, lipid-based chronic disease (3–5).

prevention of early disease in stage 3 to complications; and tertiary, or the prevention of suffering or death in stage 4 (3,4). In this chapter and recognizing the central role of insulin resistance, secondary prevention (the prevention of symptoms and complications in patients with early, asymptomatic diseases) will be interpreted in terms of CMBCD with a focus on stage 3 dysglycemia-based chronic disease (DBCD) or T2D (Figure 7.1) (3–5). In other words, the target of this discussion is the mitigation or abrogation of the progression of early T2D directly to diabetes complications and indirectly (via other metabolic syndrome traits) or directly to any stage of CVD.

A growing body of research investigating the role of behavior and personal choice has shown the beneficial impact of lifestyle medicine for the improvement, and in some cases even reversal, of T2D. As such, lifestyle medicine is a healthcare priority. One of the best-known primary prevention studies in the lifestyle medicine field is the Diabetes Prevention Program (DPP) which showed a dramatic risk reduction of T2D in people with prediabetes, particularly in those over the age of 60 years, where lifestyle changes translated into a risk reduction of 71% (6). But what about preventing the progression of the disease and emergence of complications in patients already with T2D?

7.2   EARLY OBSERVATIONS

In 1987, Wing et al. [7] published data showing that the modest achievement of weight loss through calorie restriction among patients with T2D led to improvements in hemoglobin A1c (A1C). Specifically, there was a 1% reduction in A1C for every 6.9 kg or 5% body weight loss and a 1.6% reduction in A1C in those who lost >10% of body weight from a baseline A1C of 9.9% (7). These findings and other early observations support the role of dietary modification within a comprehensive clinical approach in the management of T2D (8).

Physical activity is another potential target for disease modification in T2D (9). Combined aerobic and resistance exercise has an additive benefit and demonstrates strong evidence for lowering A1C (10). Even activities such as yoga and tai chi have been shown to not only improve balance, flexibility, and muscle strength but also A1C (11). In contrast, a sedentary lifestyle, measured by increased time spent sitting restfully, is associated with hyperglycemia, as well as a higher risk of mortality from CVD (12). Indeed, cardiovascular events, such as coronary artery disease, myocardial infarction, cardiomyopathy, arrhythmias, stroke, and sudden death, represent the leading cause of mortality among patients with T2D (13). Specifically, the incidence of CVD is approximately two-fold higher in patients with T2D compared to those without diabetes (13).

7.3 THE LOOK AHEAD TRIAL

Look AHEAD (Action for Health in Diabetes) is a landmark trial and the first large-scale study to investigate lifestyle interventions in subjects with T2D (14). Modeled after the DPP, Look AHEAD is the longest and largest randomized controlled trial that examined whether an intensive lifestyle intervention (ILI) for weight loss would decrease cardiovascular morbidity and mortality in subjects who were already diagnosed with T2D (14). Look AHEAD included 5,145 subjects with obesity/overweight and T2D. Subjects were randomly assigned to either ILI that includes a diet with decreased caloric intake and increased physical activity (175 minutes of moderate intensity per week) with monthly educational sessions or simply a diabetes support and education group (DSE) that met three times in the first 4 years and once annually afterward (15). All subjects had an A1C <11%, with a mean age of 60 years and a mean body mass index (BMI) of 36.0 kg/m². Subjects with and without CVD were included to increase the generalizability of the results, and the trial had a maximal follow-up of approximately 11 years. The primary outcome was death from CVD, non-fatal myocardial infarction, non-fatal stroke, and hospitalization from angina. Subjects randomized to the ILI group were instructed to follow a strict caloric intake through weekly counseling with a target of 1,200–1,800 kcal per day, depending on baseline weight, and a goal of achieving 7% weight loss. This goal was set based on earlier studies that demonstrated significant metabolic effects of modest (5%–10%) weight loss (16–19). A structured curriculum focusing on portion control, meal plans, and calorie counting was critical for success (15). All subjects attended annual visits for the assessment of T2D and complications (15).

7.3.1 Look AHEAD: Primary Outcome

While the final results did not find significant differences in the primary endpoint of cardiovascular mortality and morbidity between the two study groups under the prespecified intention-to-treat analysis (a neutral finding), it did show that participants in the ILI group achieved greater reductions in weight loss and waist circumference compared to the control group ($p < 0.001$) (19). Additionally and perhaps contributing to the controversy of this initial finding, a *post hoc* analysis of the Look AHEAD trial data that included patients who successfully lost weight within the intensive group showed an approximate 15% reduction in cardiovascular outcomes for every 7% of body weight loss achieved (19). This significant improvement is suggestive of a CVD benefit with a successful ILI.

Another *post hoc* analysis of the Look AHEAD trial using causal forest analysis to detect hidden heterogeneous treatment effects identified a subgroup experiencing reduced CVD events after the ILI aimed at weight loss. Specifically, subjects enrolled in the ILI group with an A1C ≥6.8% or an A1C <6.8% but a Short Form Health Survey (SF-36) general health score of ≥48 (positive perception of health status) had a 3.46% absolute risk reduction for the primary cardiovascular outcome (20). In contrast, subjects with A1C <6.8% and SF-36 <48 (negative perception of health status) had a 7.41% absolute risk increase for the primary outcome (20). The net effect of these relationships may have contributed to the neutral overall study primary outcome (20).

Multiple authors have commented on these findings and that there may have been bias toward a healthier cohort in the Look AHEAD trial (13). Enrollees had to commit themselves to a long follow-up period suggesting that a more health-conscious population emerged than typically observed in patients with T2D. Moreover, there was a lower-than-expected number of cardiovascular events during the trial period, which further supports that there may have been a relatively healthier cohort than was anticipated (21). Still, the primary endpoint may have been reached with adequate power of the study if this increased health status was taken into account (21). In short, ILI provides great benefits in terms of secondary prevention of CVD in patients with T2D and increased adiposity (22).

7.3.2 LOOK AHEAD: SECONDARY OUTCOMES

At the end of the trial, the mean weight loss from baseline was 6.0% in the intervention group and 3.5% in the control group. Risk factors for CVD, such as A1C and blood pressure, were reduced in the intervention group, most significantly after 1 year (15). Fitness levels and physical activity were measured by having participants perform an exercise test and questionnaire, respectively. Changes in fitness and physical activity were statistically greater in the ILI group and also correlated with reductions in weight (23). These findings suggest that lifestyle intervention programs should ideally implement regular intensive exercises, good adherence to a healthy diet, and frequent follow-ups to see significant improvements in weight loss and delay the progression of T2D (24).

There are other significant benefits demonstrated by the Look AHEAD study results within the ILI group (25). First, educating patients with T2D on the importance of physical activity and diet while also facilitating engagement with healthcare professionals not only results in improvements in blood glucose levels but also serum lipids, blood pressure, renal disease, sleep apnea, and depression (16). Second, disease improvement and reduction of associated complications are noted on many fronts with ILI.

Weight loss was also shown to delay the progression of chronic kidney disease (26). Subjects in the ILI group had a 31% less risk of very-high-risk chronic kidney disease (defined as glomerular filtration rate [GFR] <30 mL/min/1.73 m², GFR <45 mL/min/1.73 m² and moderate albuminuria, or GFR <60 mL/min/1.73 m² and high microalbuminuria) as compared to the DSE group (26).

Additionally, men in the ILI and DSE groups completed an International Index of Erectile Function at baseline and 1 year (27). Those in the ILI group lost more weight, thus reporting improvements in erectile function (27). Only 8% of men in the ILI group reported worsening erectile function compared to 20% in the DSE group (27).

Other outcomes measured in the Look AHEAD study that constitute secondary prevention targets were the presence and severity of depression and quality of life. Rubin and Wadden et al. (28) found that subjects in the ILI group had a significantly reduced incidence of mild or greater depression symptoms. Subjects completed Beck's Depression Inventory (BDI), a self-report of depression symptoms, at baseline and years 1, 2, 3, 4, and 8. BDI scores greater than or equal to 10 were consistent with significant depressive symptoms. The ILI group was found to have significant reductions in mild or greater depression compared to the DSE group (HR = 0.85; 95% CI 0.75–0.97; $p = 0.0145$). Those subjects in the ILI group with BDI scores less than 10 (not in the depressed range) were found to have a 15% reduction in developing depression compared to their DSE counterparts (28). The ILI group also reported improvement in somatic and cognitive symptoms of depression at year 1 (28). As another assessment of mental health and health-related quality of life, participants completed a Medical Outcomes Study Short Form 36 (SF-36) twice annually for the first 4 years and then annually until year 10. This report generated a physical component summary (PCS). Previous studies have found that SF-36 PCS scores are overall lower in individuals with T2D compared to the general U.S. population (29). PCS scores in the Look AHEAD analysis were significantly higher in the ILI group over the 10-year period ($p < 0.001$) (29).

Diabetic peripheral neuropathy (DPN) was another outcome assessed. Using the Michigan Neuropathy Screening Instrument (MNSI) questionnaire, subjects in the ILI group were found to have a significant reduction in DPN (30). Specifically, the average percentage of subjects with an MNSI score greater than or equal to 4 was significantly lower in the ILI group than in the DSE group (OR 0.89, $p = 0.026$), suggesting an improvement in DPN (30).

Obstructive sleep apnea (OSA) was yet another outcome evaluated in the study. Home polysomnograms were performed at baseline and at 1, 2, 4, and 10 years, and apnea–hypopnea indices were measured (31). Approximately three times as many Look AHEAD study subjects with OSA in the ILI group compared to those with OSA in the DSE group had total remission of their OSA. Additionally, the prevalence of severe OSA was half that in the ILI group compared to the DSE group (31).

Another analysis of the Look AHEAD trial demonstrates improvement in urinary incontinence among men with overweight/obesity and T2D at 1 year (32). The prevalence of urinary incontinence decreased from 11.3% to 9.0% in the ILI group, whereas it increased in the DSE group. The ILI group also had higher odds of urinary incontinence completely resolving (32).

Enrolled patients with T2D who lost >8% of their body weight in the ILI group demonstrated a successful reduction of hepatic steatosis and the risk of non-alcoholic fatty liver disease (NAFLD) (33). By using proton magnetic resonance spectroscopy, a greater improvement in fatty liver disease was seen in those who lost more weight, further recommending weight loss as the first-line treatment for NAFLD (33,34).

Another outcome assessed in the Look AHEAD trial was the need for a total knee replacement (TKR). Osteoarthritis, which is accelerated by T2D, has the potential to limit physical activity which can lead to an exacerbation of T2D in a vicious cycle. When severe, osteoarthritis may be treated with TKR. Subjects in the Look AHEAD trial without prior TKR provided a self-report of knee pain by using the Visual Analog Scale and Western Ontario McMaster University Osteoarthritis Index questionnaire (35). Six-month follow-up questionnaires were collected from subjects in the ILI and DSE groups. It was noted that in subjects without knee pain at baseline, there was a 29% reduced risk of TKR in the ILI group compared to the DSE group. Intentional weight loss prior to the development of knee pain has a significant impact on the prevention of TKR in this population (35).

Physical disability was another outcome reviewed. Using SF-36s, the ILI group was found to have a significant delay in the development of moderate or severe disability and an increase in the number of non-disabled years ($p < 0.005$) compared to the DSE group (36). Healthcare-related costs, such as hospitalizations and medications, significantly declined in the ILI group compared to the DSE group (37).

7.4   THE EUROASPIRE TRIALS

The EUROASPIRE trials (37) focused on CVD risk factors. EUROASPIRE I trial set the stage for establishing the risk factors that are now known to be associated with coronary heart disease. The aim of EUROASPIRE I was to assess the secondary prevention of coronary heart disease, with the goal of reducing cardiovascular morbidity and mortality. This study was conducted in two stages: a retrospective query and a prospective interview. A retrospective survey of patient data from medical records from 1991 to 1995 was obtained from hospitals in nine European countries (38). Patients were ≥70 years old and had been diagnosed with or had been treated for coronary heart disease. Of the 3,569 participants with complete records who were interviewed, 18% reported a diagnosis of diabetes, 19.4% reported current tobacco use, 25.3% had obesity, 60.6% had elevated blood pressure, and 57.7% had elevated cholesterol. Almost half of the subjects in the study had a family history of coronary heart disease. Subjects with T2D were found to have high rates of modifiable risk factors, including abnormalities in cholesterol, hypertension, and central obesity, all of which were believed to be responsive to lifestyle changes (38).

EUROASPIRE II was another survey undertaken in 1999–2000 that assessed if the Joint European Societies' recommendations on coronary artery prevention were being taken. Twenty percent of interviewed subjects had T2D, with the majority demonstrating poor glycemic control (39). Overall, the survey indicated that there were many unhealthy lifestyles among study subjects, and more effective lifestyle changes were required to address modifiable risk factors and reduce cardiovascular morbidity and mortality (39). Similarly, EUROASPIRE III and IV also involved large proportions of patients with coronary heart disease who did not reach targets for reducing cardiovascular disease, despite the state-of-the-art routine care (40). Consequently, more comprehensive and multidisciplinary approaches to lifestyle intervention are deemed necessary for secondary prevention and risk reduction in patients with CMBCD (40).

7.5 NUTRITIONAL APPROACHES FOR SECONDARY PREVENTION

Nutritional therapy is crucially important in improving T2D and its complications (41). Education and support delivered by a certified diabetes educator have been shown to improve diabetes outcomes, which include macro- and microvascular complications, including CVD. Studies specifically show improvement among patients who use carbohydrate counting or the modified plate method (42). The plate method provides portion control by dividing the plate into sections on a 9-inch-sized plate (42). This method was originally developed to make it easier for patients with T2D to restrict their carbohydrate intake without calculating specific portions (42). Additionally, a whole-food plant-based diet has been shown to be particularly beneficial in preventing and even reversing T2D, as well as demonstrating a favorable effect on body weight, cholesterol, and blood pressure. Plant-based diets are high in fiber and consist of whole grains, legumes, vegetables, fruits, nuts, and seeds. Consumption of processed foods and animal products, particularly those that favor the development of obesity, insulin resistance, T2D, dyslipidemia, hypertension, CVD, and cancer, should be eliminated or greatly reduced (43–51).

The Canadian Diabetes Association recommends plant-based diets for the management of T2D based on the analysis of data from 13 studies (52). Several large cohort studies have shown the benefits of a predominantly whole-food plant-based diet with regard to reducing the prevalence and incidence of T2D; these include the EPIC-Oxford, the California Seventh-day Adventists study, and the Adventist Health Study-2 (53–55). A whole-food plant-based diet was consistently associated with improvement of A1C, weight loss, low serum cholesterol, and blood pressure (53–55).

Nicholson et al. (56) demonstrated that subjects with T2D who followed a low-fat vegan diet compared to a conventional low-fat diet had a greater reduction in fasting serum glucose levels and body weight so much so that hypoglycemic drugs were either reduced or discontinued in the low-fat vegan group but not in the control group. The cumulative positive effect of a whole-food plant-based diet on these parameters reduces the risk of CVD in people living with diabetes.

A low-fat plant-based diet is the only dietary pattern to date that has shown significant reductions and reversal of macro- and microvascular complications of prediabetes/T2D (methodological controversies over the PREDIMED trial notwithstanding) (57). The Lifestyle Heart Study demonstrated a significant regression in coronary artery stenosis in patients with coronary artery disease by the implementation of a low-fat plant-based diet in addition to exercise, stress management, and smoking cessation (58). After 5 years, there was a reduction in atherosclerotic stenosis among subjects in the plant-based group, whereas a progression of atherosclerosis, leading to coronary angioplasty or bypass surgery, was observed in the control group (58).

7.6   CONCLUSION

Patients with T2D have an inherently higher risk of atherosclerotic cardiac disease. Within the context of the CMBCD model, secondary prevention strategies, such as ILI, yields significant improvement in the risk of vascular complications, microvascular disease, and associated conditions. Education by clinicians and frequent follow-ups are keys to the implementation of these strategies. Studies show that an overall intensive lifestyle of moderate regular physical activity and especially consumption of whole plant-based foods reduces the development and progression of CMBCD risk factors in patients with T2D.

REFERENCES

1. Caspersen CJ, Thomas GD, Boseman LA, Beckles GL, Albright AL. Aging, diabetes, and the public health system in the United States. *Am J Public Health*. 2012;102 (8):1482–1497. doi:10.2105/AJPH.2011.300616
2. Ley SH, Hamdy O, Mohan V, Hu FB. Prevention and management of type 2 diabetes: dietary components and nutritional strategies. *Lancet*. 2014;383(9933):1999–2007. doi:10.1016/S0140-6736(14)60613-9
3. Mechanick JI, Farkouh ME, Newman JD, Garvey WT. Cardiometabolic-based chronic disease, adiposity and dysglycemia drivers: JACC state-of-the-art review. *J Am Coll Cardiol*. 2020 Feb 11;75(5):525–538. doi: 10.1016/j.jacc.2019.11.044
4. Mechanick JI, Farkouh ME, Newman JD, Garvey WT. Cardiometabolic-based chronic disease, addressing knowledge and clinical practice gaps: JACC state-of-the-art review. *J Am Coll Cardiol*. 2020 Feb 11;75(5):539–555. doi: 10.1016/j.jacc.2019.11.046
5. Mechanick JI, Garber AJ, Grunberger G, Handelsman Y, Garvey WT. Dysglycemia-based chronic disease: an American Association of Clinical Endocrinologists position statement. *Endocr Pract*. 2018 Nov;24(11):995–1011. doi: 10.4158/PS-2018-0139
6. Knowler WC, Barrett-Connor E, Fowler SE, et al. Reduction in the incidence of type 2 diabetes with lifestyle intervention or metformin. *N Engl J Med*. 2002;346(6):393–403. doi:10.1056/NEJMoa012512
7. Wing RR, Koeske R, Epstein LH, Nowalk MP, Gooding W, Becker D. Long-term effects of modest weight loss in type II diabetic patients. *Arch Intern Med*. 1987;147(10): 1749–1753.
8. American Diabetes Association. 2. Classification and diagnosis of diabetes: standards of medical care in diabetes-2021. *Diabetes Care*. 2021;44(Suppl 1):S15–S33. doi:10.2337/dc21-S002
9. Kirwan JP, Sacks J, Nieuwoudt S. The essential role of exercise in the management of type 2 diabetes. *Cleve Clin J Med*. 2017;84(7 Suppl 1):S15–S21. doi:10.3949/ccjm.84. s1.03
10. Colberg SR, Sigal RJ, Fernhall B, et al. Exercise and type 2 diabetes: the American College of Sports Medicine and the American Diabetes Association: joint position statement. *Diabetes Care*. 2010;33(12):e147–e167. doi:10.2337/dc10-9990
11. Colberg SR, Sigal RJ, Yardley JE, et al. Physical activity/exercise and diabetes: a position statement of the American Diabetes Association. *Diabetes Care*. 2016;39 (11):2065–2079. doi:10.2337/dc16-1728

12. Katzmarzyk PT, Church TS, Craig CL, Bouchard C. Sitting time and mortality from all causes, cardiovascular disease, and cancer. *Med Sci Sports Exerc.* 2009;41(5):998–1005. doi:10.1249/MSS.0b013e3181930355

13. Pi-Sunyer X. The Look AHEAD Trial: a review and discussion of its outcomes. *Curr Nutr Rep.* 2014;3(4):387–391. doi:10.1007/s13668-014-0099-x

14. Salvia MG. The Look AHEAD trial: translating lessons learned into clinical practice and further study. *Diabetes Spectr.* 2017;30(3):166–170. doi:10.2337/ds17-0016

15. Look AHEAD Research Group, Wing RR, Bolin P, et al. Cardiovascular effects of intensive lifestyle intervention in type 2 diabetes. *N Engl J Med.* 2013;369(2):145–154. doi:10.1056/NEJMoa1212914

16. Look AHEAD Research Group, Wadden TA, West DS, et al. The Look AHEAD study: a description of the lifestyle intervention and the evidence supporting it. *Obesity.* 2006; 14(5):737–752. doi:10.1038/oby.2006.84

17. Guare JC, Wing RR, Grant A. Comparison of obese NIDDM and nondiabetic women: short- and long-term weight loss. *Obes Res.* 1995;3(4):329–335. doi:10.1002/j.1550-8528 .1995.tb00158.x

18. Pascale RW, Wing RR, Butler BA, Mullen M, Bononi P. Effects of a behavioral weight loss program stressing calorie restriction versus calorie plus fat restriction in obese individuals with NIDDM or a family history of diabetes. *Diabetes Care.* 1995;18(9):1241–1248. doi:10.2337/diacare.18.9.1241

19. Wing RR, Marcus MD, Salata R, Epstein LH, Miaskiewicz S, Blair EH. Effects of a very-low-calorie diet on long-term glycemic control in obese type 2 diabetic subjects. *Arch Intern Med.* 1991;151(7):1334–1340.

20. Baum A, Scarpa J, Bruzelius E, Tamler R, Basu S, Faghmous J. Targeting weight loss interventions to reduce cardiovascular complications of type 2 diabetes: a machine learning-based post-hoc analysis of heterogeneous treatment effects in the Look AHEAD trial. *Lancet Diabetes Endocrinol.* 2017;5(10):808–815. doi:10.1016/S2213-8587(17)30176-6

21. Meleady R. Intensive lifestyle intervention in type 2 diabetes. *N Engl J Med.* 2013 Dec 12;369(24):2356. doi: 10.1056/NEJMc1312802

22. Garvey WT. Long-term health benefits of intensive lifestyle intervention in the Look AHEAD study. *Obesity.* 2021;29(8):1242–1243. doi:10.1002/oby.23198

23. Jakicic, JM, Jaramillo SA, Balasubramanyam A et al. Effect of a lifestyle intervention on change in cardiorespiratory fitness in adults with type 2 diabetes: results from the Look AHEAD Study. *Int. J. Obes. 2009*; 33(3):305–316. doi:10.1038/ijo.2008.280

24. Franz MJ, MacLeod J, Evert A, et al. Academy of nutrition and dietetics nutrition practice guideline for type 1 and type 2 diabetes in adults: systematic review of evidence for medical nutrition therapy effectiveness and recommendations for integration into the nutrition care process. *J Acad Nutr Diet.* 2017;117(10):1659–1679. doi:10.1016/j.jand.2017.03.022.

25. Wing RR; Look AHEAD Research Group. Does lifestyle intervention improve health of adults with overweight/obesity and type 2 diabetes? Findings from the Look AHEAD Randomized Trial. *Obesity* 2021;29(8):1246–1258. doi:10.1002/oby.23158

26. Look AHEAD Research Group. Effect of a long-term behavioural weight loss intervention on nephropathy in overweight or obese adults with type 2 diabetes: a secondary analysis of the Look AHEAD randomised clinical trial. *Lancet Diabetes Endocrinol.* 2014;2(10):801–809. doi:10.1016/S2213-8587(14)70156-1

27. Wing RR, Rosen RC, Fava JL, et al. Effects of weight loss intervention on erectile function in older men with type 2 diabetes in the Look AHEAD trial. *J Sex Med.* 2010;7(1 Pt 1):156–165. doi:10.1111/j.1743-6109.2009.01458.x

28. Rubin RR, Wadden TA, Bahnson JL, et al. Impact of intensive lifestyle intervention on depression and health-related quality of life in type 2 diabetes: the Look AHEAD Trial. *Diabetes Care.* 2014;37(6):1544–1553. doi:10.2337/dc13-1928

29. Norris SL, McNally TK, Zhang X, et al. Published norms underestimate the health-related quality of life among persons with type 2 diabetes. *J Clin Epidemiol.* 2011;64 (4):358–365. doi:10.1016/j.jclinepi.2010.04.016

30. Look AHEAD Research Group. Effects of a long-term lifestyle modification programme on peripheral neuropathy in overweight or obese adults with type 2 diabetes: the Look AHEAD study. *Diabetologia.* 2017 Jun;60(6):980–988. doi: 10.1007/s00125-017-4253-z.

31. Foster GD, Borradaile KE, Sanders MH, et al. A randomized study on the effect of weight loss on obstructive sleep apnea among obese patients with type 2 diabetes: the Sleep AHEAD study. *Arch Intern Med.* 2009;169(17):1619–1626. doi:10.1001/archinternmed.2009.266

32. Breyer BN, Phelan S, Hogan PE, et al. Intensive lifestyle intervention reduces urinary incontinence in overweight/obese men with type 2 diabetes: results from the Look AHEAD trial. *J Urol.* 2014;192(1):144–149. doi:10.1016/j.juro.2014.02.036

33. Lazo M, Solga SF, Horska A, et al. Effect of a 12-month intensive lifestyle intervention on hepatic steatosis in adults with type 2 diabetes. *Diabetes Care.* 2010;33(10):2156–2163. doi:10.2337/dc10-0856

34. Cusi K, Isaacs S, Barb D, et al. American Association of Clinical Endocrinology clinical practice guideline for the diagnosis and management of nonalcoholic fatty liver disease in primary care and endocrinology clinical settings: co-sponsored by the American Association for the Study of Liver Diseases (AASLD). *Endocr Pract.* 2022 May;28(5):528–562. doi: 10.1016/j.eprac.2022.03.010

35. Richey PA, Johnson KC, Neiberg RH, et al. Association of the intensive lifestyle intervention with total knee replacement in the look AHEAD (Action for Health in Diabetes) clinical trial. *J Arthroplasty.* 2020;35(6):1576–1582. doi:10.1016/j.arth.2020.01.057

36. Gregg EW, Lin J, Bardenheier B, et al. Impact of intensive lifestyle intervention on disability-free life expectancy: the Look AHEAD Study. *Diabetes Care.* 2018;41(5):1040–1048. doi:10.2337/dc17-2110

37. Espeland MA, Glick HA, Bertoni A, et al. Impact of an intensive lifestyle intervention on use and cost of medical services among overweight and obese adults with type 2 diabetes: the action for health in diabetes. *Diabetes Care.* 2014;37(9):2548–2556. doi:10.2337/dc14-0093

38. EUROASPIRE. A European Society of Cardiology survey of secondary prevention of coronary heart disease: principal results. EUROASPIRE Study Group. European Action on Secondary Prevention through Intervention to Reduce Events. *Eur Heart J.* 1997;18(10):1569–1582. doi:10.1093/oxfordjournals.eurheartj.a015136

39. EUROASPIRE. Euro Heart Survey Programme. Life style and risk factor management and use of drug therapies in coronary patients from 15 countries; principal results from EUROASPIRE II Euro Heart Survey Programme. *Eur Heart J.* 2001;22(7):554–572. doi:10.1053/euhj.2001.2610

40. Kotseva K, Wood D, Backer GD, Bacquer DD, Pyörälä K, Keil U. EUROASPIRE III: a survey on the lifestyle, risk factors and use of cardioprotective drug therapies in coronary patients from 22 European countries. *Eur J Cardiovasc Prev Rehabil.* 2009;16 (2):121–137. doi:10.1097/HJR.0b013e3283294b1d

41. American Diabetes Association. 5. Lifestyle management: standards of medical care in diabetes-2019. *Diabetes Care.* 2019;42(Suppl 1):S46–S60. doi:10.2337/dc19-S005

42. Bowen ME, Cavanaugh KL, Wolff K, et al. The diabetes nutrition education study randomized controlled trial: a comparative effectiveness study of approaches to nutrition in diabetes self-management education. *Patient Educ Couns.* 2016;99(8):1368–1376. doi:10.1016/j.pec.2016.03.017

43. Dinu M, Abbate R, Gensini GF, Casini A, Sofi F. Vegetarian, vegan diets and multiple health outcomes: a SYSTEMATIC review with meta-analysis of observational studies. *Crit Rev Food Sci Nutr.* 2017;57(17):3640–3649. doi:10.1080/10408398.2016.1138447

44. Aune D, Norat T, Romundstad P, Vatten LJ. Whole grain and refined grain consumption and the risk of type 2 diabetes: a systematic review and dose-response meta-analysis of cohort studies. *Eur J Epidemiol.* 2013;28(11):845–858. doi:10.1007/s10654-013-9852-5

45. Pan A, Sun Q, Bernstein AM, et al. Red meat consumption and risk of type 2 diabetes: 3 cohorts of US adults and an updated meta-analysis. *Am J Clin Nutr.* 2011;94(4):1088–1096. doi:10.3945/ajcn.111.018978

46. Tucker LA, LeCheminant JD, Bailey BW. Meat intake and insulin resistance in women without type 2 diabetes. *J Diabetes Res.* 2015;2015:174742. doi:10.1155/2015/174742

47. Barnard N, Levin S, Trapp C. Meat consumption as a risk factor for type 2 diabetes. *Nutrients.* 2014;6(2):897–910. doi:10.3390/nu6020897

48. Ley SH, Hamdy O, Mohan V, Hu FB. Prevention and management of type 2 diabetes: dietary components and nutritional strategies. *Lancet.* 2014;383(9933):1999–2007. doi:10.1016/S0140-6736(14)60613-9

49. Forouhi NG, Wareham NJ. The EPIC-InterAct study: a study of the interplay between genetic and lifestyle behavioral factors on the risk of type 2 diabetes in European populations. *Curr Nutr Rep.* 2014;3(4):355–363. doi:10.1007/s13668-014-0098-y

50. Fretts AM, Follis JL, Nettleton JA, et al. Consumption of meat is associated with higher fasting glucose and insulin concentrations regardless of glucose and insulin genetic risk scores: a meta-analysis of 50,345 Caucasians. *Am J Clin Nutr.* 2015;102(5):1266–1278. doi:10.3945/ajcn.114.101238

51. Feskens EJ, Sluik D, van Woudenbergh GJ. Meat consumption, diabetes, and its complications. *Curr Diab Rep.* 2013;13(2):298–306. doi:10.1007/s11892-013-0365-0

52. Rinaldi S, Campbell EE, Fournier J, O'Connor C, Madill J. A comprehensive review of the literature supporting recommendations from the Canadian Diabetes Association for the use of a plant-based diet for management of type 2 diabetes. *Can J Diabetes.* 2016;40(5):471–477. doi:10.1016/j.jcjd.2016.02.011

53. Tonstad S, Butler T, Yan R, Fraser GE. Type of vegetarian diet, body weight, and prevalence of type 2 diabetes. *Diabetes Care.* 2009;32(5):791–796. doi:10.2337/dc08-1886

54. InterAct Consortium. Dietary fibre and incidence of type 2 diabetes in eight European countries: the EPIC-InterAct study and a meta-analysis of prospective studies. *Diabetologia.* 2015;58(7):1394–1408. doi:10.1007/s00125-015-3585-9

55. Vang A, Singh PN, Lee JW, Haddad EH, Brinegar CH. Meats, processed meats, obesity, weight gain and occurrence of diabetes among adults: findings from Adventist Health Studies. *Ann Nutr Metab.* 2008;52(2):96–104. doi:10.1159/000121365

56. Nicholson AS, Sklar M, Barnard ND, Gore S, Sullivan R, Browning S. Toward improved management of NIDDM: a randomized, controlled, pilot intervention using a lowfat, vegetarian diet. *Prev Med.* 1999;29(2):87–91. doi:10.1006/pmed.1999.0529

57. Estruch R, Ros E, Salas-Salvadó J, et al. Primary prevention of cardiovascular disease with a mediterranean diet supplemented with extra-virgin olive oil or nuts. *N Engl J Med.* 2018;378(25):e34. doi:10.1056/NEJMoa1800389

58. Ornish D, Scherwitz LW, Billings JH, et al. Intensive lifestyle changes for reversal of coronary heart disease. *JAMA.* 1998;280(23):2001–2007. doi:10.1001/jama.280.23.2001

8 Tertiary Prevention Using Lifestyle Medicine for Cardiometabolic-Based Chronic Disease

Dushyanthy Arasaratnam and Michael A. Via
Icahn School of Medicine at Mount Sinai

Jeffrey I. Mechanick
Kravis Center for Cardiovascular Health at Mount Sinai Heart
Icahn School of Medicine at Mount Sinai

CONTENTS

DOI: 10.1201/9781003206637-8

8.1   INTRODUCTION

Tertiary prevention is implemented in symptomatic patients with advanced disease to reduce the severity of the disease burden by mitigating the progression of disease-related complications, preventing or at least managing suffering and impairments on quality of life, lowering the risk for mortality, and improving overall clinical outcomes. Specifically, the primary target for tertiary prevention depends on the clinical phenotype in terms of organ system impairment or complications (e.g., cardiovascular disease [CVD] with chest pain, diabetic neuropathy with pain in the feet, and hypertension with headache). For context, secondary prevention reduces the progression of early, asymptomatic disease to later symptomatic disease due to complications (1). The primary target for secondary prevention is control, "reversal," and even "remission" of drivers of chronic disease, so in the case of type 2 diabetes (T2D) and CVD, this would correspond to mitigating insulin resistance and β-cell defects (leading to hyperglycemia), which impel development of macro- and micro-vascular diabetes complications, respectively. It is important to note that the same intervention (e.g., healthy nutrition or physical activity) can have both secondary and tertiary prevention effects, depending on the particular clinical status of the patient at a given time. For instance, following a cardiac event, both healthy nutrition and judicious, supervised physical activity can improve quality of life, healing, and symptoms (tertiary prevention), while also mitigating the underlying metabolic drivers that could incite a subsequent event or new cardiometabolic complication (secondary prevention).

From a teleological perspective, tertiary prevention, which historically and even currently commands the overwhelming bulk of healthcare efforts across the world, is an uphill battle since it requires some element of mitigation of tenacious pathophysiological events, decades in the making with strong, complicated, and networked underpinnings. Therefore, tertiary prevention can be costly, risky, and mostly unsuccessful. This tenet is the principal incentive to relying on driver-based chronic disease models (e.g., adiposity-based chronic disease [ABCD], dysglycemia-based chronic disease [DBCD], and cardiometabolic-based chronic disease [CMBCD]) to guide early interventions that pose less cost, risk, and chance of failure (i.e., primordial, primary, and secondary prevention strategies). In each of these models, stage 1 is "risk" (managed with primordial prevention), stage 2 is "predisease" (managed with primary prevention), stage 3 is "disease" (managed with secondary prevention), and stage 4 is "complications" (managed with tertiary prevention).

Lifestyle medicine is a necessary component of preventive care medicine and, due to the high prevalence of later CMBCD stages in the population, must be implemented as early as possible for a sustainable and successful effect. No doubt that, by the time complications set in, pharmacological and procedural therapies become vital, but this does not obviate the need for ongoing preventive care to avert further disease burden. To this end, healthcare professionals should routinely identify champions for each patient's care in the tertiary prevention setting, organize and form efficient teams for multi-disciplinary approaches, leverage technology (e.g., wearables) for nudges and sustainability, adapt to the ways of life for different ethnocultural populations, and lastly, devise protocols to ensure success. This chapter will be organized by CMBCD and DBCD complications, and their respective context and lifestyle interventions, to best illustrate how tertiary prevention can be implemented (Table 8.1).

8.2   COMPLICATION 1: CARDIOVASCULAR DISEASE

In the CMBCD model, ABCD and DBCD stage 4 correspond to adiposity- and dysglycemia-related complications, of which CVD is the most impactful in terms of morbidity and mortality (2,3). The three main types of CVD with metabolic drivers are atherosclerosis, HF, and atrial fibrillation. For each of these CVD types, relevant and predominant metabolic drivers are identified, and then notwithstanding indicated pharmacological and procedural interventions, targeted lifestyle recommendations are made, endpoints delineated, and resources provided for successful implementation.

8.2.1   ATHEROSCLEROSIS

8.2.1.1   Context

Atherosclerotic CVD, which includes myocardial infarction, cardiac ischemia, and stroke, is the leading cause of death and significant morbidity among patients with T2D (DBCD stage 3) (4), although declines in CVD mortality have been noted recently (5). Patients with insulin resistance (DBCD stage 1) and prediabetes (DBCD stage 2) also demonstrate increased the risk for atherosclerosis (6,7). One meta-analysis demonstrates a 46% increase in the risk for atherosclerotic CVD for every standard deviation increase in insulin resistance as measured by homeostasis model assessment of insulin resistance (8).

With regard to cardiometabolic risk, T2D has been considered a "CVD equivalent" (9). This has been proposed following publication of population studies demonstrating that a patient with T2D exhibits the same risk for a major cardiovascular event as a person without T2D who already had a major cardiovascular event (10,11). Although more recent published data call this association into question and suggest CVD risk may be somewhat overestimated in patients with T2D (12,13), it is clear there is widespread atherosclerotic disease among patients with T2D (14). Indeed, a meta-analysis of 57 studies, representing approximately 4.5 million patients with T2D across the globe, demonstrates a 32% prevalence for clinically apparent CVD

TABLE 8.1

Summary of Lifestyle Modifications in Patients with Cardiometabolic Complications

	Dietary pattern	Physical activity	Behavior
Atherosclerotic disease	Mediterranean dietary pattern (24) Plant-based dietary pattern (27)	150–300 minutes moderate-intensity activity weekly or 70–150 minutes high-intensity activity weekly (31,48)	Tobacco cessation (52)
Heart failure	Mediterranean-style dietary pattern (61,62,64) DASH diet (68,70)	70–90 minutes weekly, as tolerated (92). Overall benefit to regular exercise (91)	Mindfulness-based stress reduction (100,102)
Atrial fibrillation	Calorie restriction (114) Mediterranean-style dietary pattern (117)	Moderate physical activity 2–4 hours per week (121) Consider avoidance of extreme fitness (121)	Abstinence of alcohol consumption (126) Moderate coffee consumption is permissible and possibly beneficial (1–3 cups daily) (128) Psychological stress reduction, possibly through physical activity (129)
Renal Insufficiency	Reduced red meat, normoproteic diet (138) Sodium intake under 2,300 mg/day (151)	Moderate physical activity, 3–5 sessions weekly 45–60 minutes each (160)	No strong evidence for recommendation
End-stage renal disease	Avoidance of malnutrition (145)	Individualized low-intensity activity (162)	No strong evidence for recommendation
Diabetic neuropathy	Alpha lipoic acid (171) or Vitamin B1/B6 supplementation (174, 175)	150–300 minutes moderate-intensity activity weekly or 70–150 minutes high-intensity activity weekly (166)	Mindfulness-based stress reduction (187)
Diabetic retinopathy	Mediterranean dietary pattern (199)	No strong evidence for recommendation	Tobacco cessation (204) Regular dilated eye examinations (203)

Abbreviations: DASH, dietary approaches to stop hypertension.

(8). Subclinical atherosclerosis was demonstrated by coronary calcium scores in 75% of a cohort ($N=2,162$) with T2D (15). Similarly, patients with T2D demonstrate a greater degree of increased carotid artery intima media thickness (CA-IMT) than patients without T2D, suggesting again a high amount of atherosclerotic disease in this population (16). Peripheral atherosclerotic disease is also common, with a reported prevalence of 15%–17% among patients with T2D (17,18). By these observations, studies investigating lifestyle interventions that include patients at any stage of DBCD will include a sizeable portion of patients with subclinical or clinically apparent atherosclerotic disease, depending on specific inclusion criteria. In fact, the observation that atherosclerotic CVD risk remains increased in patients with advanced DBCD or CMBCD, despite optimal medical therapies to treat component risk factors (e.g., blood sugar, blood pressure, serum cholesterol, excess body weight, tobacco, unhealthy eating patterns, and physical inactivity), is referred to as "residual risk," prompting the need for lifestyle medicine as part of comprehensive tertiary prevention (2,3,19).

8.2.1.2 Lifestyle Interventions

8.2.1.2.1 Nutrition

Nutrition is defined as the interaction of diet and metabolism and is a critical component of lifestyle medicine. Although many nutritional studies have focused on individual foods or nutrients, there are theoretical, pragmatic, and evidentiary justifications to direct attention to dietary patterns – the aggregate effect of all nutrients consumed over a specified time period (20). Due to the high prevalence of both subclinical and clinically apparent atherosclerotic disease among patients with prediabetes and T2D, nutritional interventional trials include many patients with macrovascular complications. Overall findings and subset analyses suggest many of the interventions that prove beneficial in CMBCD, and DBCD stages 1, 2, and 3 may also be applied to patients with CMBCD or DBCD stage 4.

8.2.1.2.1.1 Mediterranean Diets The beneficial aspects of the many Mediterranean diets corresponding to specific geographic regions and cultures are believed to derive from antithrombotic, anti-inflammatory, and antioxidant effects, particularly related to polyphenols and olive oil products (21,22). Patients following a Mediterranean dietary pattern demonstrate reductions in blood pressure and endothelial dysfunction (21,23). The Prevención con Dieta Mediterránea (PREDIMED) multicenter trial, conducted in Spain, included participants at high cardiovascular risk (but with no history of CVD) who were randomized in a 1:1:1 fashion to a Mediterranean diet supplemented with extra-virgin olive oil [EVOO]), a Mediterranean diet with mixed nuts, or a low-fat control diet (24). Both Mediterranean diet groups had a lower risk of the primary composite endpoint of myocardial infarction, stroke, or death. The EVOO and mixed nuts groups had hazard ratios (HR) of 0.69 (95% CI 0.53–0.91) and 0.71 (95% CI 0.54–0.95), each compared with the control group (24).

A subset of patients enrolled in the PREDIMED trial were evaluated for CA-IMT. After an average of 2.4 years of follow-up, patients in the control group had an increase in CA-IMT by 0.188 mm (95% CI 0.077–0.299) compared to a decrease in CA-IMT in the mixed nuts group of −0.084 mm (95% CI −0.206–0.023) (25). These findings suggest potential for atherosclerotic plaque regression in patients following a Mediterranean diet. Additionally, markers of plaque inflammation were improved in the Mediterranean diet groups (26). These include a 35%–45% reduction in C-reactive protein (CRP), a 90%–95% reduction in interleukin-6, and a 19%–27% reduction in endothelial P-selectin expression compared to low-fat controls (26). A 34% reduction in monocyte CD40 surface expression was also noted in the mixed nuts group, and a 50% reduction in soluble intracellular adhesion molecule expression was noted in the EVOO group (26). Each of these molecular changes is expected to improve atherosclerotic plaque stability and, together with evidence of plaque regression (25), suggest benefit of a Mediterranean diet among patients with cardiovascular disease.

8.2.1.2.1.2 Plant-Based Diets A plant-based dietary pattern (vegetarian [allowing for limited amounts of animal products] or vegan [not allowing animal products]) reduces/eliminates the intake of dietary cholesterol and has beneficial effects on systemic inflammation, gastrointestinal microflora, and improvement in cardiovascular risk factors, including hypertension, central adipose distribution, and atherosclerotic plaque stability (27). In a sense, plant-based dietary patterns are similar to Mediterranean diets, in that they are rich in vegetables, fruits, whole grains, legumes, and nuts, with an obvious reduction of animal protein and fats depending on the specific level of dietary restriction. Clinical trials demonstrate that a plant-based dietary pattern results in greater weight loss by approximately 5 kg than a low-fat, calorie-restricted diet (28,29). A 14 mg/dL reduction in total cholesterol, a 13 mg/dL reduction in low-density lipoprotein cholesterol, a reduction in systolic blood pressure by 4.8 mm Hg, and a reduction in diastolic blood pressure by 2.2 mm Hg are observed in patients following plant-based diets compared to simple calorie restriction diets (28,29). Moreover, a *post hoc* analysis of the PREDIMED trial stratified patients enrolled in the Mediterranean diet groups according to quintile of meat intake. The findings demonstrate a 42% (95% CI 20–67) reduction in all-cause mortality in the lowest meat intake quintile compared to the highest quintile (30).

8.2.1.2.1.3 Calorie Restriction A restriction in calorie intake has been the traditional recommendation for weight loss and reduced risk of CVD (31). In primary prevention trials, calorie restriction appears to improve cardiac risk factors, although sustainability over the long term is questionable, and trials with cardiovascular events as endpoints have not been published (32,33).

The Action for Health in Diabetes (Look AHEAD) trial enrolled patients with T2D and a body mass index of 25 kg/m² and compared usual care to an intensive lifestyle intervention that included calorie restriction and 175 minutes of moderate physical activity weekly (34). Among approximately 14% of the enrolled patients who had known atherosclerotic disease at baseline, there was no benefit and even a trend toward an increase in the number of cardiovascular events with this intensive lifestyle intervention over a median 9.6 year follow-up (34). Other small trials (<100 participants) with known atherosclerotic disease have suggested a reduction in cardiometabolic risk factors through caloric restriction; however, these studies are underpowered and have insufficient follow-up to demonstrate reduction in cardiovascular events (35–37).

8.2.1.2.2   Physical Activity

Both engagement in regular physical activity and a patient's overall fitness present as means for significant improvement in cardiometabolic risk, including among patients with known atherosclerotic disease (38,39). Studies consistently demonstrate cardiometabolic improvement with physical activity (40–43). In a 1-year trial, reductions in central adiposity (7.6 kg weight loss; 6.6 cm waist circumference reduction) and CRP by 35% were observed following an intervention of 48 minutes of aerobic exercise performed three times weekly in 73 patients with CVD (40). A meta-analysis of nine small trials, totaling 206 patients with coronary artery disease (CAD), suggested that physical activity with aerobic exercise improves fitness and is well tolerated. The Stabilization of Atherosclerotic Plaque by Initiation of Darapladib (STABILITY) trial included 15,486 patients in 39 countries with stable CVD (43). The initial intent of this trial was to investigate the use of darapladib treatment in patients with CVD; however, as an offshoot of the original study, enrolled patients were evaluated for physical activity by questionnaire at baseline and followed for 3.8 years (43). Compared to the least active tertile (14 ± 12 metabolic equivalent of task [MET] hour/week), the intermediate active (40 ± 14 MET hour/week) and most active (90 ± 52 MET hour/week) patients had reductions in all-cause mortality by 25% and 30%, as well as cardiovascular mortality by 11% and 29%, respectively (43). In addition, the most active patients had a reduction in cardiovascular events by 19% (43).

The beneficial effects of physical activity after development of CVD are also observed among patients older than 65 years, as well as in patients who commenced exercise late in life (44,45). By contrast, a sedentary lifestyle appears to yield excess risk, in addition to simply foregoing the cardiometabolic benefits of exercise (44,46). Physical inactivity in adults, defined as less than 150 minutes of moderate physical activity weekly, is the hallmark of a sedentary lifestyle pattern and has been identified as the fourth leading cause of death worldwide (47). On this basis, 150–300 minutes of moderate physical activity or 70–150 minutes of vigorous activity weekly are recommended for patients with atherosclerotic disease, which represents approximately 7.5–30 MET hour/week (31). Efforts to minimize sedentary activity are also recommended (48).

8.2.1.2.3   Behavior

Outside of dietary choice and physical activity, behavioral changes, especially smoking cessation, are recommended to reduce cardiovascular risk in patients with known atherosclerotic disease (31). Studies on patients with CAD who quit smoking demonstrate an approximate 50% reduction in the risk of major cardiovascular events and a 40%–50% reduction in overall mortality compared to those who continue to smoke (49–51). These reductions are observed relatively quickly, within 2–3 years of cessation (49,51).

One potentially detrimental and commonly observed cardiometabolic effect following smoking cessation is weight gain. In a review of the Nurses' Health Study, patients who quit smoking gained an average of 2.74 kg in the first 2 years, 1.32 kg by 4 years, and 0.98 kg by 6 years on average, with 10% gaining 18 kg or more (52). A temporary increase in the risk for incident T2D was observed among patients who gained any weight (15% increased risk for a gain up to 5 kg; 36% for 5–10 kg; and 59% for >10 kg), compared to those with no weight gain (52). This risk for T2D peaked at 5–7 years after quitting and diminished afterward (52). Still, an approximate 60% reduction in risk of cardiovascular mortality and an approximate 50% reduction in overall mortality were observed after smoking cessation, regardless of weight gain (53). Among patients who quit smoking, a concomitant increase in physical activity was associated with reduced weight gain. For every 10-MET hour/week increase in activity, a reduction of 0.13 kg in weight gained was observed after quitting smoking (52). Based on this finding, the authors recommended a comprehensive lifestyle approach with dietary changes and regular exercise to mitigate the phenomenon of weight gain after tobacco cessation (52).

8.2.2   HEART FAILURE

8.2.2.1   Context

Heart failure has been reported to affect 2%–3% of people in the United States (54). Heart failure is primarily a disease of the older population, with prevalence rates increasing by age such that by 80 years of age or older, almost 12% of men and women have HF (3). The 5-year mortality rate from HF is as high as 50% after an HF hospitalization (54). Heart failure is classified in terms of the ejection fraction (EF): preserved (HFpEF; EF ≥ 50%), mid-range (HFmrEF; EF 40%–49%), and reduced (HFrEF; EF < 40%) (53). Practically speaking, available lifestyle management strategies that define tertiary prevention in HF focus on symptomatic relief and lowering the risk for mortality, as opposed to secondary prevention of detriment from metabolic drivers that can advance disease from early, asymptomatic forms.

8.2.2.2   Lifestyle Interventions

8.2.2.2.1   Nutrition

Traditionally, dietary advice for patients with HF has focused on individual nutrients. In particular, sodium has been extensively studied with consensus recommendations widely implemented. However, there is mounting evidence that dietary patterns may also contribute to the prevention and treatment of HF. It is important to note that a majority of these studies have evaluated the effects of nutrition therapy on HFrEF and therefore may not be applicable to those with HFmrEF or HFpEF (55).

Two popular nutritional therapies for HF include the Mediterranean and the dietary approach to stop hypertension (DASH) dietary patterns (56). These dietary patterns share a common approach – to promote fruits, vegetables, whole grains, and legumes, while limiting saturated fatty acids. The DASH diet emphasizes increased potassium intake, with decreased total fat and sodium (56). The DASH diet is also moderately high in protein and low in fat dairy (57). By contrast, Mediterranean diets emphasize greater intake of mono- and polyunsaturated fats, such as those found in oily fish, olive oil, canola oil, and nuts, as well as foods typically consumed by those living in Mediterranean regions, especially olive products and other polyphenol-rich plants (nuts, grapes/wine, pulses, grains, fruits/vegetables, etc.) (56).

8.2.2.2.1.1   Mediterranean Diets   Two large Swedish observational studies with over 30,000 participants and a median 10-year follow-up demonstrated a reduction in the HF incidence in both men (relative risk [RR] 0.69 [95% CI 0.57–0.83]) and women (RR 0.79 [95% CI 0.68–0.93]) with strict adherence to a Mediterranean diet (58,59). A mortality benefit for HF was also seen in men (RR 0.55 [95% CI 0.31, 0.98]) with HF adhering to this dietary pattern (58).

A large German cohort study of over 24,000 subjects was unable to demonstrate a significant reduction in the HF incidence in patients with high adherence to a Mediterranean diet, except when milk products were excluded (60). Interestingly, the authors also found that low meat, moderate alcohol, and high fish intakes were inversely associated with HF risk, suggesting that primary prevention of HF could be achieved with simple dietary changes (60).

In the PREDIMED trial, despite demonstrating benefit for major cardiovascular events in the groups assigned to a Mediterranean diet, there was no significant difference in HF incidence compared to controls over 4.8 years (61). This observation may be attributable to a low overall incidence of HF events in the study, or possibly the early termination of the trial, which was initially planned for 6 years (61). Specifically, out of a total 7,403 participants without HF, there were 29 new cases of HF from the EVOO group, 22 in the mixed nuts group, and 32 in the control group. These relatively small numbers likely reflect the study being underpowered (61). Interestingly, in a subset of participants tested for N-terminal pro-brain natriuretic peptide (NT-proBNP, an HF biomarker), there were significantly reduced levels in both the EVOO and mixed nuts groups, compared to the control diet, after a 1-year follow-up (62).

In a cross-sectional study of a healthy, multi-ethnic population, food questionnaires were used to calculate Mediterranean diet scores and then correlate them with cardiac MRI findings (63). A higher score was found to be associated with higher LV mass and volume, EF, and stroke volume, ultimately equating to a modest improvement in the LV structure and function (63).

Chryssohoou et al. (21) examined subjects with acute coronary syndrome and found that a Mediterranean diet was associated with a lower risk of developing LV systolic dysfunction, less likelihood of remodeling, and less likelihood of recurrent cardiovascular events at 2-year follow-up. Unlike the studies described previously which explored the value of a Mediterranean diet in subjects without HF, some subjects in this cohort did have pre-existing LV systolic dysfunction. In addition, a prospective study of patients admitted with acute HF with a mean follow-up of 2.1 years found that patients adherent to the Mediterranean diet had a significant reduction in rehospitalization from HF (HR: 0.74, 95% CI 0.61–0.90) compared with those who were not adherent (64). However, there was no significant difference in those who were adherent vs. not adherent in terms of mortality (64).

8.2.2.2.1.2   The DASH Diet   As most of the dietary recommendations for patients with HF are largely based on data from populations without HF, Levitan et al. (57) sought to explore the impact of Mediterranean and DASH diet scores on mortality among post-menopausal women from the Women's Health Initiative after hospitalization for HF. These diet scores were calculated from food frequency questionnaires. Participants were followed up for a median of 4.6 years, during which 43.1% of participants died. The highest quartile of adherence of a Mediterranean diet was associated with a non-significant trend toward reduction in death from HF (HR 0.85 [95% CI 0.70–1.02]), while adherence to the highest quartile of adherence of the DASH diet was associated with a significantly lower risk of death from HF (HR 0.84 [95% CI 0.70–1.00]).

The DASH diet, as the name suggests, was originally devised and validated for use in the management of hypertension, a frequent comorbidity in patients with HF. In a 21-day pilot study of 13 subjects with HFpEF, the DASH diet combined with sodium restriction resulted in improved time on the 6-minute walk test (6MWT), reduced clinic blood pressure measurements, and reduced 24 hours blood pressure measurements compared to baseline (65). Similarly, improvements in the 6MWT and quality of life were seen in 48 subjects with chronic, symptomatic HF who undertook 3 months of the DASH diet, despite no difference in sodium intake between the groups (66). Interestingly, in patients following the DASH dietary pattern, a greater blood pressure lowering effect for the same level of salt reduction was seen in those who already had a dietary intake of sodium at the recommended level (less than 2.3 g of sodium or 5.8 g of sodium chloride daily) (67).

There has also been increasing interest in the use of the DASH diet to prevent as well as to treat HF. Increasing DASH scores have been shown to have a linear relationship with the development of HF over a 7-year follow-up in >35,000 Swedish women (68). For women in the highest quartile of the DASH diet score, they had a 37% lower risk of HF than the lowest quartile (HR 0.63 [95% CI 0.48–0.81]) (68). Similar findings were made in a cohort study of close to 39,000 Swedish male participants who were followed up for 9 years, where men in the top quartile of adherence to the DASH diet demonstrated a significant reduction in risk for HF (HR 0.78 [95% CI 0.65–0.95]) (69). A recent sub-analysis of the Reasons for Geographic and Racial Differences in Stroke (REGARDS) cohort, evaluating over 18,000 participants, also supported the finding that DASH diet adherence was inversely associated with the incidence of HF (70). One study was published that does not support use of the DASH diet, showing no significant effects on the development of HF over a 21.5-year follow-up among almost 5,000 male and female subjects (71). However, this particular trial only administered food frequency questionnaires at baseline and 5 years, making interpretation of adherence to the DASH diet questionable (71).

8.2.2.2.1.3 Sodium Restriction   The correlation between increased salt intake and elevated blood pressure is clear and in large part based on studies that demonstrate benefits of the DASH diet (67,72). However, the evaluation of dietary sodium intake in patients with HF yields conflicting results, specifically with limited clinical evidence to suggest it is beneficial (56). There has been no consensus on the optimal level of sodium intake among patients with HF with published recommendations varying from <1,500 mg/day to <3,000 mg/day (56,73–75). Most guidelines cite expert opinion and level C evidence when referring to sodium intake and HF management (73–75). Nevertheless, sodium restriction remains one of the most commonly used lifestyles and nutritional strategies for patients with HF.

Increased activation of the renin–angiotensin–aldosterone system (RAAS) due to renal hypoperfusion, with a concurrent increase in vasopressin levels, increases sodium and fluid retention in HF (76). Sodium restriction is believed to confer benefit through reduced fluid retention; however, it has been argued that sodium restriction actually activates the RAAS system, thereby worsening fluid retention (56). Another important consideration in any form of restrictive diet is the potential to inadvertently restrict caloric and/or macro- or micronutrient intake. In a series of 216 patients with HF who recorded dietary intake over a 4-day period, approximately half (107) had insufficient water-soluble vitamin intake (77). Those with vitamin deficiencies had lower quality of life scores and increased cardiac mortality (HR 1.3 [1.025–1.640]) (77).

Arcand et al. (78) found that in a cohort of patients with HF, consisting primarily of patients with New York Heart Association (NYHA), classes I and II, an intake of ≥2,800 mg/day of sodium resulted in a 25% increase in acute decompensated HF events and increased risk for all-cause hospitalization and mortality. An intake of ≥3,800 mg of sodium daily was associated with an approximate four-fold increase in HF decompensation, hospitalization, and HF-related mortality. This suggests that intake below a threshold of approximately 2,800 mg daily could help prevent these adverse events. However, in a separate cohort study, Lennie et al. (79) found that there was a significant increase in hospital visits, readmissions, and mortality in NYHA class I and II patients who consumed <3,000 mg/day of sodium, while those with NYHA class III and IV HF who consumed <3,000 mg/day sodium had better outcomes. Adverse events, including HF and non-HF readmissions, and mortality rates were higher with low-sodium diets in some studies (80,81). The challenge in comparing studies evaluating the impact of sodium intake on HF derives from variances in protocols, fluid restriction, method of assessing the dietary sodium content, and the degree of adherence to dietary sodium restriction (82). Another confounding factor is that those who adhere to reduced sodium intake often have a poor nutritional status due to reduced calorie intake (76)

8.2.2.2.1.4 Dietary Supplements Patients requiring treatment for HF, particularly those on diuretics, may develop vitamin and micronutrient deficiencies. This is multifactorial, due to decreased dietary intake, altered absorption, and adverse effects of pharmacological therapies, such as diuretics, as well as increased requirements due to oxidative stress and myocardial dysfunction (55). Dietary supplements such as coenzyme Q10, carnitine, taurine, and antioxidants have been proposed for the treatment of HF (74). However, there has been no documentation of improved survival with replacement of these nutrients. There is heterogeneity in the data supporting reduced hospitalizations, dyspnea, and edema in patients receiving coenzyme Q10 (74).

Positive cardiac remodeling, with reduced LV end-diastolic and end-systolic volumes and improved LVEF, was seen in a double-blind, randomized controlled trial of micronutrient supplementation, including calcium, magnesium, zinc, copper, selenium, B-vitamins, vitamins A, C, D, and E, as well as coenzyme Q10 versus placebo in 32 older adults with HFrEF (55). No changes in inflammatory markers or 6MWT were seen. Exercise therapy was not utilized in these patients (55). This suggests there may be a role for micronutrient supplementation. However, the small size of the study and the potential for confounders given the broad range of micronutrients supplemented make it difficult to derive conclusions based on this study alone. Thiamine has similarly been shown to improve LVEF and may provide symptomatic improvements in patients with HFrEF (55). Additionally, as a water-soluble vitamin, thiamine is cleared renally and diuretic use, including osmotic, thiazide, and loop diuretic therapy, has been demonstrated to increase urinary thiamine losses in a dose-dependent fashion (83). Still, higher quality studies are required to corroborate routine supplementation of thiamine in patients with HF (55).

Gotsman et al. (84) reported a high prevalence of vitamin D deficiency in patients with HF and found this deficiency state to also be an independent predictor of increased mortality in this group. Vitamin D deficiency has also been associated with increased risk of hospitalizations and poor outcomes (85). Of note, lifestyle factors may explain these inverse associations with vitamin D deficiency, merely representing an incidental finding. It is also unclear whether vitamin D supplementation, as an adjunct to standard care, provides any true benefit, despite these inverse associations. A recent literature review did not find that there was strong evidence supporting daily, high-dose vitamin D supplementation weekly or monthly in reducing hospitalizations or mortality in patients with CHF (85). Limitations to interpreting these findings included small sample size and duration of short follow-up, with most trials having less than a follow-up of 1 year. Longer term studies are required to explore the potential benefits of vitamin D replacement in HF. Overall, the potential for drug interactions and adverse effects needs to be weighed against the potential benefit of any nutritional supplement. To date, the data do not support their use in HF, unless a true deficiency state is demonstrated (74,86).

8.2.2.2.2 Physical Activity

Exercise-based cardiac rehabilitation programs for patient with CVD have been shown to reduce deaths from heart disease by 31% (87). Training in patients with cardiac dysfunction has been shown to result in increases in exercise duration and improved functional class (88,89). Sullivan et al. (90) were among the first to demonstrate that a significant improvement in central hemodynamic adaptations could be achieved with a program of exercise conditioning in patients with chronic HF. A 2004 meta-analysis concluded that exercise training was not harmful for patients with HF and could reduce mortality (91). In a multicenter, randomized controlled trial of over 2,300 participants with HFrEF, exercise training did not result in significant reductions in the primary endpoint of all-cause mortality or hospitalizations (92). However, after adjustment for highly prognostic baseline characteristics predictive of the primary outcome, exercise training for a median of 95 minutes per week was associated with a significant, although modest, reduction in both all-cause mortality or hospitalization, as well as cardiovascular mortality or HF hospitalization (92). In this trial, activity time in the exercise group decreased to a median of 74 minutes per week by month 10.

Peak oxygen consumption (VO_2) is considered the gold standard in assessing prognosis in HF (93). There are numerous trials examining the benefit of exercise training in patients with HF that have demonstrated improvements in peak VO_2. Changes in peak VO_2 have ranged from 12% to 31%, depending on the setting, type of activity, duration, and intensity (94). A systematic review evaluating exercise training in 228 patients with HFpEF found that training enhanced exercise capacity and health-related quality of life (95).

In advanced cases, the use of a left ventricular assist device (LVAD) improves exercise tolerance, an effect that is maximally seen at 12 weeks post-implantation and can continue even after explantation of the device (96). Exercise training in patients with a LVAD has been demonstrated to improve VO_2 (97). The use of cardiac rehabilitation programs for patients with LVAD devices has been shown to result in statistically and clinically significant improvements in exercise capacity and quality of life (98,99).

8.2.2.2.3 Behavior

Heart failure has been associated with significant psychological distress including anxiety and depression, partially due to changes in the functional level impacting work status and relationships (100). Significant depression is common and related to a higher rate of functional decline (100). Among hospitalized patients with HF, significant depression is associated with a 2.5-fold increase in mortality at 3 months and a three-fold increase in hospital admission at 1 year, independent of age, NYHA class, baseline EF, and ischemic etiology of HF (101).

The Support, Education, and Research in Chronic Heart Failure (SEARCH) trial, a prospective cohort study that examined the effects of an 8-week psychoeducational mindfulness-based intervention (MBI) on depression, anxiety, quality of life, symptoms, and outcomes in patients with HF (100), showed that despite patients in the treatment group having more severe HF (by NYHA class) and more severe psychological distress (Center of Epidemiology – Depression, Profile of Mood States; $p < 0.05$), the intervention reduced anxiety and depression significantly in the first 3 and 6 months post-intervention. Although this effect on depressive symptoms was attenuated at the 12-month visit, the treatment improved symptoms of HF and clinical scores at 12 months compared with controls (100). A systematic review of five studies that examined MBI in adults with HF found that these interventions could significantly reduce depression and anxiety and improve health-related quality of life (102). Physical function was only evaluated in one study, with non-significant changes reported (102).

Stress has been shown to increase hospital readmissions in patients with HF (103). Moreover, among patients with CAD, mental stress is associated with ischemia more frequently in patients with severe LV dysfunction than in those with normal LV function (104). The mechanism of stress-related exacerbation of HF likely relates to increased catecholamines, activation of the RAAS system, decreased threshold for ventricular fibrillation, and increases in blood pressure and heart rate (103). Transcendental meditation, as a means to address these pathophysiological mechanisms, has been shown to prevent progression of increased LV mass (105). In a small study examining the effects of a transcendental meditation stress reduction program in African Americans, both functional capacity (as assessed by a 6MWT) and quality of life significantly improved over a 6-month follow-up period (103).

8.2.3   ATRIAL FIBRILLATION

8.2.3.1   Context

Compared to the general population, patients with T2D are at 35%–60% increased risk for development of atrial fibrillation (AF) (106). In the subset of patients with both T2D and AF, development of HF increased by 68%, cardiovascular mortality increased by 77%, and overall mortality increased by 61% compared to patients with T2D without AF (107). Although the incidence of AF is associated with A1C severity (108), no benefit in AF risk reduction was noted among patients with T2D who underwent intensive glycemic control and improvement in A1C (109). It may be that factors associated with T2D, such as hypertension, hyperlipidemia, and obesity, are responsible for the increased risk of AF (110,111). Mechanisms of atrial remodeling, fibrosis, and left atrial stretch are observed in patients with T2D (112). Pericardial fat accumulation, a form of ectopic fat seen in ABCD, is also observed in patients with T2D and associated with the development of AF (113).

8.2.3.2   Lifestyle Interventions

8.2.3.2.1   Nutrition

Results of the Action for Health in Diabetes (Look AHEAD) trial did not demonstrate a reduction in AF among patients with T2D and either overweight or obesity who underwent an intensive lifestyle intervention (114). Authors attribute this finding to the modest weight loss attained, which was insufficient for a demonstrable benefit (114). By contrast, several other studies that achieved greater degrees of weight loss showed benefit for AF. For example, a 12-kg weight loss through calorie restriction over 1 year among 150 patients with obesity and AF demonstrated an 88% reduction in the AF symptom score, a diminished left atrium area by 46%, and a 0.5-mm reduction in intraventricular septal thickness compared to a control group without dietary intervention (115). Another study investigating weight loss by calorie restriction also demonstrated reduction in the AF symptom score as well as the greatest degree of arrythmia-free survival in the group that lost >10% of body weight (116). Lastly, in the PREDIMED trial, patients who were randomized to a Mediterranean diet with extra-virgin olive oil demonstrated a 38% reduction in risk of AF compared to the control group (117).

8.2.3.2.2   Physical Activity

Clinical guidance for participation in exercise or other forms of physical activity among patients with AF is controversial (118). Although physical activity may reduce many of the cardiometabolic and dysglycemic risks associated with AF, extensive endurance exercise over the long term is associated with an increase in risk for AF development (119). In one study comparing 252 marathon runners to 305 age- and gender-matched sedentary patients who served as controls, a hazard ratio for AF development was found to be 8.8 (95% CI 1.2–61) in the group of marathon runners (120). An observed increase in the left atrial size may explain this finding. Other potential mechanisms include fibrosis and autonomic activation through exercise seen in animal models of chronic intense exercise (118). Other studies investigating the AF incidence among middle-aged elite athletes demonstrate similar findings

(119). However, it is recognized that under 5% of the population meets criteria as non-professional elite athletes (>6 hours intense exercise per week) (118). Additionally, these small trials represent relatively weak evidence for a true increase in risk and may not be generalizable to the majority of the population (118).

A majority of cases of AF are associated with underlying cardiometabolic disease such as T2D, hypertension, dyslipidemia, and CVD. The adverse effects of these metabolic drivers on AF risk are mitigated by regular physical activity, as supported by various clinical studies (118). In one Norwegian study ($N = 20,484$ adults), the association of AF risk with physical activity (assessed by questionnaire) was represented by a J-shaped curve, in which moderately active (2–4 hours per week of moderately vigorous activity such as walking or cycling) individuals had a 19% lower risk for AF than both highly active (>4 hours per week intense training and competition) and inactive persons (mainly sedentary activities such as reading or watching television) (121). In fact, the highly active and inactive groups had similar AF incidence in the study. By contrast, some published studies showed a direct relationship of improvement in AF risk with physical activity (122–124). However, these studies generally had low thresholds for "physically active," and they did not distinguish high-intensity training or elite endurance athletes from moderate physical activity. Accordingly, a moderate approach to physical activity, such as 2–4 hours per week, may be best for prevention of AF (118). Careful monitoring during and after physical activity among patients who already have developed AF is recommended, as well as more clinical studies to define safe and efficacious protocols (125).

8.2.3.2.3 *Behavior*

Several other factors that influence AF risk include alcohol consumption, tobacco use, and obstructive sleep apnea (OSA). Approximately 5%–10% of cases of AF are attributable to alcohol consumption, in a dose-dependent manner (126). Complete abstinence of alcohol is associated with reduced risk of AF incidence, as well as a 58% reduction in AF recurrence among patients with at least one prior episode of AF compared to patients who do not abstain (126). Abstinence from tobacco is also recommended to reduce AF risk (31). The use of continuous airway pressure devices for OSA treatment reduces risk of AF incidence by 42% (127). Of note, coffee consumption is commonly mentioned by healthcare professionals as an inciting factor for AF. However, and somewhat surprising to many, one published cohort study demonstrated that consumption of 1–3 cups of coffee daily is associated with a 15% reduction in incidence of AF in comparison to people who abstain from coffee (128). Psychological stress has also been associated with increased risk for AF, which is decreased by physical activity (129).

8.3 COMPLICATION 2: DIABETIC NEPHROPATHY

8.3.1 Context

Diabetic kidney disease (DKD) is the leading cause of chronic kidney disease and makes up the largest group of patients starting renal replacement therapy (130,131).

Diabetic kidney disease affects up to 50% of patients with type 1 diabetes (T1D) and T2D and is associated with an increased risk of cardiovascular morbidity and mortality (130,131).

Diabetic nephropathy is defined by increased urinary albumin excretion in the absence of other types of renal disease. It can be categorized into stages from micro-albuminuria (≥30 mg/day or 20 µg/minute of urinary albumin excretion [UAE]) to macroalbuminuria (UAE ≥300 mg/24 hour or ≥200 µg/minute) (130,131). This process may eventually lead to a decline in the glomerular filtration rate (GFR), which occurs in association with an increase in blood pressure, ultimately leading to end-stage renal disease (132). For patients who have developed diabetic nephropathy, the goal is to prevent progression of the disease from microalbuminuria to macroalbuminuria and an eventual decline in renal function, as well as reduce the significant associated cardiovascular morbidity and mortality.

Type 2 diabetes itself is a risk factor for high blood pressure, which speeds the progression of DKD and increases the risk of cardiovascular events, including strokes and heart attacks (133). It has been well demonstrated that lowering blood pressure reduces the progression of DKD (132). Long-term follow-up of people with diabetes, but no hypertension or renal disease, demonstrates a blood pressure-dependent decline in the GFR (132). Moreover, subjects with a blood pressure of <130/80 mmHg rarely develop microalbuminuria and show an annual decline in the eGFR close to that of an age-matched normal population. By contrast, patients with T2D and a blood pressure 130/80–140/90 mmHg have a greater decline in the GFR, with 30% developing microalbuminuria or proteinuria over the subsequent 12–15 years (132). In patients with early evidence of diabetic nephropathy, successful treatment of hypertension produces a beneficial effect on albuminuria (132).

8.3.2   Lifestyle Interventions

8.3.2.1   Nutrition

8.3.2.1.1   Low-Protein Diet in Early Diabetic Kidney Disease

The American Diabetes Association guidelines suggest that the total daily dietary protein intake should not exceed 0.8 g/kg/day for people with non-dialysis-dependent DKD (134), although the evidence for this is controversial. The goal of protein restriction is to reduce the progression of CKD while preserving a healthy nutritional status (135). A 2008 meta-analysis was unable to find a significant association between a low-protein diet and change in the GFR or creatinine clearance rate. However, maintaining dietary protein intake at this level did improve albuminuria (136). On the contrary, a dietary protein intake of >1.3g/kg/day or >20% of daily calories from protein has been associated with increased albuminuria, more rapid kidney function loss, and CVD mortality (134,137). Taken together, reducing dietary protein to below 0.8 g/kg/day is not recommended as it does not provide benefits in terms of glycemic measures, cardiovascular measures, or the course of GFR decline (134).

There are alternatives to a low-protein diet. Replacing red meat with chicken in a normoproteic diet for 4 weeks reduced the urinary albumin excretion rate and lipid levels in patients with T2D (138). Furthermore, when comparing a chicken-based diet versus treatment with enalapril, there was a similar reduction in the urine albumin excretion ratio in patients with T2D and microalbuminuria over a 12-month follow-up period (139). It is important to note these two studies were small (only 28 subjects in each) and of limited duration, although the findings endorse the design and use of the food questionnaire methodology (140). In a large, community-based cohort study of middle-aged adults with normal renal function, participants with the highest red meat and processed meat consumption had a higher risk of incident CKD compared with those who had a higher consumption of nuts, legumes, and low-fat dairy products (140).

8.3.2.1.2 Low Protein in Advanced Diabetic Kidney Disease

Klahr et al. (141) assessed the impact of differences in dietary protein intake and blood pressure on the rate of GFR decline in patients with moderate to severe renal impairment. In one trial, patients with moderate renal insufficiency (GFR 25–55 mL/min/1.73 m^2) were randomized to either a usual protein diet (1.3 g/kg/day) or low-protein diet (0.58 g/kg/day), and then further classified into usual- or low-blood pressure groups. Results after 2 years showed no difference in GFR decline in either protein intake or blood pressure groups. Interestingly, at 4 months, the low-protein group and the low-blood pressure group had a more rapid decline in the GFR, followed by a slower decline thereafter, although no overall difference was seen (141).

In a second study, 255 patients with more severe renal impairment (GFR 13–24 mL/min/1.73 m^2) were randomized to a low-protein diet (0.58 g/kg/day) or a very low-protein diet (0.28 g/day/day) group, with incorporation of a keto acid–amino acid supplement and further subgrouping into usual- or low-blood pressure groups (141). In this trial, again no differences were seen, although patients with more severe renal impairment who were placed on a very low-protein exhibited a trend toward a marginally slower decline in the GFR than the low-protein group. In both studies, the low-blood pressure group had more pronounced proteinuria at baseline and had a significantly lower rate of decline in the GFR (141). Based on these results, the role of protein restriction for renal protection in patients with stages 1–4 DKD cannot be recommended (134,137). However, this evidence-based recommendation may not be generalizable to all people since Western diets commonly have greater protein intake than the commonly recommended target of 0.8 mg/kg/day (134,137).

As DKD is a catabolic state, the potential pitfalls of implementing a low-protein diet include increased risk for essential amino acid deficiencies, low energy intake, sarcopenia, and protein wasting. A meta-analysis published in 2022 examined 11 studies in which ketoacid analogs of essential amino acids (KAs) were supplemented along with a low-protein diet or very low-protein diet in adults with DKD. Results suggested that KA use in DKD was favorable for renal, metabolic, and nutritional outcomes (135). Specifically, progression of DKD was attenuated by approximately 10%, urinary protein excretion reduced by an average of 1.4 g/day, fasting glycemia improved by an average of 27 mg/dL, and systolic blood pressure reduced by 10 mm Hg (135). Consideration for alternative protein sources has been proposed for patients with advanced renal disease. While patients with DKD and macroalbuminuria may benefit from a dietary change to soy-based protein sources to improve cardiovascular risk factors, there does not appear to be improvement in proteinuria or renal disease progression (136).

8.3.2.1.3   Malnutrition in End-Stage Renal Disease

In end-stage renal disease, metabolic waste products are not adequately removed, leading to progressive loss of skeletal mass and strength. Protein energy wasting – a form of malnutrition – has been observed in 28%–54% of patients receiving chronic hemodialysis (142). Dietary protein ingestion is essential to allow muscle and lean tissue maintenance. This is important since during hemodialysis, the protein equivalent of a meal is extracted from the circulation. Additionally, through recommendations to limit potassium and phosphate intake in patients with stage 5 chronic kidney disease, 97% of patients do not achieve recommended fiber intake (25 g/day), and patients also have low vitamin C, lycopene, carotenoid, and antioxidant intake (143). In addition to protein and micronutrient malnutrition, the uremic and acidotic environment induces macrophage release of TNFα, further driving systemic inflammation and anorexia secondary to central appetite suppression (144). Taken together, malnutrition, inflammation, and atherosclerosis, known as MIA syndrome, are associated with reduced quality of life and increased mortality among patients with end-stage renal disease (144). Some authors suggest liberalizing dietary intake to prevent MIA syndrome within this group of patients, although scientific debate on this topic continues (145).

The nutritional status of patients at the onset of chronic dialysis therapy is a strong predictor of their nutritional status during the course of dialysis treatment, as well as of their subsequent morbidity and mortality (146). The nutritional status prior to development of end-stage renal disease and establishment of healthy nutrition while on chronic dialysis are therefore very important. Poor dietary protein intake has been associated with protein energy wasting, which, in turn, has been linked to increased mortality in dialysis patients (147).

8.3.2.1.4   Sodium Restriction

Aggressive blood pressure control in patients with diabetes has been shown to reduce progression from normoalbuminuria to microalbuminuria, and microalbuminuria to overt albuminuria, irrespective of the baseline blood pressure or the agent used to achieve that control (148). In proteinuric DKD, there is a progressively greater rate of GFR decline at higher systolic blood pressures (149). A strong correlation has been demonstrated between dietary sodium intake and increased blood pressure in patients with DKD, regardless of whether blood pressure levels are normal or raised at baseline (133). A low-sodium diet can assist with achieving blood pressure control, which is critical in preventing the progression of DKD.

MacGregor et al. (150) demonstrated the impact of variations in sodium intake on blood pressure. They randomized 15 patients with essential hypertension on captopril and a low-sodium diet to either placebo or sodium tablets. The combination treatment of moderate sodium restriction with an angiotensin-converting enzyme inhibitor was effective in decreasing blood pressure in patients with hypertension. However, with the reintroduction of sodium, compared to subjects receiving placebo, those on sodium tablets had a significantly higher mean supine blood pressure (150).

A 2010 Cochrane Review evaluated 13 studies and found that there was a large fall in blood pressure with sodium restriction to less than 5–6 g/day in patients with diabetes, similar to that of single-drug therapy (133). This effect was seen equally in patients with T1D or T2D, and despite this "reduced" level of salt intake that was still well above recommended amounts, patients also had a small reduction in creatinine clearance. There was no change in the GFR or effective renal plasma flow with this intervention. Data were limited on the impact on urinary albumin excretion and proteinuria in this study. The authors did note that a majority of studies reviewed were of short duration and required large changes in dietary salt intake, which may not be sustainable (133). Current guideline recommendations for patients with DKD recommend restriction of dietary sodium to <2,300 mg/day for blood pressure control and cardiovascular risk reduction (151).

8.3.2.2 Physical Activity

Early stages of DKD are characterized by glomerular hyperfiltration, adaptive renal hypertrophy, and microalbuminuria. The hemodynamic and metabolic changes that occur in T2D lead to extracellular matrix accumulation, oxidative stress, renal inflammation, and activation of the RAAS (152). The pathophysiological mechanism by which exercise training exerts renoprotective action in DKD is complex, multifactorial, and not well understood (152). Most available evidence is based on experimental studies and suggest exercise attenuates both metabolic and hemodynamic changes in DKD. Metabolic improvements include increased glucose uptake, reduced generation of reactive oxygen species (ROS), and reduced catabolism, thus attenuating some of the direct damage caused by diabetes effects on the glomerular basement membrane and extracellular matrix (152).

Exercise increases glucose uptake in the skeletal muscle through activation of the adenosine monophosphate-activated protein kinase pathway and increased glucose transporter type 4 (GLUT 4) expression, as well as insulin-mediated actions, together result in reduced formation of advanced glycation end products (153,154). Additionally, there is less ROS formation as a result of reduced renal lipid peroxidation, increased glutathione peroxidase activity, activation of the sirtuin 1-gamma coactivator 1-alpha pathway, and improved mitochondrial function, leading to reduced inflammation (152). Hemodynamic improvements through exercise training result from enhanced cardiac output, reduced renal vasoconstriction, and improved endothelial function, together yielding reduced extracellular matrix protein accumulation, fibrosis, and neovascularization (152).

Despite available pharmacological interventions, the incidence of DKD continues to increase (155). Thus, the potential for regular physical activity to slow the progression of DKD is an important focus of clinical research, especially for those involved in lifestyle medicine (152). Physical activity can acutely increase urinary protein excretion, especially in individuals with T2D or impaired fasting glucose (156). Studies assessing the impact of exercise training on patients with moderate to severe CKD were unable to demonstrate a significant improvement in GFR compared to control subjects (157,158). This may be attributed to animal model observations that the capacity for physical training to augment GFR is dependent upon the amount of functional tissue remaining (159).

Interestingly, aerobic exercise has been shown to reduce proteinuria in patients with CKD, including DKD (152,160,161). Specifically, in a group of patients with moderate renal impairment, twice weekly water-based exercise was shown to reduce proteinuria and serum levels of cystatin-C (161). Regular moderate-intensity aerobic physical activity (3–5 sessions per week of brisk walking lasting 45–60 minutes, targeting a maximum heart rate of 50%–70%) in a group of previously sedentary patients with overweight/obesity and T2D reduced microalbuminuria to less than 30 mg/day in five of six patients over 6 months (160).

In patients with advanced CKD receiving dialysis, resistance training has been shown to improve plasma creatinine levels and markers of inflammation (152). N-acetyl-β-D-glucosaminidase activity, a marker of tubular damage and metabolic control in T2D, also normalized with regular activity (160). This supports the hypothesis that regular moderate-intensity activity may be beneficial in slowing down the expected increment in N-acetyl-β-D-glucosaminidase in patients with T2D and reduced GFR (160). A randomized trial of 296 patients with CKD receiving dialysis assigned to a home-based low-intensity exercise program or usual care demonstrated significant improvement in 6-minute walking distance, reduced time from sitting to standing, and improved quality of life score (162). In the subgroup of patients who successfully completed the 6-month trial, those randomized to the physical activity program had a 39% ($p = 0.037$) reduction in the hospitalization rate (162).

8.3.2.3 Behavior

A meta-analysis of eight randomized control trials found that MBI had a small impact on depression, anxiety, and psychological distress in people with chronic disease (163). A 5-year prospective randomized clinical trial assessed the impact of MBI in patients with T2D and early DKD. In the first year, there was a reduction in urinary albumin-to-creatinine ratio (ACR) in the intervention arm in contrast to the control arm, where there was a rise in the ACR. However, this effect was not seen in the second or third year of the study. The initial difference in the urine ACR seen in the first year suggests it is possible that psychosocial interventions may have a role to play in early DKD, although further work is necessary to evaluate efficacy (164). Among patients receiving dialysis, MBI is effective in reducing physical and anxiety symptoms, depression symptoms, sleep disorders, and social dysfunction (165). Improvement in each of these factors can improve quality of life for this group of patients, although effects on cardiometabolic risk are unclear.

8.4   COMPLICATION 3: DIABETIC NEUROPATHY

8.4.1   Context

Diabetic neuropathy (DN) is a significant cause of diabetes-related morbidity, affecting over half of all patients with T1D or T2D (166,167). Diabetic neuropathy has a major impact on quality of life, causing pain, gait instability, and loss of protective sensation, leading to foot ulcers and amputation (166). The impact of intensive lifestyle intervention (ILI), with a focus on weight loss through caloric restriction and physical activity, on the progression/development of DN was examined in the Look AHEAD trial (168). The study found that in people with overweight/obesity and T2D, ILI resulted in a significant reduction in questionnaire-based DN, despite no changes in physical measures of DN, except light touch (168).

8.4.2   Lifestyle Interventions

8.4.2.1   Nutrition

Translational research suggests that high-fat diets can result in neuropathy in diabetes, and withdrawal of the high-fat diet can, in turn, reduce neuropathy (166). In patients with T2D either without symptoms of DN or with symptoms for <5 years, hypertriglyceridemia was found to be an independent risk factor for development of early DN (169). However, a nutritional intervention study found that following supplementation with omega-3 polyunsaturated fatty acids, which lowers triglyceride levels, subjects with T1D did not have an improvement in nerve conduction studies or sensory function, although there was no progression of clinical disease symptoms and no decline in small and large fiber sensory and functional measures (170).

The role of antioxidants in the treatment of DN is being explored as oxidative stress is believed to be a major contributor to the disease (166). Alpha lipoic acid (ALA), a dietary supplement with antioxidant properties, has been associated with symptomatic benefit. In the ALA in Diabetic Neuropathy (ALADIN) study, infusion of ALA significantly improved symptoms and in the ALADIN II study, long-term (24 months) use was found to improve nerve function (171). The DEKAN study found that in patients with T2D and cardiac autonomic neuropathy, administration of ALA reduced heart rate variability, an indicator of cardiac autonomic neuropathy (172). Over a period of 3 weeks in the SYDNEY trial, ALA was found to improve symptoms such as pain, prickling, and numbness (171). However, in the ALADIN III study, which enrolled 509 patients with diabetic neuropathy, only modest benefit was demonstrated with ALA treatment compared to placebo at 19 days, and this benefit disappeared by 7 months (173). Still, a meta-analysis of 15 randomized trials investigating ALA (300–600 mg daily) in patients with DN suggests some benefit (odds ratio for benefit 4.0; 95% CI 2.7–5.9), with little risk for harm (174). Overall, published data to date suggest that there may be some benefit to antioxidants in improving symptoms of DN, with benefits seen even after only a short duration.

Many trials have investigated the use of cobalamin (vitamin B12), which does not appear to be beneficial for the treatment of DN (175). By contrast, supplementation with combined thiamine (vitamin B1) and pyridoxine (vitamin B6) appears to confer some symptomatic reduction (175). Other vitamins and antioxidants with potential benefits in DN are listed in Table 8.2.

8.4.2.2   Physical Activity

Persistent hyperglycemia, oxidative stress, and inflammation all contribute to the pathophysiological process underlying the development of DN (166). While intensive glycemic control has been shown to reduce the risk of peripheral neuropathy in T1D, the same has not been demonstrated for T2D, hence the importance of exploring lifestyle factors that could help alleviate symptoms and stop progression (166). Aerobic exercise has been demonstrated to have beneficial effects on neuropathy through improvement in some of the major risk factors for neuropathy: obesity, glucose control, and dyslipidemia (166). Aerobic exercise has also been shown to improve hypertension, reduce lipid and protein oxidation, inhibit adipocyte production of free fatty acids and adipokines, increase end-organ perfusion, and reduce humoral inflammation (166). Studies

TABLE 8.2

Supplements with Potential Benefit in Diabetic Neuropathy

Agent	Typical dose	Efficacy	Strength of evidence
Alpha lipoic acid (174)	300–600 mg daily	Increased nerve conduction velocities and odds ratio of 4.0 for symptom improvement	Multiple randomized trials, mostly showing efficacious results
Combined B vitamins (175)	25 mg of vitamin B1 50 mg of vitamin B6	Approximately 50% reduction in pain score	Single trial showing efficacy
Turmeric (curcumin) (205)	500–2,000 mg daily	Potential for benefit	Preclinical studies show improvement
Resveratrol (206)	250–500 mg daily	Potential for benefit	Preclinical studies show improvement

have shown there may be a role for long-term aerobic exercise training in preventing the onset of peripheral DN in patients with T2D or in more general terms, modifying the natural history of DN, independent of changes in standard measures of metabolism such as body mass index, waist circumference, or lipid profile (176,177).

In patients with existing peripheral DN, it has also been shown that interventions can improve some measures of neuropathy. The Impaired Glucose Tolerance Neuropathy Trial was a 12-month study that examined the effects of diet and exercise counselling on patients with impaired glucose tolerance and DN. As DN is characterized by early injury to small unmyelinated axons, intraepidermal nerve fiber density (IENFD) is a sensitive, quantitative, and reproducible measure of early injury (177). Proximal IENFD and foot sweat volume measured by quantitative sudomotor axon reflex, as well as patient-reported scores on the visual analog pain scale, were significantly improved after 1 year in the aforementioned study (178). There were also significant improvements in weight, glucose intolerance, and lipid parameters (178). A similar study on patients with T2D and DN at the University of Kansas found that after a 10-week aerobic exercise and resistance program, subjects had a significant improvement in neuropathy symptoms; however, the improvement in IENFD was not found to be significant, likely be due to the short duration of the study (179). There are limited data regarding the impact of exercise on peripheral neuropathy in patients with T2D. Small studies have shown that exercise improves balance, walking speed, reaction time, and quality of life, but larger randomized control trials are required to determine the true impact (166).

Another serious form of DN that is of great relevance to CVD, but not well recognized and therefore typically under-reported, is cardiac autonomic neuropathy (CAN). This condition is strongly associated with morbidity and mortality due to arrhythmia and sudden death (166). The reported prevalence of CAN varies greatly, from <5% to 90% depending on the definition used (166). Typically, the presence of an abnormal cardiovagal test result and the presence of orthostatic hypotension are used in assessing the severity, although the first clinical sign is usually a reduction in heart rate variability (166). Obesity and T2D are characterized by sympathetic overactivity due to a gradual loss of parasympathetic tone (180). Hyperglycemia activates the metabolic and/or redox state of the cell, which contributes to the development and progression of CAN when combined with impaired vascular perfusion of nerves (180). Aerobic exercise training can increase parasympathetic predominance, thereby partially attenuating the impact of diabetes on the cardiac nervous system. Patients with CAN need to rely on their perceived exertion (e.g., on the Borg scale) and not on heart rate to avoid dangerous levels of exercise intensity (180). Moderate endurance and aerobic exercise training in both T1D and T2D have been shown to improve heart rate variability and cardiac autonomic function, even in the absence of significant changes in body weight, glucose and blood pressure control, and diabetes duration (180–185). However, it is unclear whether these effects are sustained after discontinuation of exercise (104). For patients with diabetes and more severe, established CAN, a longer/more intense intervention is required to detect benefit (166,180). This supports the critical nature of early identification and intervention in altering the disease course in patients with T1D and T2D who have already developed CAN.

8.4.2.3   Behavior

Painful diabetic peripheral neuropathy (PDPN) has been associated with reduced quality of life, depression, and sleep disruption (186). Pharmacological therapies typically only provide partial relief (187). A pilot study on subjects with T2D older than 50 years with PDPN found that subjects with instruction in mindfulness-based stress reduction (MBSR) did not significantly differ from the control group in any of the pain-related parameters measured (186). However, as this was a pilot study, it was only of 4 weeks duration, which may not have been long enough to find a statistically significant difference. A randomized control trial of 66 participants found that MBSR was effective in reducing pain intensity, pain catastrophizing, depression, and perceived stress, while improving quality of life, with many of these measures showing continued improvement 2–12 weeks after the course (187).

8.5   COMPLICATION 4: DIABETIC RETINOPATHY

8.5.1   CONTEXT

Retinopathy represents another form of microvascular complication that may develop in patients with diabetes. Approximately 5%–15% of patients with T2D have vision-threatening retinopathy (188–190), and the presence of any retinopathy is noted among 40% of patients with T2D (191). Diabetic retinopathy represents the most common cause for visual impairment and blindness in patients older than 65 years (190,192). Hyperglycemia, hypertension, and localized generation of both ROS and advanced glycation end products contribute to the pathophysiology of retinopathy (193). Consequently, neurodegeneration, disruption of the blood–retina barrier with protein leakage, microaneurysms, and hard exudate formation disrupt retinal function (193). Localized hypoxia within the retina drives production of growth factors, especially vascular endothelial growth factor and platelet-derived growth factor, which contribute to neovascularization, further leakage, and the potential for vitreous hemorrhage (192).

The presence of diabetes retinopathy is associated with diabetic nephropathy (193), long QT syndrome (194), and macrovascular disease, which includes a two- to three-fold increase in the incidence of cardiovascular events (195,196).

8.5.2 LIFESTYLE INTERVENTIONS

8.5.2.1 Nutrition

Since diabetic retinopathy is associated with the duration of diabetes and level of glycemic control, dietary interventions that improve glucose levels are expected to benefit retinopathy development and progression (197). However, very few studies have investigated this complication specifically. Preclinical animal models demonstrate regression of diabetes retinopathy with the use of a low-glycemic index diet (198). In one clinical study, the PREDIMED trial demonstrated a 41% reduction in the incidence of diabetic retinopathy in subjects with T2D who were assigned to a Mediterranean compared with control diet (199).

8.5.2.2 Physical Activity

Patients with T2D who develop retinopathy demonstrate lower fitness and lower peak VO2 consumption (200). Glycemic and hypertensive control represent important factors in retinopathy that are improved with regular physical activity. While physical activity can improve both of these, cross-sectional studies do not demonstrate a clear reduction in retinopathy with increased physical activity (201). Moreover, regular physical activity increases retinal blood flow, but it is unclear whether this mitigates retinopathy progression (201). Autonomic neuropathy that may develop can lead to inefficient vasoconstriction among retinal arteries, which may not be overcome through physical activity (202).

8.5.2.3 Behavior

Regular screening is recommended for case detection and surveillance of existing retinopathy (203). Tobacco use is associated with higher risk of retinopathy, and cessation is recommended, although there is insufficient evidence confirming this specific benefit (204).

8.6 CONCLUSION

The management of complex chronic diseases and their sequelae requires a multimodal approach to both reduce the severity of disease and mitigate disease-related complications. This applies to the ABCD, DBCD, and CMBCD care models with lifestyle medicine as the centerpiece, not only for early prevention but also in later stages of disease where complications manifest and symptoms dominate the clinical picture. The principal components of lifestyle modification in tertiary prevention for managing CMBCD complications include the healthy modification of dietary patterns with judicious and evidence-based utilization of dietary supplements, routine incorporation of physical activity and exercise therapy, and mindfulness-based therapies to manage unhealthy behaviors. These lifestyle interventions should be employed in conjunction with pharmacological and/or appropriate procedural treatments. At advanced stages of CMBCD, goals of care may shift toward achievable improvements. Still, lifestyle interventions demonstrate benefits for slowing the progression of chronic diseases and their complications, as well as improvement in quality of life.

Disclosures:
Jeffrey I. Mechanick received honoraria from Abbott Nutrition for lectures and serves on the Advisory Boards for Aveta.Life and Twin Health.

REFERENCES

1. Kisling LA, Das M. *Prevention Strategies. StatPearls.* StatPearls Publishing, Treasure Island, FL; 2022.
2. Mechanick JI, Farkouh ME, Newman JD, Garvey WT. Cardiometabolic-based chronic disease, adiposity and dysglycemia drivers: JACC state-of-the-art review. *J Am Coll Cardiol.* 2020;75(5):525–38.
3. Mechanick JI, Farkouh ME, Newman JD, Garvey WT. Cardiometabolic-based chronic disease, addressing knowledge and clinical practice gaps: JACC state-of-the-art review. *J Am Coll Cardiol.* 2020;75(5):539–55.
4. Einarson TR, Acs A, Ludwig C, Panton UH. Prevalence of cardiovascular disease in type 2 diabetes: a systematic literature review of scientific evidence from across the world in 2007–2017. *Cardiovasc Diabetol.* 2018;17(1):83.
5. Pearson-Stuttard J, Bennett J, Cheng YJ, Vamos EP, Cross AJ, Ezzati M, et al. Trends in predominant causes of death in individuals with and without diabetes in England from 2001 to 2018: an epidemiological analysis of linked primary care records. *Lancet Diabetes Endocrinol.* 2021;9(3):165–73.
6. Howard G, O'Leary DH, Zaccaro D, Haffner S, Rewers M, Hamman R, et al. Insulin sensitivity and atherosclerosis. The Insulin Resistance Atherosclerosis Study (IRAS) Investigators. *Circulation.* 1996;93(10):1809–17.
7. Isomaa B, Almgren P, Tuomi T, Forsen B, Lahti K, Nissen M, et al. Cardiovascular morbidity and mortality associated with the metabolic syndrome. *Diabetes Care.* 2001;24(4):683–9.
8. Gast KB, Tjeerdema N, Stijnen T, Smit JW, Dekkers OM. Insulin resistance and risk of incident cardiovascular events in adults without diabetes: meta-analysis. *PLoS One.* 2012;7(12):e52036.
9. Laakso M. Diabetes as a 'cardiovascular disease equivalent': implications for treatment. *Nat Clin Pract Cardiovasc Med.* 2008;5(11):682–3.
10. Dawber TR, Meadors GF, Moore FE, Jr. Epidemiological approaches to heart disease: the Framingham Study. *Am J Public Health Nations Health.* 1951;41(3):279–81.
11. Feinleib M, Kannel WB, Garrison RJ, McNamara PM, Castelli WP. The Framingham Offspring Study. Design and preliminary data. *Prev Med.* 1975;4(4):518–25.
12. Kuusisto J, Laakso M. Update on type 2 diabetes as a cardiovascular disease risk equivalent. *Curr Cardiol Rep.* 2013;15(2):331.
13. Pylypchuk R, Wells S, Kerr A, Poppe K, Harwood M, Mehta S, et al. Cardiovascular risk prediction in type 2 diabetes before and after widespread screening: a derivation and validation study. *Lancet.* 2021;397(10291):2264–74.
14. Viigimaa M, Sachinidis A, Toumpourleka M, Koutsampasopoulos K, Alliksoo S, Titma T. Macrovascular complications of type 2 diabetes mellitus. *Curr Vasc Pharmacol.* 2020;18(2):110–6.

15. Lei MH, Wu YL, Chung SL, Chen CC, Chen WC, Hsu YC. Coronary artery calcium score predicts long-term cardiovascular outcomes in asymptomatic patients with type 2 diabetes. *J Atheroscler Thromb.* 2021;28(10):1052–62.

16. Joseph TP, Kotecha NS, Kumar HBC, Jain N, Kapoor A, Kumar S, et al. Coronary artery calcification, carotid intima-media thickness and cardiac dysfunction in young adults with type 2 diabetes mellitus. *J Diabetes Complicat.* 2020;34(8):107609.

17. Arora E, Maiya AG, Devasia T, Bhat R, Kamath G. Prevalence of peripheral arterial disease among type 2 diabetes mellitus in coastal Karnataka. *Diabetes Metab Syndr.* 2019;13(2):1251–3.

18. Eshcol J, Jebarani S, Anjana RM, Mohan V, Pradeepa R. Prevalence, incidence and progression of peripheral arterial disease in Asian Indian type 2 diabetic patients. *J Diabetes Complicat.* 2014;28(5):627–31.

19. Di Pino A, DeFronzo RA. Insulin resistance and atherosclerosis: implications for insulin-sensitizing agents. *Endocr Rev.* 2019;40(6):1447–67.

20. Zhao S, Mechanick JI, Jacques PF. Eating patterns. In: Mechanick JI, Via MA, Zhou S, editors. *Molectular Nutrition.* Washington DC: Endocrine Press; 2015. pp. 53–64.

21. Chrysohoou C, Panagiotakos DB, Aggelopoulos P, Kastorini CM, Kehagia I, Pitsavos C, et al. The Mediterranean diet contributes to the preservation of left ventricular systolic function and to the long-term favorable prognosis of patients who have had an acute coronary event. *Am J Clin Nutr.* 2010;92(1):47–54.

22. Russo M, Perrone GA, Polese M, Mechanick JI, Fini M, Tafani M. Molecular nutrient targeting with Mediterranean diets. In: Mechanick JI, Via MA, Zhou S, editors. *Molecular Nutrition.* Washington, DC: Endocrine Press; 2015. pp. 63–79.

23. Esposito K, Marfella R, Ciotola M, Di Palo C, Giugliano F, Giugliano G, et al. Effect of a Mediterranean-style diet on endothelial dysfunction and markers of vascular inflammation in the metabolic syndrome: a randomized trial. *JAMA.* 2004;292(12):1440–6.

24. Estruch R, Ros E, Salas-Salvado J, Covas MI, Corella D, Aros F, et al. Primary prevention of cardiovascular disease with a Mediterranean diet supplemented with extra-virgin olive oil or nuts. *N Engl J Med.* 2018;378(25):e34.

25. Sala-Vila A, Romero-Mamani ES, Gilabert R, Nunez I, de la Torre R, Corella D, et al. Changes in ultrasound-assessed carotid intima-media thickness and plaque with a Mediterranean diet: a substudy of the PREDIMED trial. *Arterioscler Thromb Vasc Biol.* 2014;34(2):439–45.

26. Casas R, Sacanella E, Urpi-Sarda M, Chiva-Blanch G, Ros E, Martinez-Gonzalez MA, et al. The effects of the Mediterranean diet on biomarkers of vascular wall inflammation and plaque vulnerability in subjects with high risk for cardiovascular disease. A randomized trial. *PLoS One.* 2014;9(6):e100084.

27. Kahleova H, Levin S, Barnard N. Cardio-metabolic benefits of plant-based diets. *Nutrients.* 2017;9(8):848.

28. Wang F, Zheng J, Yang B, Jiang J, Fu Y, Li D. Effects of vegetarian diets on blood lipids: a systematic review and meta-analysis of randomized controlled trials. *J Am Heart Assoc.* 2015;4(10):e002408.

29. Barnard ND, Levin SM, Yokoyama Y. A systematic review and meta-analysis of changes in body weight in clinical trials of vegetarian diets. *J Acad Nutr Diet.* 2015;115(6): 954–69.

30. Martinez-Gonzalez MA, Sanchez-Tainta A, Corella D, Salas-Salvado J, Ros E, Aros F, et al. A provegetarian food pattern and reduction in total mortality in the Prevencion con Dieta Mediterranea (PREDIMED) study. *Am J Clin Nutr.* 2014;100(Suppl 1): 320S–8S.

31. Arnett DK, Blumenthal RS, Albert MA, Buroker AB, Goldberger ZD, Hahn EJ, et al. 2019 ACC/AHA guideline on the primary prevention of cardiovascular disease: a report

of the American College of Cardiology/American Heart Association task force on clinical practice guidelines. *Circulation.* 2019;140(11):e596–e646.

32. Huffman KM, Parker DC, Bhapkar M, Racette SB, Martin CK, Redman LM, et al. Calorie restriction improves lipid-related emerging cardiometabolic risk factors in healthy adults without obesity: distinct influences of BMI and sex from CALERIE a multicentre, phase 2, randomised controlled trial. *EClinicalMedicine.* 2022;43:101261.

33. Kristensson FM, Andersson-Assarsson JC, Svensson PA, Carlsson B, Peltonen M, Carlsson LMS. Effects of bariatric surgery in early- and adult-onset obesity in the prospective controlled swedish obese subjects study. *Diabetes Care.* 2020;43(4):860–6.

34. Look ARG, Wing RR, Bolin P, Brancati FL, Bray GA, Clark JM, et al. Cardiovascular effects of intensive lifestyle intervention in type 2 diabetes. *N Engl J Med.* 2013;369(2):145–54.

35. Oshakbayev K, Dukenbayeva B, Otarbayev N, Togizbayeva G, Tabynbayev N, Gazaliyeva M, et al. Weight loss therapy for clinical management of patients with some atherosclerotic diseases: a randomized clinical trial. *Nutr J.* 2015;14:120.

36. Pedersen LR, Olsen RH, Jurs A, Astrup A, Chabanova E, Simonsen L, et al. A randomised trial comparing weight loss with aerobic exercise in overweight individuals with coronary artery disease: the CUT-IT trial. *Eur J Prev Cardiol.* 2015;22(8):1009–17.

37. Pedersen LR, Olsen RH, Jurs A, Anholm C, Fenger M, Haugaard SB, et al. A randomized trial comparing the effect of weight loss and exercise training on insulin sensitivity and glucose metabolism in coronary artery disease. *Metabolism.* 2015;64(10):1298–307.

38. Lechner K, von Schacky C, McKenzie AL, Worm N, Nixdorff U, Lechner B, et al. Lifestyle factors and high-risk atherosclerosis: pathways and mechanisms beyond traditional risk factors. *Eur J Prev Cardiol.* 2020;27(4):394–406.

39. Eckel RH, Jakicic JM, Ard JD, de Jesus JM, Houston Miller N, Hubbard VS, et al. 2013 AHA/ACC guideline on lifestyle management to reduce cardiovascular risk: a report of the American College of Cardiology/American Heart Association Task Force on Practice Guidelines. *Circulation.* 2014;129(25 Suppl 2):S76–99.

40. Pedersen LR, Olsen RH, Anholm C, Astrup A, Eugen-Olsen J, Fenger M, et al. Effects of 1 year of exercise training versus combined exercise training and weight loss on body composition, low-grade inflammation and lipids in overweight patients with coronary artery disease: a randomized trial. *Cardiovasc Diabetol.* 2019;18(1):127.

41. Pedersen LR, Olsen RH, Anholm C, Walzem RL, Fenger M, Eugen-Olsen J, et al. Weight loss is superior to exercise in improving the atherogenic lipid profile in a sedentary, overweight population with stable coronary artery disease: a randomized trial. *Atherosclerosis.* 2016;246:221–8.

42. Pattyn N, Coeckelberghs E, Buys R, Cornelissen VA, Vanhees L. Aerobic interval training vs. moderate continuous training in coronary artery disease patients: a systematic review and meta-analysis. *Sports Med.* 2014;44(5):687–700.

43. Stewart RAH, Held C, Hadziosmanovic N, Armstrong PW, Cannon CP, Granger CB, et al. Physical activity and mortality in patients with stable coronary heart disease. *J Am Coll Cardiol.* 2017;70(14):1689–700.

44. Marzetti E, Calvani R, Tosato M, Cesari M, Di Bari M, Cherubini A, et al. Physical activity and exercise as countermeasures to physical frailty and sarcopenia. *Aging Clin Exp Res.* 2017;29(1):35–42.

45. Fiuza-Luces C, Santos-Lozano A, Joyner M, Carrera-Bastos P, Picazo O, Zugaza JL, et al. Exercise benefits in cardiovascular disease: beyond attenuation of traditional risk factors. *Nat Rev Cardiol.* 2018;15(12):731–43.

46. Young DR, Hivert MF, Alhassan S, Camhi SM, Ferguson JF, Katzmarzyk PT, et al. Sedentary behavior and cardiovascular morbidity and mortality: a science advisory from the American Heart Association. *Circulation.* 2016;134(13):e262–79.

47. Kohl HW, 3rd, Craig CL, Lambert EV, Inoue S, Alkandari JR, Leetongin G, et al. The pandemic of physical inactivity: global action for public health. *Lancet.* 2012;380(9838): 294–305.

48. Piercy KL, Troiano RP, Ballard RM, Carlson SA, Fulton JE, Galuska DA, et al. The physical activity guidelines for Americans. *JAMA.* 2018;320(19):2020–8.

49. Aberg A, Bergstrand R, Johansson S, Ulvenstam G, Vedin A, Wedel H, et al. Cessation of smoking after myocardial infarction. Effects on mortality after 10 years. *Br Heart J.* 1983;49(5):416–22.

50. Salonen JT. Stopping smoking and long-term mortality after acute myocardial infarction. *Br Heart J.* 1980;43(4):463–9.

51. Vlietstra RE, Kronmal RA, Oberman A, Frye RL, Killip T, 3rd. Effect of cigarette smoking on survival of patients with angiographically documented coronary artery disease. Report from the CASS registry. *JAMA.* 1986;255(8):1023–7.

52. Hu Y, Zong G, Liu G, Wang M, Rosner B, Pan A, et al. Smoking cessation, weight change, type 2 diabetes, and mortality. *N Engl J Med.* 2018;379(7):623–32.

53. Savarese G, Stolfo D, Sinagra G, Lund LH. Heart failure with mid-range or mildly reduced ejection fraction. *Nat Rev Cardiol.* 2022;19(2):100–16.

54. Inamdar AA, Inamdar AC. Heart failure: diagnosis, management and utilization. *J Clin Med.* 2016;5(7):62.

55. Billingsley H, Rodriguez-Miguelez P, Del Buono MG, Abbate A, Lavie CJ, Carbone S. Lifestyle interventions with a focus on nutritional strategies to increase cardiorespiratory fitness in chronic obstructive pulmonary disease, heart failure, obesity, sarcopenia, and frailty. *Nutrients.* 2019;11(12):2849.

56. Billingsley HE, Hummel SL, Carbone S. The role of diet and nutrition in heart FAILURE: a state-of-the-art narrative review. *Prog Cardiovasc Dis.* 2020;63(5):538–51.

57. Levitan EB, Lewis CE, Tinker LF, Eaton CB, Ahmed A, Manson JE, et al. Mediterranean and DASH diet scores and mortality in women with heart failure: the Women's Health Initiative. *Circ Heart Fail.* 2013;6(6):1116–23.

58. Tektonidis TG, Akesson A, Gigante B, Wolk A, Larsson SC. Adherence to a Mediterranean diet is associated with reduced risk of heart failure in men. *Eur J Heart Fail.* 2016;18(3):253–9.

59. Tektonidis TG, Akesson A, Gigante B, Wolk A, Larsson SC. A Mediterranean diet and risk of myocardial infarction, heart failure and stroke: a population-based cohort study. *Atherosclerosis.* 2015;243(1):93–8.

60. Wirth J, di Giuseppe R, Boeing H, Weikert C. A Mediterranean-style diet, its components and the risk of heart failure: a prospective population-based study in a non-Mediterranean country. *Eur J Clin Nutr.* 2016;70(9):1015–21.

61. Papadaki A, Martinez-Gonzalez MA, Alonso-Gomez A, Rekondo J, Salas-Salvado J, Corella D, et al. Mediterranean diet and risk of heart failure: results from the PREDIMED randomized controlled trial. *Eur J Heart Fail.* 2017;19(9):1179–85.

62. Fito M, Estruch R, Salas-Salvado J, Martinez-Gonzalez MA, Aros F, Vila J, et al. Effect of the Mediterranean diet on heart failure biomarkers: a randomized sample from the PREDIMED trial. *Eur J Heart Fail.* 2014;16(5):543–50.

63. Levitan EB, Ahmed A, Arnett DK, Polak JF, Hundley WG, Bluemke DA, et al. Mediterranean diet score and left ventricular structure and function: the Multi-Ethnic Study of Atherosclerosis. *Am J Clin Nutr.* 2016;104(3):595–602.

64. Miro O, Estruch R, Martin-Sanchez FJ, Gil V, Jacob J, Herrero-Puente P, et al. Adherence to Mediterranean diet and all-cause mortality after an episode of acute heart failure: results of the MEDIT-AHF study. *JACC Heart Fail.* 2018;6(1):52–62.

65. Hummel SL, Seymour EM, Brook RD, Kolias TJ, Sheth SS, Rosenblum HR, et al. Low-sodium dietary approaches to stop hypertension diet reduces blood pressure, arterial

stiffness, and oxidative stress in hypertensive heart failure with preserved ejection fraction. *Hypertension*. 2012;60(5):1200–6.

66. Rifai L, Pisano C, Hayden J, Sulo S, Silver MA. Impact of the DASH diet on endothelial function, exercise capacity, and quality of life in patients with heart failure. *Proc (Bayl Univ Med Cent)*. 2015;28(2):151–6.

67. Sacks FM, Svetkey LP, Vollmer WM, Appel LJ, Bray GA, Harsha D, et al. Effects on blood pressure of reduced dietary sodium and the dietary approaches to stop hypertension (DASH) diet. DASH-Sodium Collaborative Research Group. *N Engl J Med*. 2001;344(1):3–10.

68. Levitan EB, Wolk A, Mittleman MA. Consistency with the DASH diet and incidence of heart failure. *Arch Intern Med*. 2009;169(9):851–7.

69. Levitan EB, Wolk A, Mittleman MA. Relation of consistency with the dietary approaches to stop hypertension diet and incidence of heart failure in men aged 45 to 79 years. *Am J Cardiol*. 2009;104(10):1416–20.

70. Goyal P, Balkan L, Ringel JB, Hummel SL, Sterling MR, Kim S, et al. The dietary approaches to stop hypertension (DASH) diet pattern and incident heart failure. *J Card Fail*. 2021;27(5):512–21.

71. Del Gobbo LC, Kalantarian S, Imamura F, Lemaitre R, Siscovick DS, Psaty BM, et al. Contribution of major lifestyle risk factors for incident heart failure in older adults: the cardiovascular health study. *JACC Heart Fail*. 2015;3(7):520–8.

72. Intersalt: An International Study of Electrolyte Excretion and Blood Pressure. Results for 24 hour urinary sodium and potassium excretion. Intersalt Cooperative Research Group. *BMJ*. 1988;297(6644):319–28.

73. Heart Failure Society of America, Lindenfeld J, Albert NM, Boehmer JP, Collins SP, Ezekowitz JA, et al. HFSA 2010 comprehensive heart failure practice guideline. *J Card Fail*. 2010;16(6):e1–194.

74. Yancy CW, Jessup M, Bozkurt B, Butler J, Casey DE, Jr., Drazner MH, et al. 2013 ACCF/AHA guideline for the management of heart failure: a report of the American College of Cardiology Foundation/American Heart Association Task Force on Practice Guidelines. *J Am Coll Cardiol*. 2013;62(16):e147–239.

75. Whelton PK, Appel LJ, Sacco RL, Anderson CA, Antman EM, Campbell N, et al. Sodium, blood pressure, and cardiovascular disease: further evidence supporting the American Heart Association sodium reduction recommendations. *Circulation*. 2012;126(24):2880–9.

76. Khan MS, Jones DW, Butler J. Salt, no salt, or less salt for patients with heart failure? *Am J Med*. 2020;133(1):32–8.

77. Lee KS, Moser DK, Park JH, Lennie TA. The association of deficiencies of water-soluble vitamin intake with health-related quality of life and prognosis in patients with heart failure. *Qual Life Res*. 2021;30(4):1183–90.

78. Arcand J, Ivanov J, Sasson A, Floras V, Al-Hesayen A, Azevedo ER, et al. A high-sodium diet is associated with acute decompensated heart failure in ambulatory heart failure patients: a prospective follow-up study. *Am J Clin Nutr*. 2011;93(2):332–7.

79. Lennie TA, Song EK, Wu JR, Chung ML, Dunbar SB, Pressler SJ, et al. Three gram sodium intake is associated with longer event-free survival only in patients with advanced heart failure. *J Card Fail*. 2011;17(4):325–30.

80. Paterna S, Gaspare P, Fasullo S, Sarullo FM, Di Pasquale P. Normal-sodium diet compared with low-sodium diet in compensated congestive heart failure: is sodium an old enemy or a new friend? *Clin Sci*. 2008;114(3):221–30.

81. Paterna S, Parrinello G, Cannizzaro S, Fasullo S, Torres D, Sarullo FM, et al. Medium term effects of different dosage of diuretic, sodium, and fluid administration on neurohormonal and clinical outcome in patients with recently compensated heart failure. *Am J Cardiol*. 2009;103(1):93–102.

82. Gupta D, Georgiopoulou VV, Kalogeropoulos AP, Dunbar SB, Reilly CM, Sands JM, et al. Dietary sodium intake in heart failure. *Circulation*. 2012;126(4):479–85.

83. Sica DA. Loop diuretic therapy, thiamine balance, and heart failure. *Congest Heart Fail*. 2007;13(4):244–7.

84. Gotsman I, Shauer A, Zwas DR, Hellman Y, Keren A, Lotan C, et al. Vitamin D deficiency is a predictor of reduced survival in patients with heart failure; vitamin D supplementation improves outcome. *Eur J Heart Fail*. 2012;14(4):357–66.

85. Busa V, Dardeir A, Marudhai S, Patel M, Valaiyaduppu Subas S, Ghani MR, et al. Role of vitamin D supplementation in heart failure patients with vitamin D deficiency and its effects on clinical outcomes: a literature review. *Cureus*. 2020;12(10):e10840.

86. Mechanick JI, Brett EM, Chausmer AB, Dickey RA, Wallach S, American Association of Clinical Endocrinologists. American Association of Clinical Endocrinologists medical guidelines for the clinical use of dietary supplements and nutraceuticals. *Endocr Pract*. 2003;9(5):417–70.

87. Fahey T, Schroeder K. Cardiology. *Br J Gen Pract*. 2004;54(506):695–702.

88. Conn EH, Williams RS, Wallace AG. Exercise responses before and after physical conditioning in patients with severely depressed left ventricular function. *Am J Cardiol*. 1982;49(2):296–300.

89. Lee AP, Ice R, Blessey R, Sanmarco ME. Long-term effects of physical training on coronary patients with impaired ventricular function. *Circulation*. 1979;60(7):1519–26.

90. Sullivan MJ, Higginbotham MB, Cobb FR. Exercise training in patients with severe left ventricular dysfunction. Hemodynamic and metabolic effects. *Circulation*. 1988;78(3):506–15.

91. Piepoli MF, Davos C, Francis DP, Coats AJ, ExTra MC. Exercise training meta-analysis of trials in patients with chronic heart failure (ExTraMATCH). *BMJ*. 2004;328(7433):189.

92. O'Connor CM, Whellan DJ, Lee KL, Keteyian SJ, Cooper LS, Ellis SJ, et al. Efficacy and safety of exercise training in patients with chronic heart failure: HF-ACTION randomized controlled trial. *JAMA*. 2009;301(14):1439–50.

93. Arena R, Myers J, Aslam SS, Varughese EB, Peberdy MA. Peak VO$_2$ and VE/VCO$_2$ slope in patients with heart failure: a prognostic comparison. *Am Heart J*. 2004;147(2):354–60.

94. Pina IL, Apstein CS, Balady GJ, Belardinelli R, Chaitman BR, Duscha BD, et al. Exercise and heart failure: a statement from the American Heart Association Committee on exercise, rehabilitation, and prevention. *Circulation*. 2003;107(8):1210–25.

95. Taylor RS, Davies EJ, Dalal HM, Davis R, Doherty P, Cooper C, et al. Effects of exercise training for heart failure with preserved ejection fraction: a systematic review and meta-analysis of comparative studies. *Int J Cardiol*. 2012;162(1):6–13.

96. Alsara O, Perez-Terzic C, Squires RW, Dandamudi S, Miranda WR, Park SJ, et al. Is exercise training safe and beneficial in patients receiving left ventricular assist device therapy? *J Cardiopulm Rehabil Prev*. 2014;34(4):233–40.

97. Cattadori G, Segurini C, Picozzi A, Padeletti L, Anza C. Exercise and heart failure: an update. *ESC Heart Fail*. 2018;5(2):222–32.

98. Amstad T, Taeymans J, Englberger L, Mohacsi P, Steiner D, Wilhelm MJ, et al. Cardiac rehabilitation in patients with ventricular assist device. *J Cardiopulm Rehabil Prev*. 2022;42(2):97–102.

99. Kerrigan DJ, Williams CT, Ehrman JK, Saval MA, Bronsteen K, Schairer JR, et al. Cardiac rehabilitation improves functional capacity and patient-reported health status in patients with continuous-flow left ventricular assist devices: the Rehab-VAD randomized controlled trial. *JACC Heart Fail*. 2014;2(6):653–9.

100. Sullivan MJ, Wood L, Terry J, Brantley J, Charles A, McGee V, et al. The Support, Education, and Research in Chronic Heart Failure Study (SEARCH): a mindfulness-based psychoeducational intervention improves depression and clinical symptoms in patients with chronic heart failure. *Am Heart J*. 2009;157(1):84–90.

101. Jiang W, Alexander J, Christopher E, Kuchibhatla M, Gaulden LH, Cuffe MS, et al. Relationship of depression to increased risk of mortality and rehospitalization in patients with congestive heart failure. *Arch Intern Med*. 2001;161(15):1849–56.
102. Zou H, Cao X, Geng J, Chair SY. Effects of mindfulness-based interventions on health-related outcomes for patients with heart failure: a systematic review. *Eur J Cardiovasc Nurs*. 2020;19(1):44–54.
103. Jayadevappa R, Johnson JC, Bloom BS, Nidich S, Desai S, Chhatre S, et al. Effectiveness of transcendental meditation on functional capacity and quality of life of African Americans with congestive heart failure: a randomized control study. *Ethn Dis*. 2007;17(1):72–7.
104. Akinboboye O, Krantz DS, Kop WJ, Schwartz SD, Levine J, Del Negro A, et al. Comparison of mental stress-induced myocardial ischemia in coronary artery disease patients with versus without left ventricular dysfunction. *Am J Cardiol*. 2005;95(3):322–6.
105. Schneider RH, Myers HF, Marwaha K, Rainforth MA, Salerno JW, Nidich SI, et al. Stress reduction in the prevention of left ventricular hypertrophy: a randomized controlled trial of transcendental meditation and health education in hypertensive African Americans. *Ethn Dis*. 2019;29(4):577–86.
106. Huxley RR, Alonso A, Lopez FL, Filion KB, Agarwal SK, Loehr LR, et al. Type 2 diabetes, glucose homeostasis and incident atrial fibrillation: the atherosclerosis risk in communities study. *Heart*. 2012;98(2):133–8.
107. Du X, Ninomiya T, de Galan B, Abadir E, Chalmers J, Pillai A, et al. Risks of cardiovascular events and effects of routine blood pressure lowering among patients with type 2 diabetes and atrial fibrillation: results of the ADVANCE study. *Eur Heart J*. 2009;30(9):1128–35.
108. Dublin S, Glazer NL, Smith NL, Psaty BM, Lumley T, Wiggins KL, et al. Diabetes mellitus, glycemic control, and risk of atrial fibrillation. *J Gen Intern Med*. 2010;25(8):853–8.
109. Fatemi O, Yuriditsky E, Tsioufis C, Tsachris D, Morgan T, Basile J, et al. Impact of intensive glycemic control on the incidence of atrial fibrillation and associated cardiovascular outcomes in patients with type 2 diabetes mellitus (from the action to control cardiovascular risk in diabetes study). *Am J Cardiol*. 2014;114(8):1217–22.
110. Schoen T, Pradhan AD, Albert CM, Conen D. Type 2 diabetes mellitus and risk of incident atrial fibrillation in women. *J Am Coll Cardiol*. 2012;60(15):1421–8.
111. Wang TJ, Parise H, Levy D, D'Agostino RB, Sr., Wolf PA, Vasan RS, et al. Obesity and the risk of new-onset atrial fibrillation. *JAMA*. 2004;292(20):2471–7.
112. Packer M. Disease-treatment interactions in the management of patients with obesity and diabetes who have atrial fibrillation: the potential mediating influence of epicardial adipose tissue. *Cardiovasc Diabetol*. 2019;18(1):121.
113. Wanahita N, Messerli FH, Bangalore S, Gami AS, Somers VK, Steinberg JS. Atrial fibrillation and obesity--results of a meta-analysis. *Am Heart J*. 2008;155(2):310–5.
114. Alonso A, Bahnson JL, Gaussoin SA, Bertoni AG, Johnson KC, Lewis CE, et al. Effect of an intensive lifestyle intervention on atrial fibrillation risk in individuals with type 2 diabetes: the Look AHEAD randomized trial. *Am Heart J*. 2015;170(4):770–7 e5.
115. Abed HS, Wittert GA, Leong DP, Shirazi MG, Bahrami B, Middeldorp ME, et al. Effect of weight reduction and cardiometabolic risk factor management on symptom burden and severity in patients with atrial fibrillation: a randomized clinical trial. *JAMA*. 2013;310(19):2050–60.
116. Pathak RK, Middeldorp ME, Meredith M, Mehta AB, Mahajan R, Wong CX, et al. Long-term effect of goal-directed weight management in an atrial fibrillation cohort: a long-term follow-up study (LEGACY). *J Am Coll Cardiol*. 2015;65(20):2159–69.
117. Martinez-Gonzalez MA, Toledo E, Aros F, Fiol M, Corella D, Salas-Salvado J, et al. Extravirgin olive oil consumption reduces risk of atrial fibrillation: the PREDIMED (Prevencion con Dieta Mediterranea) trial. *Circulation*. 2014;130(1):18–26.

118. Morseth B, Lochen ML, Ariansen I, Myrstad M, Thelle DS. The ambiguity of physical activity, exercise and atrial fibrillation. *Eur J Prev Cardiol*. 2018;25(6):624–36.

119. Sanchis-Gomar F, Perez-Quilis C, Lippi G, Cervellin G, Leischik R, Lollgen H, et al. Atrial fibrillation in highly trained endurance athletes - description of a syndrome. *Int J Cardiol*. 2017;226:11–20.

120. Molina L, Mont L, Marrugat J, Berruezo A, Brugada J, Bruguera J, et al. Long-term endurance sport practice increases the incidence of lone atrial fibrillation in men: a follow-up study. *Europace*. 2008;10(5):618–23.

121. Morseth B, Graff-Iversen S, Jacobsen BK, Jorgensen L, Nyrnes A, Thelle DS, et al. Physical activity, resting heart rate, and atrial fibrillation: the Tromso Study. *Eur Heart J*. 2016;37(29):2307–13.

122. Mozaffarian D, Furberg CD, Psaty BM, Siscovick D. Physical activity and incidence of atrial fibrillation in older adults: the cardiovascular health study. *Circulation*. 2008; 118(8):800–7.

123. Drca N, Wolk A, Jensen-Urstad M, Larsson SC. Physical activity is associated with a reduced risk of atrial fibrillation in middle-aged and elderly women. *Heart*. 2015;101(20): 1627–30.

124. Williams PT, Franklin BA. Reduced incidence of cardiac arrhythmias in walkers and runners. *PLoS One*. 2013;8(6):e65302.

125. Keteyian SJ, Ehrman JK, Fuller B, Pack QR. Exercise testing and exercise rehabilitation for patients with atrial fibrillation. *J Cardiopulm Rehabil Prev*. 2019;39(2):65–72.

126. Voskoboinik A, Kalman JM, De Silva A, Nicholls T, Costello B, Nanayakkara S, et al. Alcohol abstinence in drinkers with atrial fibrillation. *N Engl J Med*. 2020;382(1):20–8.

127. Shukla A, Aizer A, Holmes D, Fowler S, Park DS, Bernstein S, et al. Effect of obstructive sleep apnea treatment on atrial fibrillation recurrence: a meta-analysis. *JACC Clin Electrophysiol*. 2015;1(1–2):41–51.

128. Bodar V, Chen J, Gaziano JM, Albert C, Djousse L. Coffee consumption and risk of atrial fibrillation in the physicians' health study. *J Am Heart Assoc*. 2019;8(15):e011346.

129. O'Keefe EL, O'Keefe JH, Lavie CJ. Exercise counteracts the cardiotoxicity of psychosocial stress. *Mayo Clin Proc*. 2019;94(9):1852–64.

130. Gross JL, de Azevedo MJ, Silveiro SP, Canani LH, Caramori ML, Zelmanovitz T. Diabetic nephropathy: diagnosis, prevention, and treatment. *Diabetes Care*. 2005;28(1): 164–76.

131. Selby NM, Taal MW. An updated overview of diabetic nephropathy: diagnosis, prognosis, treatment goals and latest guidelines. *Diabetes Obes Metab*. 2020;22(Suppl 1):3–15.

132. Giunti S, Barit D, Cooper ME. Mechanisms of diabetic nephropathy: role of hypertension. *Hypertension*. 2006;48(4):519–26.

133. Suckling RJ, He FJ, Macgregor GA. Altered dietary salt intake for preventing and treating diabetic kidney disease. *Cochrane Database Syst Rev*. 2010;12:CD006763.

134. American Diabetes Association. 11. Microvascular complications and foot care: standards of medical care in diabetes-2020. *Diabetes Care*. 2020;43(Suppl 1):S135–S51.

135. Bellizzi V, Garofalo C, Ferrara C, Calella P. Ketoanalogue supplementation in patients with non-dialysis diabetic kidney disease: a systematic review and meta-analysis. *Nutrients*. 2022;14(3):441.

136. Evert AB, Dennison M, Gardner CD, Garvey WT, Lau KHK, MacLeod J, et al. Nutrition therapy for adults with diabetes or prediabetes: a consensus report. *Diabetes Care*. 2019;42(5):731–54.

137. KDOQI. KDOQI clinical practice guidelines and clinical practice recommendations for diabetes and chronic kidney disease. *Am J Kidney Dis*. 2007;49(2 Suppl 2):S12–154.

138. Gross JL, Zelmanovitz T, Moulin CC, De Mello V, Perassolo M, Leitao C, et al. Effect of a chicken-based diet on renal function and lipid profile in patients with type 2 diabetes: a randomized crossover trial. *Diabetes Care.* 2002;25(4):645–51.

139. de Mello VD, Zelmanovitz T, Azevedo MJ, de Paula TP, Gross JL. Long-term effect of a chicken-based diet versus enalapril on albuminuria in type 2 diabetic patients with microalbuminuria. *J Ren Nutr.* 2008;18(5):440–7.

140. Haring B, Selvin E, Liang M, Coresh J, Grams ME, Petruski-Ivleva N, et al. Dietary protein sources and risk for incident chronic kidney disease: results from the atherosclerosis risk in communities (ARIC) study. *J Ren Nutr.* 2017;27(4):233–42.

141. Klahr S, Levey AS, Beck GJ, Caggiula AW, Hunsicker L, Kusek JW, et al. The effects of dietary protein restriction and blood-pressure control on the progression of chronic renal disease. Modification of Diet in Renal Disease Study Group. *N Engl J Med.* 1994;330(13):877–84.

142. Carrero JJ, Thomas F, Nagy K, Arogundade F, Avesani CM, Chan M, et al. Global prevalence of protein-energy wasting in kidney disease: a meta-analysis of contemporary observational studies from the international society of renal nutrition and metabolism. *J Ren Nutr.* 2018;28(6):380–92.

143. Kalantar-Zadeh K, Kopple JD, Deepak S, Block D, Block G. Food intake characteristics of hemodialysis patients as obtained by food frequency questionnaire. *J Ren Nutr.* 2002;12(1):17–31.

144. Maraj M, Kusnierz-Cabala B, Dumnicka P, Gala-Bladzinska A, Gawlik K, Pawlica-Gosiewska D, et al. Malnutrition, inflammation, atherosclerosis syndrome (MIA) and diet recommendations among end-stage renal disease patients treated with maintenance hemodialysis. *Nutrients.* 2018;10(1): 69.

145. Biruete A, Jeong JH, Barnes JL, Wilund KR. Modified nutritional recommendations to improve dietary patterns and outcomes in hemodialysis patients. *J Ren Nutr.* 2017;27(1):62–70.

146. Kopple JD. Dietary protein and energy requirements in ESRD patients. *Am J Kidney Dis.* 1998;32(6 Suppl 4):S97–104.

147. Murray DP, Young L, Waller J, Wright S, Colombo R, Baer S, et al. Is dietary protein intake predictive of 1-year mortality in dialysis patients? *Am J Med Sci.* 2018;356(3):234–43.

148. Schrier RW, Estacio RO, Esler A, Mehler P. Effects of aggressive blood pressure control in normotensive type 2 diabetic patients on albuminuria, retinopathy and strokes. *Kidney Int.* 2002;61(3):1086–97.

149. Leehey DJ, Zhang JH, Emanuele NV, Whaley-Connell A, Palevsky PM, Reilly RF, et al. BP and renal outcomes in diabetic kidney disease: the veterans affairs nephropathy in diabetes trial. *Clin J Am Soc Nephrol.* 2015;10(12):2159–69.

150. MacGregor GA, Markandu ND, Singer DR, Cappuccio FP, Shore AC, Sagnella GA. Moderate sodium restriction with angiotensin converting enzyme inhibitor in essential hypertension: a double blind study. *Br Med J (Clin Res Ed).* 1987;294(6571):531–4.

151. American Diabetes Association Professional Practice Committee, Draznin B, Aroda VR, Bakris G, Benson G, Brown FM, et al. 11. Chronic kidney disease and risk management: standards of medical care in diabetes-2022. *Diabetes Care.* 2022;45(Suppl 1):S175–S84.

152. Amaral LSB, Souza CS, Lima HN, Soares TJ. Influence of exercise training on diabetic kidney disease: a brief physiological approach. *Exp Biol Med.* 2020;245(13):1142–54.

153. Holten MK, Zacho M, Gaster M, Juel C, Wojtaszewski JF, Dela F. Strength training increases insulin-mediated glucose uptake, GLUT4 content, and insulin signaling in skeletal muscle in patients with type 2 diabetes. *Diabetes.* 2004;53(2):294–305.

154. Wojtaszewski JF, Birk JB, Frosig C, Holten M, Pilegaard H, Dela F. 5'AMP activated protein kinase expression in human skeletal muscle: effects of strength training and type 2 diabetes. *J Physiol*. 2005;564(Pt 2):563–73.

155. Afkarian M, Zelnick LR, Hall YN, Heagerty PJ, Tuttle K, Weiss NS, et al. Clinical manifestations of kidney disease among US adults with diabetes, 1988–2014. *JAMA*. 2016;316(6):602–10.

156. Brzezinski RY, Friedensohn L, Shapira I, Zeltser D, Rogowski O, Berliner S, et al. Exercise-induced albuminuria increases over time in individuals with impaired glucose metabolism. *Cardiovasc Diabetol*. 2020;19(1):90.

157. Eidemak I, Haaber AB, Feldt-Rasmussen B, Kanstrup IL, Strandgaard S. Exercise training and the progression of chronic renal failure. *Nephron*. 1997;75(1):36–40.

158. Greenwood SA, Koufaki P, Mercer TH, MacLaughlin HL, Rush R, Lindup H, et al. Effect of exercise training on estimated GFR, vascular health, and cardiorespiratory fitness in patients with CKD: a pilot randomized controlled trial. *Am J Kidney Dis*. 2015;65(3):425–34.

159. Averbukh Z, Marcus E, Berman S, Shiloah E, Horn T, Weissgarten J, et al. Effect of exercise training on glomerular filtration rate of mice with various degrees of renal mass reduction. *Am J Nephrol*. 1992;12(3):174–8.

160. Lazarevic G, Antic S, Vlahovic P, Djordjevic V, Zvezdanovic L, Stefanovic V. Effects of aerobic exercise on microalbuminuria and enzymuria in type 2 diabetic patients. *Ren Fail*. 2007;29(2):199–205.

161. Pechter U, Ots M, Mesikepp S, Zilmer K, Kullissaar T, Vihalemm T, et al. Beneficial effects of water-based exercise in patients with chronic kidney disease. *Int J Rehabil Res*. 2003;26(2):153–6.

162. Manfredini F, Mallamaci F, D'Arrigo G, Baggetta R, Bolignano D, Torino C, et al. Exercise in patients on dialysis: a multicenter, randomized clinical trial. *J Am Soc Nephrol*. 2017;28(4):1259–68.

163. Bohlmeijer E, Prenger R, Taal E, Cuijpers P. The effects of mindfulness-based stress reduction therapy on mental health of adults with a chronic medical disease: a meta-analysis. *J Psychosom Res*. 2010;68(6):539–44.

164. Kopf S, Oikonomou D, Hartmann M, Feier F, Faude-Lang V, Morcos M, et al. Effects of stress reduction on cardiovascular risk factors in type 2 diabetes patients with early kidney disease - results of a randomized controlled trial (HEIDIS). *Exp Clin Endocrinol Diabetes*. 2014;122(6):341–9.

165. Moosavi Nejad M, Shahgholian N, Samouei R. The effect of mindfulness program on general health of patients undergoing hemodialysis. *J Educ Health Promot*. 2018;7:74.

166. Zilliox LA, Russell JW. Physical activity and dietary interventions in diabetic neuropathy: a systematic review. *Clin Auton Res*. 2019;29(4):443–55.

167. Ghavami H, Radfar M, Soheily S, Shamsi SA, Khalkhali HR. Effect of lifestyle interventions on diabetic peripheral neuropathy in patients with type 2 diabetes, result of a randomized clinical trial. *Agri*. 2018;30(4):165–70.

168. Look ARG. Effects of a long-term lifestyle modification programme on peripheral neuropathy in overweight or obese adults with type 2 diabetes: the Look AHEAD study. *Diabetologia*. 2017;60(6):980–8.

169. Smith AG, Singleton JR. Obesity and hyperlipidemia are risk factors for early diabetic neuropathy. *J Diabetes Complicat*. 2013;27(5):436–42.

170. Lewis EJH, Perkins BA, Lovblom LE, Bazinet RP, Wolever TMS, Bril V. Effect of omega-3 supplementation on neuropathy in type 1 diabetes: a 12-month pilot trial. *Neurology*. 2017;88(24):2294–301.

171. Johansen JS, Harris AK, Rychly DJ, Ergul A. Oxidative stress and the use of antioxidants in diabetes: linking basic science to clinical practice. *Cardiovasc Diabetol*. 2005;4:5.

172. Ziegler D, Schatz H, Conrad F, Gries FA, Ulrich H, Reichel G. Effects of treatment with the antioxidant alpha-lipoic acid on cardiac autonomic neuropathy in NIDDM patients. A 4-month randomized controlled multicenter trial (DEKAN Study). Deutsche Kardiale Autonome Neuropathie. *Diabetes Care*. 1997;20(3):369–73.

173. Ziegler D, Hanefeld M, Ruhnau KJ, Hasche H, Lobisch M, Schutte K, et al. Treatment of symptomatic diabetic polyneuropathy with the antioxidant alpha-lipoic acid: a 7-month multicenter randomized controlled trial (ALADIN III Study). ALADIN III Study Group. Alpha-lipoic acid in diabetic neuropathy. *Diabetes Care*. 1999;22(8):1296–301.

174. Han T, Bai J, Liu W, Hu Y. A systematic review and meta-analysis of alpha-lipoic acid in the treatment of diabetic peripheral neuropathy. *Eur J Endocrinol*. 2012;167(4):465–71.

175. Karaganis S, Song XJ. B vitamins as a treatment for diabetic pain and neuropathy. *J Clin Pharm Ther*. 2021;46(5):1199–212.

176. Balducci S, Iacobellis G, Parisi L, Di Biase N, Calandriello E, Leonetti F, et al. Exercise training can modify the natural history of diabetic peripheral neuropathy. *J Diabetes Complicat*. 2006;20(4):216–23.

177. Singleton JR, Marcus RL, Jackson JE, K. Lessard M, Graham TE, Smith AG. Exercise increases cutaneous nerve density in diabetic patients without neuropathy. *Ann Clin Transl Neurol*. 2014;1(10):844–9.

178. Smith AG, Russell J, Feldman EL, Goldstein J, Peltier A, Smith S, et al. Lifestyle intervention for pre-diabetic neuropathy. *Diabetes Care*. 2006;29(6):1294–9.

179. Kluding PM, Pasnoor M, Singh R, Jernigan S, Farmer K, Rucker J, et al. The effect of exercise on neuropathic symptoms, nerve function, and cutaneous innervation in people with diabetic peripheral neuropathy. *J Diabetes Complicat*. 2012;26(5):424–9.

180. Voulgari C, Pagoni S, Vinik A, Poirier P. Exercise improves cardiac autonomic function in obesity and diabetes. *Metabolism*. 2013;62(5):609–21.

181. Chen SR, Lee YJ, Chiu HW, Jeng C. Impact of glycemic control, disease duration, and exercise on heart rate variability in children with type 1 diabetes mellitus. *J Formos Med Assoc*. 2007;106(11):935–42.

182. Madden KM, Lockhart C, Potter TF, Cuff D. Aerobic training restores arterial baroreflex sensitivity in older adults with type 2 diabetes, hypertension, and hypercholesterolemia. *Clin J Sport Med*. 2010;20(4):312–7.

183. Simmonds MJ, Minahan CL, Serre KR, Gass GC, Marshall-Gradisnik SM, Haseler LJ, et al. Preliminary findings in the heart rate variability and haemorheology response to varied frequency and duration of walking in women 65–74 yr with type 2 diabetes. *Clin Hemorheol Microcirc*. 2012;51(2):87–99.

184. Sridhar B, Haleagrahara N, Bhat R, Kulur AB, Avabratha S, Adhikary P. Increase in the heart rate variability with deep breathing in diabetic patients after 12-month exercise training. *Tohoku J Exp Med*. 2010;220(2):107–13.

185. Vanninen E, Uusitupa M, Lansimies E, Siitonen O, Laitinen J. Effect of metabolic control on autonomic function in obese patients with newly diagnosed type 2 diabetes. *Diabet Med*. 1993;10(1):66–73.

186. Teixeira E. The effect of mindfulness meditation on painful diabetic peripheral neuropathy in adults older than 50 years. *Holist Nurs Pract*. 2010;24(5):277–83.

187. Nathan HJ, Poulin P, Wozny D, Taljaard M, Smyth C, Gilron I, et al. Randomized trial of the effect of mindfulness-based stress reduction on pain-related disability, pain intensity, health-related quality of life, and A1C in patients with painful diabetic peripheral neuropathy. *Clin Diabetes*. 2017;35(5):294–304.

188. Lin KD, Hsu CC, Ou HY, Wang CY, Chin MC, Shin SJ. Diabetes-related kidney, eye, and foot disease in Taiwan: an analysis of nationwide data from 2005 to 2014. *J Formos Med Assoc*. 2019;118(Suppl 2):S103–S10.

189. Song SJ, Han K, Choi KS, Ko SH, Rhee EJ, Park CY, et al. Trends in diabetic retinopathy and related medical practices among type 2 diabetes patients: results from the National Insurance Service Survey 2006–2013. *J Diabetes Investig.* 2018;9(1):173–8.

190. Centers for Disease Control and Prevention. Correctable visual impairment among persons with diabetes--United States, 1999–2004. *MMWR Morb Mortal Wkly Rep.* 2006; 55(43):1169–72.

191. Raymond NT, Varadhan L, Reynold DR, Bush K, Sankaranarayanan S, Bellary S, et al. Higher prevalence of retinopathy in diabetic patients of South Asian ethnicity compared with white Europeans in the community: a cross-sectional study. *Diabetes Care.* 2009;32(3):410–5.

192. Lin KY, Hsih WH, Lin YB, Wen CY, Chang TJ. Update in the epidemiology, risk factors, screening, and treatment of diabetic retinopathy. *J Diabetes Investig.* 2021;12(8):1322–5.

193. Wong TY, Cheung CM, Larsen M, Sharma S, Simo R. Diabetic retinopathy. *Nat Rev Dis Primers.* 2016;2:16012.

194. Kobayashi S, Nagao M, Asai A, Fukuda I, Oikawa S, Sugihara H. Severity and multiplicity of microvascular complications are associated with QT interval prolongation in patients with type 2 diabetes. *J Diabetes Investig.* 2018;9(4):946–51.

195. Cheung N, Rogers S, Couper DJ, Klein R, Sharrett AR, Wong TY. Is diabetic retinopathy an independent risk factor for ischemic stroke? *Stroke.* 2007;38(2):398–401.

196. Cheung N, Wang JJ, Klein R, Couper DJ, Sharrett AR, Wong TY. Diabetic retinopathy and the risk of coronary heart disease: the atherosclerosis risk in communities study. *Diabetes Care.* 2007;30(7):1742–6.

197. Francisco SG, Smith KM, Aragones G, Whitcomb EA, Weinberg J, Wang X, et al. Dietary patterns, carbohydrates, and age-related eye diseases. *Nutrients.* 2020;12(9).

198. Rowan S, Jiang S, Chang ML, Volkin J, Cassalman C, Smith KM, et al. A low glycemic diet protects disease-prone Nrf2-deficient mice against age-related macular degeneration. *Free Radic Biol Med.* 2020;150:75–86.

199. Salas-Salvado J, Bullo M, Estruch R, Ros E, Covas MI, Ibarrola-Jurado N, et al. Prevention of diabetes with Mediterranean diets: a subgroup analysis of a randomized trial. *Ann Intern Med.* 2014;160(1):1–10.

200. Estacio RO, Regensteiner JG, Wolfel EE, Jeffers B, Dickenson M, Schrier RW. The association between diabetic complications and exercise capacity in NIDDM patients. *Diabetes Care.* 1998;21(2):291–5.

201. Gale J, Wells AP, Wilson G. Effects of exercise on ocular physiology and disease. *Surv Ophthalmol.* 2009;54(3):349–55.

202. Lanigan LP, Clark CV, Allawi J, Hill DW, Keen H. Responses of the retinal circulation to systemic autonomic stimulation in diabetes mellitus. *Eye.* 1989;3(Pt 1):39–47.

203. American Diabetes Association Professional Practice Committee, Draznin B, Aroda VR, Bakris G, Benson G, Brown FM, et al. 12. Retinopathy, neuropathy, and foot care: standards of medical care in diabetes-2022. *Diabetes Care.* 2022;45(Suppl 1):S185–S94.

204. Chaturvedi N, Stephenson JM, Fuller JH. The relationship between smoking and microvascular complications in the EURODIAB IDDM complications study. *Diabetes Care.* 1995;18(6):785–92.

205. Parsamanesh N, Moossavi M, Bahrami A, Butler AE, Sahebkar A. Therapeutic potential of curcumin in diabetic complications. *Pharmacol Res.* 2018;136:181–93.

206. Huang DD, Shi G, Jiang Y, Yao C, Zhu C. A review on the potential of resveratrol in prevention and therapy of diabetes and diabetic complications. *Biomed Pharmacother.* 2020;125:109767.

9 The Mediterranean Diet

Alexa Yuen and Reshmi Srinath
Icahn School of Medicine at Mount Sinai Hospital
Division of Endocrinology, Diabetes and Bone Disease

CONTENTS

9.1 HISTORICAL CONTEXT

Mediterranean diets typically refer to various eating patterns found in the Mediterranean region, first recognized in the late 1950s and early 1960s before the era of mass scale food production and globalization of ultra-processed foods.[1] In the 1950s, physiologist Dr. Ancel Keys noted that the poor population of small towns in southern Italy was much healthier than wealthy citizens of New York City. Keys believed that this was due to food choices and consequently began to study the foods that made up the diet of these populations. This led to the "Seven Countries Study," which documented the relationship between lifestyles, nutrition, and cardiovascular disease (CVD) in 14 regions across the countries of Finland, Holland, Italy, the United States, Greece, Japan, and Yugoslavia.[2] This study concluded that populations consuming a Mediterranean diet in Crete, Greece, and rural villages in Southern Italy, among others, displayed low rates of hyperlipidemia and coronary artery disease.[3] Later, at the International Conference on the Diets of the Mediterranean in 1993, the term "Mediterranean diet pattern" was defined as the dietary practice found in olive-growing areas of the Mediterranean region in the early 1960s.[4]

DOI: 10.1201/9781003206637-9

The Mediterranean basin was a crossroads where many ancient civilizations and cultures interacted, influencing languages, religions, and lifestyles over centuries. Distinct eating patterns emerged in rural settlements where dietary choices were shaped by the availability of local foods, frugality, and the social practice of eating in the company of family and friends. Indeed, the etymology of the word companion translates to "one who breaks bread with another." In general, cooking styles were slow, using boiling and stewing at lower temperatures with higher moisture in the final dishes.[5,6]

The most universal and defining component of Mediterranean diets is the use of olive oil. The olive tree was originally domesticated approximately 6,000–8,000 years ago in the eastern Mediterranean and subsequently spread to regions bordering the Mediterranean Sea by the Phoenicians, Syrians, and Palestinians. The Greeks and Romans further expanded the cultivation and the use of olive products when they brought it to colonized territories.[7,8]

Mediterranean climate and agriculture also allowed for the cultivation of a wide variety of plants. The Arab world introduced crops, such as citrus, eggplant, almonds, and pomegranate, while the "New World" introduced potatoes, tomatoes, corn, peppers, and chilis.[9] These vegetables were often prepared as salads, soups, or cooked dishes.[10]

Ancient Roman culinary culture placed bread, wine, and olive oil as a central part of their diet, supplemented by cheese, vegetables, fish, and small portions of meat. Cereals, including bread, couscous, pasta, and later, polenta, were also important components of the diet due to their ability to feed the poorer social classes.[9] Meat was typically expensive in the traditional Mediterranean diets and consumed sparingly. Pigs were more often used in the northern Mediterranean versions, while sheep and goat were the typical choice in the south.[8,11] Sheep and goat were also raised to produce milk for drinking as well as yogurts and cheeses for various dishes. Fish was consumed in moderation, depending on proximity to the sea.[5]

9.2 COMPONENTS

General definitions of Mediterranean diets are similar across publications that attempt to describe them. They involved high consumption of olive oil, vegetables, fruits, cereals, nuts, and legumes with moderate ingestion of fish, meats, dairy, and wine as well as low intake of sweets and eggs.[12] Given the high intake of vegetables, nuts, and olive oil, the Mediterranean diets can be considered primarily as a plant-based eating pattern.[4]

The dominant position of olive oil in the eating pattern, which is typically consumed with large quantities of vegetables and legumes, is pervasive across the Mediterranean region. Vegetables are prepared as salads, soups, and cooked dishes, along with lemon juice, vinegar, and herbs for seasoning.[10] Nuts and seeds that are eaten in the region include almonds, hazelnuts, pine nuts, pistachios, and walnuts, which are sometimes prepared with honey, syrup, or dried fruit to make sweets. However, a formal dessert dish more commonly consists of fresh fruit.[13] Bread serves as a staple food and is consumed consistently with each meal. However, certain regions, such as Italy, incorporate starches into their meals, predominantly using durum wheat to produce products including pasta, couscous, and bulgur in addition to bread.[14,15] Excluding Muslim cultures, alcohol is consumed in moderation predominantly with meals as red wine.[16,17] Moderate alcohol consumption is defined as 2–25 g of alcohol per day for women or one to two 125 mL glasses of red wine and 10–50 g of alcohol a day for men of one to four glasses of red wine.[17,18] Fish, shellfish, crustaceans, and mollusks are incorporated depending on proximity to the sea, while meats, predominantly from goats and sheep, are used sparingly.[5,11,19]

Despite common themes, defining specific Mediterranean diets has proven to be challenging. Mediterranean countries' eating and culinary cultures reflect their individual histories and traditions, making the diet patterns quite variable. As a result, components used to calculate adherence to a particular diet are widely different and poorly correlated.[20] This has made it difficult to compare trials and understand the mechanisms that drive health benefits.[12]

Components of the Mediterranean diets have commonly been presented as food pyramids. A representative sample of pyramids include the first pyramid created by Oldways Preservation and Exchange Trust in 1993 and later revised in 2009,[12,21] the Greek Dietary Guidelines in 1999,[22] and the Mediterranean Diet Foundation in 2010.[23,24] However, the differences among definitions are interpretive. For instance, the Mediterranean Diet Foundation suggests that breads and cereals are consumed in 1–2 servings with each meal, while the 1999 Greek Dietary Guidelines calculates the frequency as eight servings daily.[12] Alternatively, the Oldways Preservation and Trust quantifies the frequency of nut consumption in terms of every meal, while the 1999 Greek Dietary Guidelines proposes that nuts are consumed in 3–4 servings weekly (Figure 9.1).[12]

To quantitatively define Mediterranean diets, Davis et al.[12] conducted a systematic review of the literature with general descriptive definitions, diet pyramids, number

Foods	Oldway's Preservation and Trust (2009) [21]	Mediterranean Diet Foundation (2011) [5]	1999 Greek Dietary Guidelines (1999) [22] [1]
Olive oil	Every meal	Every meal	Main added lipid
Vegetables	Every meal	≥2 serves every meal	6 serves daily
Fruits	Every meal	1–2 serves every meal	3 serves daily
Breads and cereals	Every meal	1–2 serves every meal	8 serves daily
Legumes	Every meal	≥2 serves weekly	3–4 serves weekly
Nuts	Every meal	1–2 serves daily	3–4 serves weekly
Fish/seafood	Often, at least two times per week	≥2 serves weekly	5–6 servings weekly
Eggs	Moderate portions, daily to weekly	2–4 serves weekly	3 servings weekly
Poultry	Moderate portions, daily to weekly	2 serves weekly	4 servings weekly
Dairy foods	Moderate portions, daily to weekly	2 serves daily	2 serves daily
Red meat	Less often	<2 serves/week	4 servings monthly
Sweets	Less often	<2 serves/week	3 servings weekly
Red wine	In moderation	In moderation and respecting social beliefs	Daily in moderation

[1] Serving sizes specified as: 25 g bread, 100 g potato, 50–60 g cooked pasta, 100 g vegetables, 80 g apple, 60 g banana, 100 g orange, 200 g melon, 30 g grapes, 1 cup milk or yoghurt, 1 egg, 60 g meat, and 100 g cooked dry beans.

FIGURE 9.1   Comparison of Mediterranean diet pyramids. (Sourced from definition of the Mediterranean diet by Davis et al.[12] and reprinted with permission from Dr. Courtney Davis.)

of servings of foods, grams of key food groups, and nutrient content. They found considerable variation in the quantity of different food groups, with olive oil consumption ranging from 15.7 to 80 mL/day, legumes from 5.5 to 60.5 g/day, vegetables from 210 to 682 g/day, and fruits and nuts from 109 to 463 g/day.[12] They also found that among studies, the nutrient content was more consistent than food quantity, suggesting some key components including consumption of fatty acids as a percentage of total energy intake, and protein, folate, β-carotene, antioxidants, or phytosterol content could be used to define the diet.[12] However, because servings of food tend to be better received than nutrients or grams, they calculated the portion sizes based on observational studies: a Mediterranean diet consists of approximately seven servings of bread, four servings of cereal, five servings of vegetables, 1.5 servings of potato, 1.5 servings of fruit, 0.5–0.75 servings of meat, 0.5 servings of cheese, and one serving of dairy per day, along with one serving of nuts and three servings of legumes and fish per week.[12] These findings differed from popular Mediterranean diet pyramids, which, for example, recommend 3–4 servings of nuts and three daily servings of fruit. The research team hypothesized that this mismatch between recommendations created from Cretan, Greek, and Southern Italian dietary patterns in the 1960s and what is practiced today reflect the influence of globalization and the spread of the Western diet [12]

To better understand the impact of Mediterranean diets on health, various questionnaires have been developed. These questionnaires typically document food frequency and portion size and convert answers into a score or quantitative measure that represents adherence.[5] Trichopoulou et al.[25] designed the first food frequency questionnaire – the Mediterranean diet score – in 1995, which was subsequently revised in 2003. Points were awarded for consumption at or greater than the median quantity of food items characteristic of a Mediterranean diet, including vegetables, legumes, fruits, nuts, cereal, and fish. Points were also awarded for consuming less than median quantities of foods not commonly found in a Mediterranean diet, including meat, poultry, and dairy.[25,26] Multiple different scores have since been developed including the 14-point adherence index validated in the Prevención con Dieta Mediterránea (PREDIMED) study.[27]

9.3   MOLECULAR MECHANISMS

Adherence to a Mediterranean diet has been shown to lower the risk of CVD, cancer, and metabolic disease, but the mechanisms that drive these effects are not fully clarified. This is important for successful implementation tactics and development of comprehensive approaches to prevent chronic disease, especially those involving other aspects of lifestyle medicine. Five main categories of mechanisms to enhance longevity have been proposed: lipid-lowering effect, protection against oxidative stress and inflammation, modifications of hormones involved in the pathogenesis of cancer, alteration of nutrient-sensing pathways by amino acids, and gut microbiota metabolites' influence on metabolic health.[28] These effects appear to be the result of the high plant consumption and high intake of olive oils and nuts (Figure 9.2), which carry downstream anti-inflammatory and antioxidant effects.

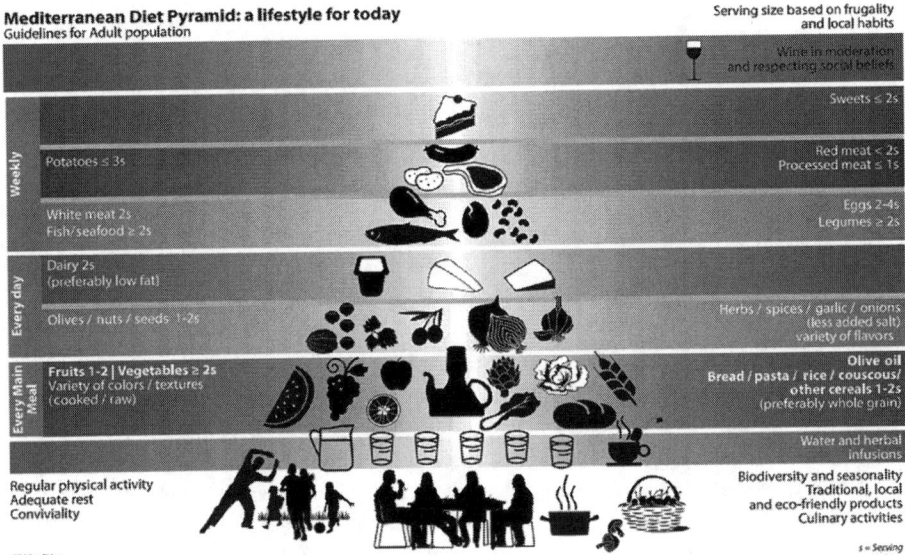

FIGURE 9.2 Mediterranean Diet Foundation Diet Pyramid. (Sourced from the Fundación Dieta Mediterránea and reprinted with permission from Ms. Jordi González Juste.[24])

9.3.1 Lipid Lowering

Atherosclerosis is the leading cause of CHD and develops in the setting of elevated cholesterol and inflammation.[29] Epidemiological studies have shown that reduced intake of saturated fatty acids (SFAs) is associated with lower cholesterol levels and reduced incidence of CHD, especially when saturated fat is substituted with polyunsaturated fatty acids (PUFAs) and monounsaturated fatty acids (MUFAs).[30]

People who incorporate a Mediterranean dietary pattern into their lifestyle have lower LDL and total cholesterol. While Mediterranean diets involve a relatively high consumption of total fat predominantly from extra virgin olive oil (EVOO) and nuts, the total intake of SFAs is low due to minimal consumption of meat, milk, and butter.[28] As a result, Mediterranean diets involve a high consumption of MUFAs and low consumption of atherogenic SFAs. This both lowers plasma levels of LDL cholesterol and reduces oxidation of LDL particles. MUFAs reduce the susceptibility of LDL to oxidize compared to LDL enriched in SFAs.[31,32] Oxidized LDL serves as a prognostic marker for subclinical atherosclerosis, and higher levels confer greater risk of acute CHD. Therefore, lowering oxidized LDL levels can be protective against heart disease.[33] MUFAs reduce blood pressure, pro-inflammatory plasma proteins, and several markers of oxidative stress as well as offer protection against the vascular aging process.[31,32,34] SFAs and MUFAs have also been shown to alter expression of genes in adipose tissue, with a high-SFA diet increasing expression of genes involved in inflammation within adipocytes.[35] Higher MUFA intake induces a more anti-inflammatory gene expression profile with a decrease in peripheral blood cell expression of oxidative phosphorylation and inflammation related processes.[31,32,34–36]

Another mechanism that may drive lower levels of cholesterol is high dietary fiber consumption. Mediterranean diets provide at least 14 g of vegetable fiber for each 1,000 kcal per day, which is more than double than is consumed in more Westernized diets. High intake of water-soluble fiber, found in high concentrations in beans and fruit, has a significant cholesterol-lowering effect, with each additional gram of fiber lowering plasma LDL cholesterol by approximately 1.12 mg/L.[37,38] Additionally, high intake of phytosterols from nuts, seeds, whole grains, vegetables, and fruit may contribute to lower cholesterol levels by competing with intestinal cholesterol absorption.[39]

9.3.2 Oxidative Stress and Inflammation

Several studies found that adherence to the Mediterranean diet affects expression of inflammatory mediators. In the PREDIMED study, after 3 months, plasma concentrations of the inflammatory markers interleukin-6 (IL-6), vascular cell adhesion molecule-1 (VCAM-1), and intercellular adhesion molecule-1 (ICAM-1) decreased in both Mediterranean diet groups, while C-reactive protein (CRP) was decreased in just the Mediterranean diet supplemented with EVOO.[40] By contrast, VCAM-1 and ICAM-1 concentrations increased after 3 months in the control, low-fat diet group.[40] Moreover, in both Mediterranean diet groups, concentrations of molecules involved in adhesion, inflammation, and atherosclerosis were lower than those found in the control group, including cluster of differentiation (CD)49d, CD11b, and CD40 expression in T-lymphocytes and monocytes.[41] One year after subjects followed their assigned diets, the plasma concentrations of IL-6, tumor necrosis factor receptor (TNFR) 60, and TNFR80 decreased in both Mediterranean diet groups, while ICAM-1, TNFR60, and TNFR80 increased in the control low-fat diet group.[42] These findings suggest that the Mediterranean diet pattern inhibits inflammatory pathways related to atherosclerosis.

Mediterranean diets typically include a copious consumption of vegetables, fruits, nuts, seeds, legumes, whole grains, and EVOO, which are rich in antioxidant vitamins and phenolic phytochemicals. These phytochemicals are bioactive non-nutrient plant compounds that have been associated with protection from various chronic diseases, including heart disease, cancer, diabetes, and hypertension.[43] For instance, the aleurone layer of wheat bran contains ferulic acid, alkylresorcinols, apigenin, lignans, and phytic acid, which have antioxidant and anticarcinogenic activities in rodent models of colon and skin cancer.[44–46] Spermidine, found in the germ of whole grains, has been shown to extend life span in flies, nematodes, rodents, and human cells, possibly by inhibiting histone acetyltransferases, resulting in higher resistance to oxidative stress, reduced subclinical inflammation, and reduced rates of cell necrosis during aging.[47] Other phytochemicals found in plants exert anti-cancer effects and include lycopene in tomatoes, capsaicin in hot pepper, sulforaphane in cruciferous vegetables, and monoterpenes in citrus fruit.[48]

The beneficial, particularly anti-inflammatory, effects of olive oil may be due to the high content of phenolic compounds, such as α-tocopherol, carotenoids, and MUFAs.[49–52] Up to 36 polyphenols in olive oil have been identified, although the collection of polyphenols found in a specific batch changes depending on the variety of olive fruit, region of production, agricultural techniques, fruit maturity at harvest, and oil-processing methods.[53] Oleuropein has been found to inhibit vascular smooth muscle cell proliferation through a cell cycle block between the G1 and S phases, inhibit lipoxygenase activity and production of leukotriene, and exhibit anti-ischemic and hypolipidemic activities.[54–56] Hydroxytyrosol has been found to attenuate tumor necrosis factor-α, inducible nitric oxide synthase, and cyclooxygenase-2 in lipopolysaccharide-induced monocytes and inhibit production of nitric oxide and prostaglandin E.[57,58] Oleocanthal possesses a similar chemical structure to ibuprofen and acts to inhibit the cyclooxygenase enzymes in the prostaglandin biosynthesis pathway, providing anti-inflammatory effects.[59] Oleic acid, the main fatty acid in olive oil, diminishes the inflammatory effects of SFAs in human aortic endothelial cells by reducing the incorporation of stearic acid into phospholipids and by decreasing nuclear factor-$\kappa\beta$ activation.[60]

9.3.3 CANCER

Calorie restriction without malnutrition has been shown to effectively reduce the incidence of cancer in animal models and reduce several metabolic and hormonal factors connected to the pathogenesis of several common cancers in humans.[61] However, even without intentionally reducing caloric intake, substituting refined and processed foods found in Western eating patterns with minimally processed plant foods, characteristic of Mediterranean eating, has been found to result in significant weight loss.[62] In a 5-month study where women were randomized to a Mediterranean diet without calorie restriction, participants lost 4 kg compared to the control group and had a reduction in fasting glucose, c-peptide, and total and free testosterone.[62] A possible mechanism of the weight loss is the increased production of gut hormones, including glucagon-like peptide-1 (GLP-1) and peptide YY, due to short-chain fatty acid (SCFA) production. These SCFAs are produced by gut microbiota metabolism of the resistant starch and oligosaccharides commonly found in foods consumed in a Mediterranean diet.[63] FFA2 and FFA3, receptors for SCFAs, are expressed in neuroendocrine tissues of the intestinal tract, pancreatic β-cells, adipocytes, and cells of the immune system.[63] The increased insulin sensitivity may be due to SCFA activity at these receptors, affecting GLP-1, PYY, and leptin production as well as diminishing systemic inflammation.[63] The weight loss that ensues may also reduce insulin resistance, which is enhanced with a higher intake of low-glycemic index foods and MUFAs.[62,64,65] As for the hormonal changes observed, the same women were also found to have increased plasma concentrations of insulin growth factor-binding protein (IGFBP)-1, IGFBP-2, and sex hormone-binding globulin. Insulin, estrogen, androgens, and IGF-1 can act as mitogens, which stimulate the development of common cancers, such as breast, colon, prostate, and endometrial histotypes; lower hormonal activity may help reduce the risk of development or progression of certain malignancies.[66] Additionally, the high fiber content of a Mediterranean diet may help increase fecal excretion of estrogens, leading to reduced plasma levels of estrone and estradiol.[67] The high fiber diet also accelerates colonic transit and may limit absorption of carcinogenic substances.[28]

9.3.4 Nutrient Sensing

Animal models have shown that moderate protein restriction can extend lifespan. The protein intake in the traditional Mediterranean diet is roughly 20% lower than that in the typical Western diet, with animal protein consumption 50%–60% lower.[68] The protein content in a Mediterranean diet derives predominantly from legumes and whole cereals.[69] Isocaloric restriction of protein or substitution of animal protein with plant protein has been found to significantly slow prostate and breast cancer growth.[68] This reduction is also associated with a decrease in serum IGF-1 levels and mechanistic target of rapamycin (mTOR) activity in human xenograft animal models.[68] mTOR is a protein kinase that regulates cell growth, survival, metabolism, and immunity, which are implicated in the development of several cancers.[70]

In an epidemiological study using the National Health and Nutrition Examination Survey (NHANES) III database, individuals aged 50–65 years with the highest protein intake, at more than 20% of their total daily calories, had a 75% increase in total mortality and a four-fold increase in cancer mortality.[71] Other epidemiological studies suggest that high protein intake is associated with a higher risk of obesity, CVD, and type 2 diabetes.[72] A randomized clinical trial recruited middle-aged, mildly obese men and separated them into an isocaloric diet restricted to 7%–9% of the daily calories from protein versus a control diet with roughly 50% more protein per day.[73] After an average of 43 days, the protein-restricted group experienced a significant decrease in body weight, fat mass, and fasting glucose levels.[73] Another controlled trial randomized postmenopausal women with obesity to one of three interventions: a weight loss group that consumed a hypocaloric diet with 0.8 g of protein per kilogram body weight per day; a weight loss and high-protein diet group that consumed a hypocaloric diet containing 1.2 g of protein per kilogram body weight per day; and a weight maintenance control group.[74] After 26–29 weeks, the participants in the weight loss groups successfully lost roughly 10% of their body weight. However, while individuals in the lower protein weight loss group had an increased glucose disposal rate, their counterparts on the weight loss diet supplemented with protein saw no significant change, suggesting that high protein intake prevented the weight loss-mediated improvement in glucose metabolism.[74]

As Mediterranean diets involve higher plant protein and lower animal protein consumption than the Western diet, the specific amino acids found in each diet differ and can affect disease processes in the human body. For example, methionine, leucine, isoleucine, valine, and tryptophan are 20%–40% lower in Mediterranean diets than in the Western diet.[28] Methionine restriction has been found to extend average and maximal lifespan, improve glucose metabolism, protect against obesity and hepatic steatosis, and reduce oxidative stress in rodents.[75] The branched-chain amino acids leucine, isoleucine, and valine have been found to modulate insulin sensitivity.[76] In insulin-resistant humans and rodents, branched-chain amino acids levels are at higher levels.[73] However, reduction of the dietary intake of these amino acids improves glucose tolerance, β-cell stress, and body composition.[73]

9.3.5 GUT MICROBIOTA

The significance of the gut microbiome on human health has become increasingly apparent, having effects on many chronic disease processes, including cancers, autoimmune conditions, and obesity.[77,78] Environmental exposures, such as maternal interactions, diet, antibiotics, and surgery, can significantly impact the composition of the gut microbiome. Moreover, specific nutrients, particularly protein and insoluble fiber, have been found to alter the gut microbiome and, as a result, play a role in human health.[28] Mediterranean diets contain significantly more fiber than a Western diet, and in the mammalian colon, resistant starches and fibers are fermented by gut microbiota to produce SCFAs, which include acetate, propionate, and butyrate.[79,80] Adherence to a Mediterranean dietary pattern supports the population of gut bacteria that more effectively produce SCFAs, including the genera *Bacteroides*, *Prevotella*, and *Faecalibacterium*.[81] Specific bacterial species in these genera, such as *Bacteroides fragilis* and *Faecalibacterium prausnitzii* have been found to induce CD4+ T cells, which secrete anti-inflammatory interleukin-10.[82,83]

SCFAs produced by the microbiota have been associated with multiple beneficial effects including reduced gut mucosal permeability, decreased rates of colon cancer, suppressed pro-inflammatory mediators, increased release of satiety hormones GLP-1 and GLP-2, and attenuated risk of autoimmune diseases.[80] These outcomes are thought to be mediated by specific G-protein-coupled receptor activation on immune cells and epigenetic effects through inhibition of histone deacetylases.[80,81] By contrast, choline and L-carnitine, found in red meats, eggs, and cheeses, are consumed at 50% greater quantities in a Western diet than in a Mediterranean diet. These compounds are metabolized to tri-methylamine N-oxide (TMAO), a compound found to increase the risk of developing CVD and exerting a prothrombotic effect in both rodent models and humans.[84,85]

9.4 CLINICAL STUDIES

9.4.1 CARDIOVASCULAR DISEASE

Mediterranean diets have consistently been associated with a lower incidence of CVD outcomes, beginning with the landmark Seven Countries study by Ancel Keys et al.[2] Subsequently, one of the largest prospective cohort studies ($N = 74,886$ female nurses without a history of CVD or diabetes, followed up from 1984 to 2004) used the NHS database to examine how a Mediterranean diet affected the risk for cardiovascular events in women.[86] Adherence to the Mediterranean diet used in the study was measured by the alternate Mediterranean diet (aMed) score, based on the initial score by Trichopoulou et al.[25,86] The study found that women in the top quintile of the Mediterranean diet score were at lower risk for CHD and CVD mortality than those in the bottom quintile (CHD RR: 0.71, CI: 0.62–0.82; CVD mortality RR: 0.61, CI: 0.49–0.76).[86] A subsequent study added 29,343 male health professionals from the Health Professionals Follow-up Study to the 50,195 women from the NHS cohort and found that an increase in the aMed score after 4 years was accompanied by a 9% lower CVD risk (95% CI: 3%–14%) over the next 20 years of follow-up.[87] Similarly, the

EPIC-Norfolk study followed up 23,902 subjects in the United Kingdom for 12 years and found an inverse association between Mediterranean diet adherence and CVD morality (HR: 0.91, 95% CI: 0.87–0.96), ischemic heart disease (HR: 0.94, CI: 0.90–0.98), and stroke (HR: 0.93, 95% CI: 0.87–0.99).[88] The EPIC-NL study followed up 34,708 participants in the Netherlands for 10–15 years and found that increased adherence was inversely associated with fatal CVD (HR: 0.78, 95% CI: 0.69–0.88) and myocardial infarction (HR: 0.86, 95% CI: 0.79–0.93).[89] A 2020 systematic review and meta-analysis by Becerra-Tomás et al.[97] included 38 cohorts and compared highest versus lowest categories of Mediterranean diet adherence. Their analysis showed inverse associations with CVD mortality (RR: 0.79; 95% CI: 0.77–0.82), CHD incidence (RR: 0.73, 95% CI: 0.62–0.86), CHD mortality (RR: 0.83, 95% CI: 0.75–0.92), stroke incidence (RR: 0.80, 95% CI: 0.71–0.90), stroke mortality (RR: 0.87, 95% CI: 0.80–0.96), and myocardial infarction incidence (RR: 0.73, 95% CI: 0.61–0.88).[90,91]

The Lyon Diet Heart Study[92] was a secondary prevention randomized control trial that examined whether a Mediterranean diet rich in alpha-linolenic acid would reduce the rate of a recurrent myocardial infarction after the first event. Six hundred five patients were recruited in France between March 1988 and March 1992 who had survived a myocardial infarction within 6 months of enrollment. These individuals were randomized to a Mediterranean-type diet or a more prudent Western diet, which served as the control group. The experimental group received counseling from a research cardiologist and dietician. The participants were advised to incorporate more bread, vegetables, fish, and fruit as well as to reduce meat consumption and replace butter and cream with provided margarine. By contrast, the control group received standard dietary advice from hospital dieticians or attending physicians. Primary endpoints were death from cardiovascular causes and non-fatal myocardial infarctions, while secondary endpoints included unstable angina, stroke, heart failure, pulmonary embolism, and peripheral embolism. Analysis of results in 1998, with a mean follow-up of 46 months per patient, found that there were significantly less events in the group directed to follow the Mediterranean diet than the control. The Mediterranean diet group had 14 events versus 44 in the control diet group (P=0.0001). When secondary endpoints were included, the Mediterranean diet group had 27 events compared to the control group, which experienced 90 events (P=0.0001).[93] This achieved a risk reduction of 0.27 (95% confidence interval: 0.12–0.59) for cardiac death and non-fatal myocardial infarction and 0.30 (95% confidence interval: 0.11–0.82) for overall mortality.[92]

The largest dietary intervention trial was the PREDIMED study, a large multicenter randomized control trial conducted in Spain to assess the effects of the Mediterranean diet on primary prevention of CVD. This study focused on specific dietary ingredients that emerged as the strongest candidates for the beneficial effects seen in the Mediterranean diet. The study recruited 7,447 participants between 55 and 80 years of age between June 2003 and June 2009 who were assigned to one of three dietary intervention groups: a Mediterranean diet supplemented with EVOO, a Mediterranean diet-supplemented with nuts, or a control low-fat diet. Eligible participants had to have no documented CVD but be at high risk of developing CVD, defined as having comorbidities including diabetes mellitus type 2, hypertension, dyslipidemia, a history of smoking, excess weight, or a family history of premature CHD. The primary endpoint was a composite of myocardial infarction, stroke, and death from cardiovascular causes. Subjects assigned to this Mediterranean diet with EVOO received 1 L of oil per week per household, with the recommendation for each person to consume at least four tablespoons of oil per day. Participants allocated to the group following the Mediterranean diet supplemented with nuts received 30 g of mixed nuts per day per person. The control group received nonfood gifts.

Participants in either of the Mediterranean diet groups received dietary training sessions, which included a 14-item dietary questionnaire, to assess adherence to the Mediterranean diet that was subsequently used to provide personalized advice to improve adherence.[94] This questionnaire set specific criteria for what is expected of adherence to the Mediterranean diet, and if these criteria were met, a point would be added to the score. Criteria included at least two servings of vegetables a day, at least four tablespoons of EVOO per day, at least seven glasses of wine per week, preferential consumption of poultry over red meats, and less than one sweetened beverage a day.[27] Participants in the control group completed the 14-item questionnaire at their baseline visit to assess their adherence to the Mediterranean diet and subsequently received a leaflet about the low-fat diet.[94] The study was structured to follow up subjects for 6 years but was prematurely stopped at a median of 4.8 years of follow-up. Interim analysis provided sufficient evidence of benefit for the two Mediterranean diets. The group following the Mediterranean diet supplemented with EVOO had 96 events (3.8%), while that assigned to a Mediterranean diet supplemented with nuts had 83 events (3.4%). 109 (4.4%) events occurred in the control group.[94] The hazard ratio for events in the group supplemented with EVOO was 0.70 (95% CI: 0.53–0.92), and the hazard ratio for the group supplemented with nuts was 0.70 (95% CI: 0.53–0.94) when compared to the control diet.[94]

Of note, the PREDIMED trial and the findings on cardiovascular outcomes were initially published in 2013[95] but retracted after an audit found irregularities in randomization of participants to study arms.[96] Instead, participants were assigned based on clinic site, and randomization tables were used inconsistently. These aberrations affected 21% of subjects.[96] After the original paper was retracted, data were re-analyzed as a non-randomized study and excluded participants who were not randomized appropriately.[96] The modified results were published in 2018.[94] Given the impaired randomization, it is unclear whether these changes to the analyses increase the validity of the results, especially as the trial design already has weaknesses including a lack of blinding and possible investigator bias.

Despite their flaws, these seminal clinical trials motivated other investigations to explore the impact of diet on CVD, including the ongoing Coronary Diet Intervention with Olive Oil Cardiovascular Prevention Study (CORDIOPREV).[97] This study enrolled 1,002 patients with a history of coronary heart disease (CHD) between July 2009 and February 2012 and randomized participants to consume either a Mediterranean diet rich in extra virgin olive oil or a low-fat diet. These groups will be followed up for 7 years to observe the effect of the diet on cardiovascular events during this time.[97]

9.4.2 OBESITY

The European Prospective Investigation into Cancer and Nutrition-Physical Activity, Nutrition, Alcohol Consumption, Cessation of Smoking, Eating Out of Home, and Obesity (EPIC-PANACEA[98]) project was an observation study that followed up

373,803 individuals from ten European countries over a median of 5 years. The investigators found that participants who had greater adherence to Mediterranean dietary patterns lost weight and were 10% less likely to become overweight or obese than their low-adherence counterparts.[98] A systematic review by Mancini et al.[99] included five randomized controlled trials with a total of 998 subjects and showed that a Mediterranean diet resulted in greater weight loss than the low-fat diet after at least 12 months of the follow-up. The subjects on the Mediterranean diet in this study had a mean weight change between −4.1 and −10.1 kg, the low-fat and/or low-carb diet had a change of −4.7 to −7.7 kg, and the control diet saw a change of +2.9 to −5.7 kg.[99] These findings affirmed that despite the high fat intake, the Mediterranean dietary pattern does not increase weight gain and can instead help with weight loss, reduce risk of developing obesity, and by extension, reduce risks of obesity-related complications.

9.4.3   Type 2 Diabetes

The ATTICA study[100] was conducted in Greece and found that individuals with higher adherence to a Greek Mediterranean diet had a lower 10-year incidence of type 2 diabetes. The study was based on a large-scale, health and nutrition-oriented, prospective design carried out from 2001 to 2002 in the province of Attica, where Athens is a major metropolis. Three thousand forty-two people without a history of CVD or atherosclerotic disease, chronic viral infections, or living in institutions were recruited and interviewed about their sociodemographic characteristics, history of hypertension, hypercholesterolemia, diabetes, family history of CVD, dietary habits, smoking, and physical activity. Their nutritional habits were evaluated using a food frequency questionnaire, and their adherence to the Greek Mediterranean diet was measured by Trichopoulou's Mediterranean diet score.[25] After removing 210 individuals with diabetes at baseline and 1,347 people without data regarding their diabetes status after 10 years, 1,485 participants were examined. During the 10-year follow-up period, 191 cases of type 2 diabetes were recorded, and the investigators found that the incidence of type 2 diabetes was 21% in participants who had poor adherence to this Mediterranean diet, 8% who had medium adherence, and 5% who had high adherence ($P < 0.001$).[100] Subgroup analysis of the participants without diabetes when initially randomized at the onset of the PREDIMED trial likewise found a reduced risk of type 2 diabetes, with a 30% risk reduction in those randomized to a Mediterranean diet when compared to the control group.[101]

9.4.4   Cancer

A comprehensive meta-analysis by Morze et al.[102] included 117 randomized controlled trials, case–control studies, and cohort studies published up to April 2020, with a total of 3,202,496 participants. Study findings demonstrated that the highest adherence to a Mediterranean diet among cancer survivors was inversely associated with cancer mortality (RR: 0.87, 95% CI: 0.82–0.92) and all-cause mortality (RR: 0.75, 95% CI: 0.66–0.86.) High adherence to a Mediterranean diet was also found to be associated with reduced risk of multiple types of cancer, including breast (RR: 0.94, 95% CI: 0.90–0.97), colorectal (RR: 0.83, 95% CI: 0.76–0.90), head and neck

(RR: 0.56, 95% CI: 0.44–0.72), respiratory (RR: 0.84, 95% CI: 0.76–0.94), gastric (RR: 0.70, 95% CI: 0.61–0.80), bladder (RR: 0.87, 95% CI: 0.76–0.98), and liver histotypes (RR: 0.64, 95% CI: 0.54–0.75).[102]

Among intervention studies, 35 of the 4,152 women in PREDIMED[103] were diagnosed with breast cancer, and the women in the Mediterranean diet arm supplemented with EVOO exhibited significant protection (hazard ratio (HR): 0.32, 95% confidence interval (CI): 0.13–0.79). In the Lyon Heart Study,[104] increased adherence to the Mediterranean diet yielded 61% reduction in cancer incidence after 4 years of follow-up. Likewise, the EPIC cohort[105] also demonstrated a lower overall cancer risk among those with a higher Mediterranean diet score, with stronger inverse associations for smoking-related cancers.

9.4.5 LONGEVITY

Trichopoulou et al.[25] conducted one of the first studies on the association between Mediterranean diets and life expectancy. 182 residents who were older than 70 years were recruited from three Greek villages, and a Mediterranean diet score was developed to assess their adherence to the Mediterranean dietary pattern. After follow-up in 1993–1994, the results showed that a higher diet score was significantly associated with a reduced risk of death: risk of death was reduced by 17% per one unit increase in diet score and by more than 50% per four-unit increases.[25] The Melbourne Collaborative Cohort Study followed up 41,513 men and women over an average of 19 years and similarly showed that adherence to a Mediterranean diet was associated with less overall and cardiovascular mortality (HR: 0.86, CI: 0.80–0.93).[106] In studies using the NHS cohort by Crous-Bou et al.,[91,107] women who more closely followed a Mediterranean diet had longer telomere lengths, suggesting an association of this dietary pattern with deceleration of the aging process. However, results from other interventional studies have not been so clear. In the PREDIMED trial,[94] Mediterranean diet interventions had no significant effect on all-cause mortality (RR: 1.01, 95% CI: 0.81–1.25). On the contrary, i the Lyon Heart Study,[91,92] the results suggested that this Mediterranean diet intervention could reduce risk of total mortality.

Disclosures:
None

REFERENCES

1. Radd-Vagenas S, Kouris-Blazos A, Singh MF, Flood VM. Evolution of mediterranean diets and cuisine: concepts and definitions. *Asia Pac J Clin Nutr.* 2017;26(5):749–763.
2. Keys A, Menotti A, Aravanis C, et al. The seven countries study: 2,289 deaths in 15 years. *Prev Med.* 1984;13(2):141–154.
3. Menotti A, Keys A, Blackburn H, et al. Comparison of multivariate predictive power of major risk factors for coronary heart diseases in different countries: results from eight nations of the Seven Countries Study, 25-year follow-up. *J Cardiovasc Risk.* 1996; 3(1):69–75.
4. Willett WC, Sacks F, Trichopoulou A, et al. Mediterranean diet pyramid: a cultural model for healthy eating. *Am J Clin Nutr.* 1995;61(6 Suppl):1402S–1406S.

5. Hidalgo-Mora JJ, Garcia-Vigara A, Sanchez-Sanchez ML, Garcia-Perez MA, Tarin J, Cano A. The mediterranean diet: a historical perspective on food for health. *Maturitas.* 2020;132:65–69.

6. Sukkar SG. Mediterranean diet? no, thanks: mediterranean lifestyle! *Med J Nutr Metab.* 2011(4): 79–81.

7. Zohary D, Hopf M, Weiss E. *Domestication of Plants in the Old World: The Origin and Spread of Cultivated Plants in Southwest Asia, Europ, and the Mediterranean Basin.* Oxford, UK: Oxford Universit Press; 2012.

8. Serra-Majem L, Román-Viñas B, Snachez-Villegas A, Guasch-Ferré M, Corella D, Vecchia CL. Benefits of the mediterranean diet: epidemiological and molecular aspects. *Mol Aspects Med.* 2019;67:1–55.

9. Altomare R, Cacciabaudo F, Damiano G, et al. The mediterranean diet: a history of health. *Iran J Public Health.* 2013;42(5):449–457.

10. Louis AF. *Feating & fasting in Crete.* Athens, Greece: Kedros Publications; 2001.

11. Wahlqvist ML, Kouris-Blazos A, Trichopolous A. The wisdom of the Greek cuisine and way of life: comparison of the food and health beliefs of elderly Greeks in Greece and Australia. *Age Nutr.* 1991(2): 163–173.

12. Davis C, Cryan J, Hodgson J, Murphy K. Definition of the mediterranean diet: a literature review. *Nutrients.* 2015;7:9139–9153.

13. Salas-Salvadi J, Papandreou C. The mediterranean diet: history, concepts and elements. In: Preedy V, Watson RR, eds. *The Mediterranean Diet: An Evidence-Based approach.* Jerusalem: Academic Press; 2015.

14. Trichopoulou A, Lagiou P. Healthy traditional mediterranean diet: an expression of culture, history, and lifestyle. *Nutr Rev.* 1997;55(11 Pt 1):383–389.

15. Rizzello CG, Cavoski I, Turk J, Ercolini D, Nionelli L, Pontonio E, De Angelis M, De Filippis F, Gobbetti M, Di Cagno R. Organic cultivation of *Triticum turgidum* subsp. *durum* is reflected in the flour-sourdough fermentation-bread axis. *Appl Environ Microbiol.* 2015 May 1;81(9):3192–3204.

16. Arnoni Y, Berry E. On the origins and evolution of the mediterranean diet. In: Preedy V, Watson RR, eds. *The Mediterranean Diet: An Evidence Based Approach.* Jerusalem: Academic Press; 2015.

17. Minzer S, Estruch R, Casas R. Wine intake in the framework of a mediterranean diet and chronic non-communicable diseases: a short literature review of the last 5 years. *Molecules.* 2020;25(21):5045.

18. Morales G, Martínez-González MA, Barbería-Latasa M, Bes-Rasstrollo M, Gea A. Mediterranean diet, alcohol-drinking pattern and their combined effect on all-cause mortality: the Seguimiento Universidad de Navarra (SUN) cohort. *European Journal of Nutrition.* 2020;60:1489–1498.

19. Topić Popović N, Benussi Skukan A, Džidara P, et al. Microbiological quality of marketed fresh and frozen seafood caught off the Adriatic coast of Croatia. *Veterinarni Medicina.* 2017;55(5):233–241.

20. Mila-Villarroel R, Bach-Faig A, Puig J, et al. Comparison and evaluation of the reliability of indexes of adherence to the mediterranean diet. *Public Health Nutr.* 2011; 14(12A):2338–2345.

21. Mediterranean Diet Pyramid. https://oldwayspt.org/traditional-diets/mediterranean-diet. Accessed 11/5/2021.

22. Varela-Moreiras G, Avila JM, Cuadrado C, del Pozo S, Ruiz E, Moreiras O. Evaluation of food consumption and dietary patterns in Spain by the Food Consumption Survey: updated information. *Eur J Clin Nutr.* 2010;64(Suppl 3): S37–43.

23. Bach-Faig A, Berry EM, Lairon D, et al. Mediterranean diet pyramid today. Science and cultural updates. *Public Health Nutr.* 2011;14(12A):2274–2284.

24. The Mediterranean Diet pyramid has adapted to the new way of life. CIHEAM - Mediterranean Agronomic Institute of Chania. http://www.mediterradiet.org/nutrition/mediterranean_diet_pyramid. Accessed 12/31/2021.

25. Trichopoulou A, Kouris-Blazos A, Wahlqvist ML, et al. Diet and overall survival in elderly people. *BMJ.* 1995;311(7018):1457–1460.

26. Trichopoulou A, Costacou T, Bamia C, Trichopoulos D. Adherence to a Mediterranean diet and survival in a Greek population. *N Engl J Med.* 2003;348(26):2599–2608.

27. Martinez-Gonzalez MA, Garcia-Arellano A, Toledo E, et al. A 14-item mediterranean diet assessment tool and obesity indexes among high-risk subjects: the PREDIMED trial. *PLoS One.* 2012;7(8):e43134.

28. Tosti V, Bertozzi B, Fontana L. Health benefits of the mediterranean diet: metabolic and molecular mechanisms. *J Gerontol A Biol Sci Med Sci.* 2018;73(3):318–326.

29. Hansson GK. Inflammation, atherosclerosis, and coronary artery disease. *N Engl J Med.* 2005;352(16):1685–1695.

30. Sacks FM, Lichtenstein AH, Wu JHY, et al. Dietary fats and cardiovascular disease: a presidential advisory from the American Heart Association. *Circulation.* 2017;136(3):e1–e23.

31. Schwingshackl L, Hoffmann G. Monounsaturated fatty acids and risk of cardiovascular disease: synopsis of the evidence available from systematic reviews and meta-analyses. *Nutrients.* 2012;4(12):1989–2007.

32. Sales-Campos H, Souza PR, Peghini BC, da Silva JS, Cardoso CR. An overview of the modulatory effects of oleic acid in health and disease. *Mini Rev Med Chem.* 2013;13(2):201–210.

33. Meisinger C, Baumert J, Khuseyinova N, Loewel H, Koenig W. Plasma oxidized low-density lipoprotein, a strong predictor for acute coronary heart disease events in apparently healthy, middle-aged men from the general population. *Circulation.* 2005;112(5):651–657.

34. Marin C, Yubero-Serrano EM, Lopez-Miranda J, Perez-Jimenez F. Endothelial aging associated with oxidative stress can be modulated by a healthy mediterranean diet. *Int J Mol Sci.* 2013;14(5):8869–8889.

35. van Dijk SJ, Feskens EJ, Bos MB, et al. A saturated fatty acid-rich diet induces an obesity-linked proinflammatory gene expression profile in adipose tissue of subjects at risk of metabolic syndrome. *Am J Clin Nutr.* 2009;90(6):1656–1664.

36. van Dijk SJ, Feskens EJ, Bos MB, et al. Consumption of a high monounsaturated fat diet reduces oxidative phosphorylation gene expression in peripheral blood mononuclear cells of abdominally overweight men and women. *J Nutr.* 2012;142(7):1219–1225.

37. Salas-Salvado J, Farres X, Luque X, et al. Effect of two doses of a mixture of soluble fibres on body weight and metabolic variables in overweight or obese patients: a randomised trial. *Br J Nutr.* 2008;99(6):1380–1387.

38. Theuwissen E, Mensink RP. Water-soluble dietary fibers and cardiovascular disease. *Physiol Behav.* 2008;94(2):285–292.

39. Abumweis SS, Barake R, Jones PJ. Plant sterols/stanols as cholesterol lowering agents: a meta-analysis of randomized controlled trials. *Food Nutr Res.* 2008;52.

40. Estruch R, Martinez-Gonzalez MA, Corella D, et al. Effects of a mediterranean-style diet on cardiovascular risk factors: a randomized trial. *Ann Intern Med.* 2006;145(1):1–11.

41. Estruch R. Anti-inflammatory effects of the mediterranean diet: the experience of the PREDIMED study. *Proc Nutr Soc.* 2010;69(3):333–340.

42. Urpi-Sarda M, Casas R, Chiva-Blanch G, et al. Virgin olive oil and nuts as key foods of the Mediterranean diet effects on inflammatory biomakers related to atherosclerosis. *Pharmacol Res.* 2012;65(6):577–583.

43. Bloch A, Thomson CA. Position of the American Dietetic Association: phytochemicals and functional foods. *J Am Diet Assoc.* 1995;95(4):493–496.

44. Ogiwara T, Satoh K, Kadoma Y, et al. Radical scavenging activity and cytotoxicity of ferulic acid. *Anticancer Res.* 2002;22(5):2711–2717.

45. Yang CS, Landau JM, Huang MT, Newmark HL. Inhibition of carcinogenesis by dietary polyphenolic compounds. *Annu Rev Nutr.* 2001;21:381–406.

46. Sang S, Ju J, Lambert JD, et al. Wheat bran oil and its fractions inhibit human colon cancer cell growth and intestinal tumorigenesis in Apc(min/+) mice. *J Agric Food Chem.* 2006;54(26):9792–9797.

47. Eisenberg T, Abdellatif M, Schroeder S, et al. Cardioprotection and lifespan extension by the natural polyamine spermidine. *Nat Med.* 2016;22(12):1428–1438.

48. Divella R, Daniele A, Savino E, Paradiso A. Anticancer effects of nutraceuticals in the mediterranean diet: an epigenetic diet model. *Cancer Genomics Proteomics.* 2020;17(4):335–350.

49. Cicerale S, Lucas LJ, Keast RS. Antimicrobial, antioxidant and anti-inflammatory phenolic activities in extra virgin olive oil. *Curr Opin Biotechnol.* 2012;23(2):129–135.

50. Massaro M, De Caterina R. Vasculoprotective effects of oleic acid: epidemiological background and direct vascular antiatherogenic properties. *Nutr Metab Cardiovasc Dis.* 2002;12(1):42–51.

51. Visioli F, Galli C. The effect of minor constituents of olive oil on cardiovascular disease: new findings. *Nutr Rev.* 1998;56(5 Pt 1):142–147.

52. Visioli F, Galli C. Antiatherogenic components of olive oil. *Curr Atheroscler Rep.* 2001; 3(1):64–67.

53. Cicerale S, Conlan XA, Sinclair AJ, Keast RS. Chemistry and health of olive oil phenolics. *Crit Rev Food Sci Nutr.* 2009;49(3):218–236.

54. Abe R, Beckett J, Abe R, et al. Olive oil polyphenol oleuropein inhibits smooth muscle cell proliferation. *Eur J Vasc Endovasc Surg.* 2011;41(6):814–820.

55. de la Puerta R, Ruiz Gutierrez V, Hoult JR. Inhibition of leukocyte 5-lipoxygenase by phenolics from virgin olive oil. *Biochem Pharmacol.* 1999;57(4):445–449.

56. Andreadou I, Sigala F, Iliodromitis EK, et al. Acute doxorubicin cardiotoxicity is successfully treated with the phytochemical oleuropein through suppression of oxidative and nitrosative stress. *J Mol Cell Cardiol.* 2007;42(3):549–558.

57. Zhang X, Cao J, Zhong L. Hydroxytyrosol inhibits pro-inflammatory cytokines, iNOS, and COX-2 expression in human monocytic cells. *Naunyn Schmiedebergs Arch Pharmacol.* 2009;379(6):581–586.

58. Richard N, Arnold S, Hoeller U, Kilpert C, Wertz K, Schwager J. Hydroxytyrosol is the major anti-inflammatory compound in aqueous olive extracts and impairs cytokine and chemokine production in macrophages. *Planta Med.* 2011;77(17):1890–1897.

59. Beauchamp GK, Keast RS, Morel D, et al. Phytochemistry: ibuprofen-like activity in extra-virgin olive oil. *Nature.* 2005;437(7055):45–46.

60. Harvey KA, Walker CL, Xu Z, et al. Oleic acid inhibits stearic acid-induced inhibition of cell growth and pro-inflammatory responses in human aortic endothelial cells. *J Lipid Res.* 2010;51(12):3470–3480.

61. Most J, Tosti V, Redman LM, Fontana L. Calorie restriction in humans: an update. *Ageing Res Rev.* 2017;39:36–45.

62. Kaaks R, Bellati C, Venturelli E, et al. Effects of dietary intervention on IGF-I and IGF-binding proteins, and related alterations in sex steroid metabolism: the diet and androgens (DIANA) randomised trial. *Eur J Clin Nutr.* 2003;57(9):1079–1088.

63. Cani PD, Delzenne NM. The role of the gut microbiota in energy metabolism and metabolic disease. *Curr Pharm Des.* 2009;15(13):1546–1558.

64. Ludwig DS. The glycemic index: physiological mechanisms relating to obesity, diabetes, and cardiovascular disease. *JAMA.* 2002;287(18):2414–2423.

65. Lovejoy JC. Dietary fatty acids and insulin resistance. *Curr Atheroscler Rep.* 1999;1(3): 215–220.

66. Longo VD, Fontana L. Calorie restriction and cancer prevention: metabolic and molecular mechanisms. *Trends Pharmacol Sci*. 2010;31(2):89–98.

67. Goldin BR, Adlercreutz H, Gorbach SL, et al. Estrogen excretion patterns and plasma levels in vegetarian and omnivorous women. *N Engl J Med*. 1982;307(25):1542–1547.

68. Lamming DW, Cummings NE, Rastelli AL, et al. Restriction of dietary protein decreases mTORC1 in tumors and somatic tissues of a tumor-bearing mouse xenograft model. *Oncotarget*. 2015;6(31):31233–31240.

69. Simpson SJ, Le Couteur DG, Raubenheimer D, et al. Dietary protein, aging and nutritional geometry. *Ageing Res Rev*. 2017;39:78–86.

70. Hua H, Kong Q, Zhang H, Wang J, Luo T, Jiang Y. Targeting mTOR for cancer therapy. *J Hematol Oncol*. 2019;12(1):71.

71. Levine ME, Suarez JA, Brandhorst S, et al. Low protein intake is associated with a major reduction in IGF-1, cancer, and overall mortality in the 65 and younger but not older population. *Cell Metab*. 2014;19(3):407–417.

72. Tinker LF, Sarto GE, Howard BV, et al. Biomarker-calibrated dietary energy and protein intake associations with diabetes risk among postmenopausal women from the Women's Health Initiative. *Am J Clin Nutr*. 2011;94(6):1600–1606.

73. Fontana L, Cummings NE, Arriola Apelo SI, et al. Decreased consumption of branched-chain amino acids improves metabolic health. *Cell Rep*. 2016;16(2):520–530.

74. Smith GI, Yoshino J, Kelly SC, et al. High-protein intake during weight loss therapy eliminates the weight-loss-induced improvement in insulin action in obese postmenopausal women. *Cell Rep*. 2016;17(3):849–861.

75. Brown-Borg HM, Buffenstein R. Cutting back on the essentials: can manipulating intake of specific amino acids modulate health and lifespan? *Ageing Res Rev*. 2017;39:87–95.

76. Lynch CJ, Adams SH. Branched-chain amino acids in metabolic signalling and insulin resistance. *Nat Rev Endocrinol*. 2014;10(12):723–736.

77. Clemente JC, Ursell LK, Parfrey LW, Knight R. The impact of the gut microbiota on human health: an integrative view. *Cell*. 2012;148(6):1258–1270.

78. Tseng CH, Wu CY. The gut microbiome in obesity. *J Formos Med Assoc*. 2019;118(Suppl 1):S3–S9.

79. Thorburn AN, Macia L, Mackay CR. Diet, metabolites, and "western-lifestyle" inflammatory diseases. *Immunity*. 2014;40(6):833–842.

80. Richards JL, Yap YA, McLeod KH, Mackay CR, Marino E. Dietary metabolites and the gut microbiota: an alternative approach to control inflammatory and autoimmune diseases. *Clin Transl Immunol*. 2016;5(5):e82.

81. Haro C, Garcia-Carpintero S, Rangel-Zuniga OA, et al. Consumption of two healthy dietary patterns restored microbiota dysbiosis in obese patients with metabolic dysfunction. *Mol Nutr Food Res*. 2017;61(12).

82. Mazmanian SK, Liu CH, Tzianabos AO, Kasper DL. An immunomodulatory molecule of symbiotic bacteria directs maturation of the host immune system. *Cell*. 2005;122(1):107–118.

83. Round JL, Mazmanian SK. Inducible Foxp3+ regulatory T-cell development by a commensal bacterium of the intestinal microbiota. *Proc Natl Acad Sci U S A*. 2010;107(27): 12204–12209.

84. Tang WH, Wang Z, Levison BS, et al. Intestinal microbial metabolism of phosphatidylcholine and cardiovascular risk. *N Engl J Med*. 2013;368(17):1575–1584.

85. Zhu W, Gregory JC, Org E, et al. Gut microbial metabolite TMAO enhances platelet hyperreactivity and thrombosis risk. *Cell*. 2016;165(1):111–124.

86. Fung TT, Rexrode KM, Mantzoros CS, Manson JE, Willett WC, Hu FB. Mediterranean diet and incidence of and mortality from coronary heart disease and stroke in women. *Circulation*. 2009;119(8):1093–1100.

87. Sotos-Prieto M, Bhupathiraju SN, Mattei J, et al. Changes in diet quality scores and risk of cardiovascular disease among US men and women. *Circulation*. 2015;132(23): 2212–2219.

88. Hoevenaar-Blom MP, Nooyens AC, Kromhout D, et al. Mediterranean style diet and 12-year incidence of cardiovascular diseases: the EPIC-NL cohort study. *PLoS One*. 2012;7(9):e45458.

89. Tong TY, Wareham NJ, Khaw KT, Imamura F, Forouhi NG. Prospective association of the Mediterranean diet with cardiovascular disease incidence and mortality and its population impact in a non-mediterranean population: the EPIC-Norfolk study. *BMC Med*. 2016;14(1):135.

90. Becerra-Tomas N, Blanco Mejia S, Viguiliouk E, et al. Mediterranean diet, cardiovascular disease and mortality in diabetes: a systematic review and meta-analysis of prospective cohort studies and randomized clinical trials. *Crit Rev Food Sci Nutr*. 2020;60(7): 1207–1227.

91. Guasch-Ferre M, Willett WC. The Mediterranean diet and health: a comprehensive overview. *J Intern Med*. 2021;290(3):549–566.

92. de Lorgeril M, Renaud S, Mamelle N, et al. Mediterranean alpha-linolenic acid-rich diet in secondary prevention of coronary heart disease. *Lancet*. 1994;343(8911):1454–1459.

93. de Lorgeril M, Salen P, Martin JL, Monjaud I, Delaye J, Mamelle N. Mediterranean diet, traditional risk factors, and the rate of cardiovascular complications after myocardial infarction: final report of the Lyon Diet Heart Study. *Circulation*. 1999;99(6):779–785.

94. Martinez-Gonzalez MA, Ros E, Estruch R. Primary prevention of cardiovascular disease with a mediterranean diet supplemented with extra-virgin olive oil or nuts. *N Engl J Med*. 2018;379(14):1388–1389.

95. Estruch R, Ros E, Salas-Salvado J, et al. Primary prevention of cardiovascular disease with a mediterranean diet. *N Engl J Med*. 2013;368(14):1279–1290.

96. Agarwal A, Ioannidis JPA. PREDIMED trial of mediterranean diet: retracted, republished, still trusted? *BMJ*. 2019;364:l341.

97. Delgado-Lista J, Perez-Martinez P, Garcia-Rios A, et al. CORonary Diet Intervention with Olive oil and cardiovascular PREVention study (the CORDIOPREV study): rationale, methods, and baseline characteristics: a clinical trial comparing the efficacy of a mediterranean diet rich in olive oil versus a low-fat diet on cardiovascular disease in coronary patients. *Am Heart J*. 2016;177:42–50.

98. Romaguera D, Norat T, Vergnaud AC, et al. Mediterranean dietary patterns and prospective weight change in participants of the EPIC-PANACEA project. *Am J Clin Nutr*. 2010;92(4):912–921.

99. Mancini JG, Filion KB, Atallah R, Eisenberg MJ. Systematic review of the mediterranean diet for long-term weight loss. *Am J Med*. 2016;129(4):407–415.

100. Koloverou E, Panagiotakos DB, Pitsavos C, et al. Adherence to mediterranean diet and 10-year incidence (2002–2012) of diabetes: correlations with inflammatory and oxidative stress biomarkers in the ATTICA cohort study. *Diabetes Metab Res Rev*. 2016;32(1):73–81.

101. Salas-Salvado J, Bullo M, Estruch R, et al. Prevention of diabetes with Mediterranean diets: a subgroup analysis of a randomized trial. *Ann Intern Med*. 2014;160(1):1–10.

102. Morze J, Danielewicz A, Przybylowicz K, Zeng H, Hoffmann G, Schwingshackl L. An updated systematic review and meta-analysis on adherence to mediterranean diet and risk of cancer. *Eur J Nutr*. 2021;60(3):1561–1586.

103. Toledo E, Salas-Salvado J, Donat-Vargas C, et al. Mediterranean diet and invasive breast cancer risk among women at high cardiovascular risk in the PREDIMED trial: a randomized clinical trial. *JAMA Intern Med*. 2015;175(11):1752–1760.

104. de Lorgeril M, Salen P, Martin JL, Monjaud I, Boucher P, Mamelle N. Mediterranean dietary pattern in a randomized trial: prolonged survival and possible reduced cancer rate. *Arch Intern Med.* 1998;158(11):1181–1187.
105. Couto E, Boffetta P, Lagiou P, et al. Mediterranean dietary pattern and cancer risk in the EPIC cohort. *Br J Cancer.* 2011;104(9):1493–1499.
106. Hodge AM, Bassett JK, Dugue PA, et al. Dietary inflammatory index or mediterranean diet score as risk factors for total and cardiovascular mortality. *Nutr Metab Cardiovasc Dis.* 2018;28(5):461–469.
107. Crous-Bou M, Fung TT, Prescott J, et al. Mediterranean diet and telomere length in Nurses' Health Study: population based cohort study. *BMJ.* 2014;349:g6674.

10 Vegan Diets for Diabetes Prevention and Management of Cardiometabolic Risk

Neal D. Barnard
George Washington University School of
Medicine and Health Sciences Physicians
Committee for Responsible Medicine

Hana Kahleova
Physicians Committee for Responsible Medicine

CONTENTS

The risk of developing type 2 diabetes is strongly related to food choices. When the disease is diagnosed, its management depends largely on food choices, as well. For both prevention and management, vegan diets have proven particularly useful.[1] In the following sections, we examine evidence from large population studies and

DOI: 10.1201/9781003206637-10

clinical trials supporting the use of such diets and present clinical strategies for their implementation.

Many patients imagine that type 2 diabetes comes from overconsumption of sugar or of carbohydrates in general. This is an understandable misinterpretation; when they consume starch or sugar, their blood glucose levels rise. However, a 2017 meta-analysis of prospective cohort studies found no association of total dietary sugars with type 2 diabetes incidence. Sucrose intake was, in fact, associated with an 11% decreased risk of developing type 2 diabetes.[2] It is important for patients to understand that their condition began as insulin resistance, that is, an impairment of insulin's ability to foster the entry of glucose into muscle and liver cells. In turn, insulin resistance is caused by accumulated fat particles in muscle and liver cells, termed intramyocellular and hepatocellular lipid, respectively.[3,4] Fat build-up inside muscle and liver cells impairs insulin's ability to work.

As insulin resistance worsens, consumption of any carbohydrate-containing food will tend to elevate blood glucose levels simply because the normal physiological mechanisms for storing glucose are impaired. These predictable blood sugar increases in response to carbohydrate intake, making it appear that sugar or starch *caused* the disease; in fact, the problem started with lipid accumulation.

Dietary fat, particularly saturated fat, has been associated with an increased risk of type 2 diabetes.[5,6] Increased fat intake increases intracellular lipid concentrations surprisingly rapidly. In a study on young normal-weight males, a high-fat diet (55%–60% of energy) increased intramyocellular lipid accumulation in the tibialis anterior muscle by 48% in 3 days (Bachman, 2001).[7] Similarly, diet changes readily reduce this accumulated fat. In lean, insulin-resistant individuals, a low-fat, energy-restricted diet (7% fat, 1,200 kcal/day) was shown to reduce intramyocellular lipid content by 30% in 9 weeks.[8]

The ability of a vegan diet to reduce intramyocellular lipid was first suggested by a case–control study that found soleus muscle intramyocellular lipid concentrations to be 31% lower in vegans than in omnivores.[9] Later, a controlled trial in overweight individuals without type 2 diabetes demonstrated that a low-fat vegan diet, consumed with no limitation on energy intake, reduced hepatocellular and intramyocellular lipid by 34.4% ($P=0.002$) and 10.4% ($P=0.03$), respectively, in 16 weeks. In turn, the changes in hepatocellular and intramyocellular lipid strongly correlated with changes in insulin resistance (both $r=0.51$; $P=0.01$).[10] These studies suggest that diet changes can dramatically modify intracellular lipid accumulation and the insulin resistance it causes, and that a low-fat vegan diet can do so without any specific caloric restriction.

10.1 OBSERVATIONAL STUDIES ON DIETARY PATTERNS AND DIABETES PREVALENCE

The pathophysiology of insulin resistance described above suggests that diets that favor plant-based foods would reduce the risk of type 2 diabetes. Indeed, the Adventist Health Study-2, including 60,903 participants, identified diabetes in 7.6% of meat eaters, but only 2.9% of those following vegan diets. Intermediate prevalence was found in those who ate meat less than once per week (6.1%), those who ate no meat other than fish (4.8%), and lacto-ovo-vegetarians (3.2%).[11] In a prospective study in this population, a similar pattern was identified for diabetes incidence. Among 15,200 men and 26,187 women from this cohort followed for 2 years, those following vegan diets were less than half as likely to develop type 2 diabetes than nonvegetarians; the odds ratio for developing diabetes among those following vegan diets was 0.304 (95% CI 0.110–0.842) for Black individuals and 0.429 (95% CI 0.249–0.740) for all other races.[12]

Conversely, meat consumption is associated with greatly increased diabetes risk. An analysis of participants in three large Harvard cohorts (26,357 men from the Health Professionals Follow-up Study, 48,709 women from the Nurses' Health Study, and 74,077 women from the Nurses' Health Study II) found that, over a 4-year period, each half serving of meat consumed per day was associated with a 48% (95% CI, 1.37–1.59) increased risk of developing type 2 diabetes (Pan, 2013).[13] Similar associations between meat consumption and type 2 diabetes risk were found in the European Prospective Investigation into Cancer and Nutrition (EPIC)-InterAct study.[14]

Even in populations consuming very little meat overall, type 2 diabetes is less prevalent among those avoiding meat altogether. In a study of 4,384 Taiwanese Buddhist volunteers, among whom overall meat consumption was modest, type 2 diabetes was 51% less prevalent in vegetarian men (OR: 0.49, 95% CI:0.28–0.89), 74% less prevalent in premenopausal vegetarian women (OR: 0.26, 95% CI: 0.06–1.21), and 75% less prevalent in postmenopausal women (OR: 0.25, 95% CI: 0.15–0.42), after adjustment for age, body mass index, family history of diabetes, education, leisure time physical activity, smoking, and alcohol. No cases of type 2 diabetes were identified in the small group ($N = 69$) of vegans in the study. (Chiu, 2014).[15] A prospective study in this population showed a strongly protective effect of avoiding meat. Among 2,918 Buddhists who were free of diabetes at baseline, risk of developing type 2 diabetes during 5 years of follow-up was 35% lower among those following vegetarian diets (HR: 0.65, 95% CI: 0.46, 0.92) and 53% lower among those who converted to a vegetarian diet (HR: 0.47, 95% CI: 0.30, 0.71) than among nonvegetarians, adjusted for age, physical activity, family history of diabetes, and baseline body mass index.[16]

These studies suggest that plant-based diets are strongly protective against developing type 2 diabetes and that meat consumed in even modest amounts increases diabetes risk. The role of meat in diabetes risk is likely due to its macronutrient content; muscle tissue is composed of protein and fat, with essentially no carbohydrate or fiber, and is a significant source of dietary fat.

10.2 CLINICAL TRIALS OF PLANT-BASED DIETARY INTERVENTIONS FOR TYPE 2 DIABETES MANAGEMENT

In individuals with type 2 diabetes, intervention trials have tested the effects of plant-based diets on diabetes management. A 1994 study used a near-vegetarian diet in 652 individuals with type 2 diabetes in a 26-day residential program.[17] The diet derived less than 10% of energy from fat and included 35–40 g of fiber per 1,000 kcal. Unfortunately, from the standpoint of isolating the effect of diet, the program also included exercise. Of those on no medications at baseline, fasting glucose fell 24%

($P < 0.001$). Of 197 participants treated with oral agents, 140 were able to discontinue their use, and their mean fasting glucose concentration decreased 17% ($P < 0.001$). Of 212 participants treated with insulin at the outset, 83 (39%) discontinued its use, yet their mean fasting glucose concentration decreased 6% ($P < 0.001$).[17]

A 2006 randomized controlled trial compared a low-fat, vegan diet and a portion-controlled diet in 99 individuals with type 2 diabetes over 22 weeks, while holding physical activity constant to the extent possible. The vegan diet included no limitations on serving sizes, carbohydrate intake, or energy intake, while the portion-controlled diet set limits on all three. Among those who made no changes to diabetes medications, hemoglobin A1c (A1c) fell 1.23 percentage points in the vegan group, compared with 0.38 points in the portion-controlled group ($P = 0.01$).[18] During a 12-month follow-up in the same population, A1c changes from baseline to last available value or last value before any medication adjustment were −0.40 in the vegan group and +0.01 in the portion-controlled group ($P = 0.03$).[19]

Other clinical trials have similarly reported improved glycemic control with plant-based diets administered without any intentional limits on energy or carbohydrate intake and without exercise, although the observed glycemic changes vary depending on baseline levels, medication changes, and other factors. A 2014 meta-analysis reported that consumption of vegetarian diets was associated with a reduction in A1c of 0.39 absolute percentage point (95% confidence interval, −0.62 to −0.15; $P = 0.001$).[1]

The marked effects of a low-fat vegan diet on glycemic control are likely attributable to reductions in intramyocellular and hepatocellular lipid. As noted earlier, a low-fat vegan diet causes rapid and significant reductions in these muscle and liver lipid levels, which correlate with changes in insulin resistance.[10] However, such diets are also associated with marked reductions in body weight and other clinically important changes, as we will see below.

10.3   NUTRITIONAL INTERVENTIONS FOR NEUROPATHY

Limited evidence suggests that dietary interventions may improve neuropathic pain associated with type 2 diabetes. A reduced-calorie, low-fat, vegan diet was used along with daily exercise (a 30-minute walk) in a 25-day residential study of individuals with type 2 diabetes and peripheral neuropathy (Crane, 1994).[20] In 17 of the 21 participants, neuropathic leg pains remitted completely in 2 weeks, and the four remaining participants had partial relief.

A 20-week controlled trial assessed the effects of a low-fat vegan diet without exercise in individuals with painful diabetic neuropathy. Compared with an untreated control group, the dietary intervention reduced neuropathic symptoms and improved nerve function as measured by electrochemical skin conductance.[21] These promising results suggest the value of further research on neuropathy and other complications of diabetes.

10.4   DIET AND TYPE 1 DIABETES

The role of vegan diets for type 1 diabetes has been less extensively studied than for type 2 diabetes. Nonetheless, evidence suggests that such diets may improve blood glucose control, reduce insulin requirements, and may reduce long-term complications in type 1 diabetes.

In a 1991 crossover study, ten individuals with type 1 diabetes began either a high-carbohydrate, high-fiber diet rich in whole grains, beans, vegetables, and fruits, with only small quantities of meat and dairy products, or a low-carbohydrate, low-fiber diet including moderate amounts of meat and dairy products for 4 weeks. Then, after a 6-week washout period, the participants began the opposite diet for an additional 4 weeks. The high-carbohydrate, high-fiber diet reduced basal insulin requirements and increased carbohydrate disposed of per unit insulin.[22]

In a 2008 controlled trial, 63 individuals with type 1 diabetes were randomly assigned either to a high-fiber, low-glycemic index diet emphasizing fruit, legumes, and vegetables or to a low-fiber, high-glycemic index diet. The high-fiber, low-glycemic index diet led to significant improvements in blood sugar control and a substantial reduction in hypoglycemic episodes.[23] This is particularly helpful clinically. While blood glucose control based on pharmaceuticals can increase the risk of hypoglycemia, a dietary approach can improve glycemic control without increasing the risk of hypoglycemia.

Diabetes management means more than reducing insulin use; reducing cardiovascular morbidity is a primary consideration. The use of low-fat vegan diets in type 1 diabetes was the subject of a 2020 case report that described not only significant increases in insulin sensitivity and reductions in insulin requirements but also improvements in cardiovascular risk factors.[24]

10.5 NUTRITION AND GESTATIONAL DIABETES

Gestational diabetes is diabetes that is diagnosed for the first time during pregnancy. The prevalence of gestational diabetes is increasing; in the United States, it occurs in as many as one in ten pregnancies.[25] Gestational diabetes increases the risk of pregnancy-related complications, such as polyhydramnios, preterm delivery, and cesarean delivery, and it also puts the fetus at a higher risk of congenital malformations, macrosomia, neonatal respiratory distress syndrome, hypoglycemia, and even intrauterine death.[26]

Dietary habits before pregnancy are important determinants of body mass index, an important risk factor for gestational diabetes.[27] However, dietary pattern changes during pregnancy also appear to affect the development of gestational diabetes. Vegetarian and vegan diets during pregnancy are associated with reduced gestational weight gain.[28] Diets characterized by high amounts of whole grains, fruits, and vegetables are associated with reduced gestational diabetes risk, while a Western diet, as well as dietary patterns that include high amounts of red and processed meat, is associated with a higher prevalence of gestational diabetes.[29,30] The data from the KOALA Birth Cohort Study that compared the dietary intakes of women with and without gestational diabetes found that, after adjustment for other relevant covariates, gestational diabetes was significantly associated with higher consumption of meat and cheese. Gestational diabetes was also associated with indirect indicators of animal product intake, namely, dietary animal-to-plant protein ratio and maternal plasma arachidonic acid.[31]

In the Nurses' Health Study II, among 13,110 eligible women with a mean follow-up of 8 years, a high fiber intake was associated with reduced gestational diabetes incidence. An increment of 10 g/day in total fiber intake was found to be associated with a 26% risk reduction in gestational diabetes and an increment of 5 g/day in cereal or fruit fiber intake was associated with a 23% or 26% reduction in gestational diabetes, respectively.[32]

Apart from the risk of gestational diabetes, dietary habits during pregnancy may also influence on the risk of maternal and neonatal complications. A longitudinal study in 238 pregnant women in the Democratic Republic of the Congo showed that preeclampsia occurred more frequently among women who rarely consumed vegetables during pregnancy (33.3%) than among women who consumed at least three servings of vegetables per day (3.7%).[33]

Vegan pregnant women may have a lower risk of preeclampsia and cesarean delivery, less postpartum depression, and lower neonatal and maternal mortality than women following omnivorous diets.[34] These benefits can be partly explained by a lower body mass index in vegans than in omnivores and greater amounts of fiber in a vegan diet.[32]

10.6 INFLUENCE ON CARDIOVASCULAR RISK FACTORS

Because the mortality and morbidity of diabetes are typically related to cardiovascular diseases, management of cardiovascular risk factors is central to diabetes management. Plant-based diets play major roles in reducing these risk factors, as described below.

10.7 BODY WEIGHT

Excess body weight is a key cardiovascular risk factor. Compared with diets containing animal products, plant-based diets are associated with healthier body weights. In the Adventist Health Study-2, body mass index declined in comparison to meat eaters (28.8 kg/m²), those eating meat less than once per week, (27.3 kg/m²), those limiting meat consumption to fish (26.3 kg/m²), lacto-ovo-vegetarians (25.7 kg/m²), and those avoiding animal products altogether (23.6 kg/m²).[11] In other words, even among Seventh-day Adventist research participants, whose dietary habits are considerably healthier than Americans overall, more than 5 kg/m² separated the average body mass index of meat eaters and vegans. A similar, although less dramatic, gradient was found in the European Prospective Investigation into Cancer and Nutrition (EPIC), in which the mean body mass indices of those avoiding animal products altogether (22.5 kg/m² in men and 22.0 kg/m² in women) were lower than those of meat eaters (24.4 kg/m² in men and 23.5 kg/m² in women).[35]

Clinical trials have confirmed the weight-reducing effects of plant-based diets. In a study of 64 overweight women randomly assigned to either a low-fat vegan diet with no limits on energy intake or to a control diet based on the guidelines of the National Cholesterol Education Program, mean weight loss was 5.8 kg in the vegan group and 3.8 kg in the control group over 14 weeks ($P = .01$).[36] Over a 2-year follow-up period, these figures were 3.1 and 0.8 kg, respectively ($P < .05$), indicating that weight loss in the vegan group was maintained over the long term.[37]

Similar weight loss has been shown in other clinical trials. In a meta-analysis of 17 intervention groups testing the effects of vegetarian diets overall, mean weight loss among study completers was 4.6 kg. Weight loss was greater among participants with higher baseline weights and smaller among those already at a healthy weight.[38] Weight loss also tends to be greater in studies using longer intervention periods and in studies for which weight loss is a study goal, as opposed to an incidental finding. Similarly, a separate meta-analysis of 12 clinical trials found that weight change among individuals following vegan diets was −2.52 kg (95% confidence interval [CI]: −3.02 to −1.98).[39]

There are two explanations for the weight loss observed with low-fat vegan diets. The primary explanation is the diet's low energy density. Carbohydrates have only four calories per gram, and fiber has effectively zero. Both of these low-calorie nutrients are abundant in whole grains, legumes, vegetables, and fruits but are absent in meat, which has substantial amounts of fat. Fat holds nine calories per gram. A diet excluding animal products therefore tends to be less energy-dense than an omnivorous diet. However, because it is high in fiber and complex carbohydrate, it is experienced as filling and satisfying.

A secondary reason for weight loss with low-fat vegan diets is a slight increase in postprandial metabolism. As nutrients are absorbed and utilized after meals, some energy is expended in what is referred to as the *thermic effect of food*. This expenditure continues for a few hours after each meal and accounts for approximately 10% of total energy expenditure.

This after-meal calorie expenditure is higher in individuals who have been following a low-fat vegan diet. In a 2005 study of overweight women, the thermic effect of food was elevated by roughly 15%,[36] a result that was confirmed in a later study in overweight men and women.[10]

The apparent explanation for the added energy expenditure that results from a low-fat vegan diet is the diet's effect on mitochondrial action.[40,41] Perhaps surprisingly, the number and activity of mitochondria—which, in turn, influence energy expenditure—are not fixed. Rather, they change depending on the diet. In a 2005 study, a high-fat (50% of energy) diet administered for just 3 days caused a significant downregulation of the genes required for mitochondrial oxidative phosphorylation in the skeletal muscle. The reduction in mitochondrial biogenesis leads to a parallel reduction in energy expenditure.[31] In other words, fat intake retards postprandial energy expenditure. Low-fat diets have the reverse effect.

Research has also suggested an additional mechanism: Some gut bacterial species produce endotoxins that can pass into the circulation and influence cellular metabolism. In a 2015 study, researchers administered a high-fat (55% of energy) diet to human volunteers, finding that the concentration of circulating endotoxin doubled within 5 days. Apparently, the ingested fat impaired the gut's ability to block the entry of endotoxin into the systemic circulation. In turn, endotoxin disrupted mitochondrial activity and impaired postprandial cellular glucose oxidation.[30]

In summary, low-fat vegan diets lead to a significant but, from the standpoint of the user, imperceptible reduction in energy intake, along with a modest increase in energy expenditure, both of which are achieved without any restrictions on food portions or exercise. The result is significant and sustained weight loss.

10.8 PLASMA LIPIDS

Elevated concentrations of plasma cholesterol, particularly low-density lipoprotein cholesterol, are a significant contributor to the risk of cardiovascular events.[1] Low-density lipoprotein cholesterol concentrations are strongly influenced by dietary saturated fat and, to a lesser extent, dietary cholesterol. In the United States, the principal sources of saturated fat are dairy products and meat. By contrast, nearly all plants are extremely low in saturated fat. These differences are not trivial, as can be seen in Table 10.1.

Two exceptions should be noted. Partially hydrogenated oils have dyslipidemic effects similar to those of animal fats. In addition, tropical oils (e.g., coconut and palm oils) are high in saturated fat and, despite being marketed as healthful alternatives to animal products, have cholesterol-raising power or their own.[42]

Dietary cholesterol has a smaller effect on blood cholesterol concentrations than saturated fat. Nonetheless, randomized trials, summarized in systematic reviews and meta-analyses, have shown that dietary cholesterol elevates both total and low-density lipoprotein cholesterol concentrations.[43–49]

Widespread confusion regarding the effects of dietary cholesterol on circulating cholesterol has been the result of concerted efforts by the egg industry to rehabilitate the image of dietary cholesterol. Nonetheless, both industry-funded and non-industry-funded studies show that dietary cholesterol tends to elevate plasma low-density lipoprotein cholesterol levels.[50]

Vegan diets typically contain very little saturated fat and essentially no cholesterol; in clinical trials, vegetarian and vegan diets typically cause sharp reductions in plasma cholesterol levels. In a 2015 meta-analysis of 11 randomized controlled trials, vegetarian diets lowered total and low-density lipoprotein cholesterol by 13.9 mg/dL (0.36 mmol/L) and 13.1 mg/dL (0.34 mmol/L), respectively (both $P < 0.001$).[51]

TABLE 10.1

Saturated Fat and Cholesterol Content of Representative Animal-Source and Plant-Source Food Products

	Cholesterol	Saturated fat (% of recommended daily allowance)
Roast beef, lean only (100 g)	83 mg	3.4 g (17%)
Chicken with skin (100 g)	88 mg	3.8 g (14%)
Chicken without skin (100 g)	89 mg	2.0 g (10%)
Chinook salmon (100 g)	85 mg	3.2 g (13%)
Cheddar cheese (2 oz)	58 mg	11.0 g (43%)
Two large eggs	362 mg	3.1 g (19%)
Black beans (100 g)	0	0.1 g (1%)
Brown rice (100 g)	0	0.2 g (1%)
Broccoli (100 g)	0	0.1 g (3%)
Sweet potato (100 g)	0	0.04 g (0.5%)

Source: National Agricultural Library, US Department of Agriculture. http://ndb.nal.usda.gov/ndb/foods.

Certain foods appear to have an additional lipid-lowering effect, apart from the absence of saturated fat and cholesterol. These include oats, barley, and beans, all of which are rich in soluble fiber, as well as almonds, soy protein, and sterol-containing margarines. A "portfolio diet" including these cholesterol-lowering foods while excluding animal-derived foods was shown to reduce low-density lipoprotein cholesterol concentrations by nearly 30% in 4 weeks.[52] Collectively, these findings suggest that because a vegan diet minimizes cholesterol and saturated fat, while containing abundant fiber, it is the regimen of choice for reducing total and low-density lipoprotein cholesterol.

10.9   BLOOD PRESSURE

High blood pressure increases cardiovascular disease risk independently of other risk factors.[53] In a 2014 meta-analysis of seven controlled trials with a total of 311 participants, consumption of vegetarian diets was associated with a reduction in the mean systolic BP of 4.8 mmHg and of the mean diastolic BP of 2.2 mmHg compared with omnivorous diets.[54] The actual reduction depends on initial blood pressure values, among other factors.

This effect may be explained by several features of the diet: they cause weight loss, are naturally high in potassium,[55] and tend to reduce blood viscosity.[56] The classic Dietary Approaches to Stop Hypertension (DASH) study was predicated on the well-known blood-pressure-lowering effect of vegetarian diets and used a semi-vegetarian regimen to demonstrate rapid changes in blood pressure caused by increasing vegetables and fruits and reducing meat and fat.[57]

The ability of low-fat vegan diets to reduce plasma lipid concentrations and blood pressure means not only that these diets reduce cardiovascular risk. It also means that individuals with diabetes, whose pharmaceutical regimens commonly include statins and antihypertensives in addition to their medications for glycemic control, may be able to reduce their use of medications and reduce the side effects and expenses associated with them.

It is noteworthy that Mediterranean diets, as that term is used in research, typically favor plant-based foods over animal-derived products. The Prevención con Dieta Mediterránea (PREDIMED) study showed that the risk of a major cardiovascular event was reduced by approximately 30% in those following a Mediterranean diet supplemented with either extra-virgin olive oil or nuts compared with an untreated control group.[58] However, a sub-analysis revealed that the more that study participants followed a plant-based dietary pattern, the lower their risk of cardiovascular events.[59] In other words, a diet that reduces animal products and substitutes plant-derived oils for animal-derived fats is better than a typical omnivorous diet. But there is substantial benefit to going further and moving toward a plant-based diet.

For control of body weight and blood pressure, low-fat vegan diets are far superior to typical Mediterranean diets. In a randomized cross-over study of 62 overweight individuals, with a Mediterranean and a vegan diet each followed for 16 weeks (the Mediterranean regimen mirrored that used in the PREDIMED study olive oil arm), the vegan diet led to a mean weight loss of 6.0 kg compared to 0.0 on the Mediterranean diet. Among participants with no medication changes, total and LDL cholesterol decreased 18.7 mg/dL (0.5 mmol/L) and 15.3 mg/dL (0.4 mmol/L), respectively, on the vegan diet, compared with 3.1 mg/dL (0.1 mmol/L) and 0.5 mg/dL (0.01 mmol/L), respectively, on the Mediterranean diet. Systolic and diastolic blood pressures decreased 9.3 and 7.3 mmHg on the Mediterranean diet compared with 3.4 and 4.1 mmHg on the vegan diet.[60]

10.10 NUTRITIONAL ADEQUACY

"So, where do you get your protein?" is a common question put to clinicians prescribing vegan diets for patients with diabetes. Other concerns about nutrient adequacy follow. It is important for clinicians and patients to understand that with a shift from omnivorous diets to vegan diets, overall nutrition typically improves significantly, as has been demonstrated using Harvard's Alternative Healthy Eating Index in individuals with diabetes.[61] This is not surprising, given that vegan diets are abundant in vegetables and fruits, high in fiber, and largely devoid of saturated fat and cholesterol.

In omnivorous diets, meat, dairy products, and eggs provide excess protein and fat, while crowding out the nutrients in plants, notably fiber, complex carbohydrates, and vitamin C. Regarding the persistent question about protein adequacy, vegan diets composed of a variety grains, legumes, vegetables, and fruits provide more than adequate protein. Specifically, they provide all essential amino acids, even without intentional food combining. The Academy of Nutrition and Dietetics reports that "Vegetarian, including vegan, diets typically meet or exceed recommended protein intakes, when caloric intakes are adequate."[62] In clinical situations with exceptional nutritional needs (e.g., end-stage renal disease or burn injuries), consultation with dietetic specialists will be required, regardless of the patient's habitual diet.

Calcium intake is often low in people following any sort of diet, whether omnivorous or plant-based. While dairy industry marketing has led many to think of dairy products as an essential calcium source, it is important to remember that cows do not synthesize calcium; rather, they consume it in plants. Humans do, too, particularly in green leafy vegetables, which provide other essential nutrients as well.

Iron intake is often higher on vegan diets than on meat-containing diets. However, plants contain *non-heme* iron, which is more absorbable when iron stores are low and less absorbable when iron stores are high, permitting healthful iron balance. By contrast, about half of the iron in red meat is *heme* iron, whose absorption is less influenced by iron status. As a result, frequent meat consumption may lead to iron overload, heart disease, Alzheimer's disease, and cancer, presumably due to iron's tendency to catalyze the formation of free radicals and carcinogens.[63,64]

Vitamin B_{12} is essential for blood cell formation and nerve function. The vitamin is produced, not by plants or animals, but by bacteria. Meat and dairy products contain B_{12} traces because intestinal bacteria in animals produce it. On a vegan diet, vitamin B_{12} must come from B_{12}-fortified foods or supplements. The recommended dietary allowance is 2.4 micrograms per day; all common supplements exceed this amount. However, many omnivores are low in B_{12}, too, as a result of insufficient stomach acid that is needed to separate B_{12} from the protein to which it is bound or the use of metformin or acid blockers, which interfere with its absorption. B_{12} deficiency also occasionally results from *Helicobacter pylori* infection and parasitism.[65]

While B_{12} supplementation is essential for those on a vegan diet, it is a reasonable recommendation for all.

Vitamin D facilitates calcium absorption and may play a role in cancer prevention. Its natural source is sunlight on the skin. Individuals who do not get regular sunlight will benefit from a supplement regardless of their dietary habits.

Some may regard a vegan diet as a modern trend, imagining that humans descended from spear-wielding "hunter-gatherers" who subsisted on meat-heavy diets. In reality, humans are great apes, in the same family as chimpanzees, gorillas, orangutans, and bonobos, all of whom consume largely plant-based diets. True carnivores compensate for the diet's deficiencies by producing their own vitamin C, which humans cannot. They also expel carcinogenic compounds from their naturally short colons. Humans, like other great apes, are physiologically suited for diets based on plants.

In the 1970s, Alan Walker of Johns Hopkins University presented strong evidence of fruit as a dietary staple among early humans, rather like that of other great apes, and showed substantial dietary variability.[66] In addition to fruit, foods rich in starch were also important in human nutrition to cover high glucose demands of the brain, red blood cells, and the developing fetus.[67] As Louis Leakey and others have written, meat-eating probably began as scavenging, which was not possible until the Stone Age provided tools that allowed the efficient removal of muscle tissue from animal bones.[66] Because the remains of plant-derived foods quickly deteriorate, the archeologic record has been distorted by the more persistent remnants of animal bones that have accumulated since the advent of hunting.

Hunter-gatherer societies subsisting on large quantities of animal products have not done well from the standpoint of cardiovascular health, as evidenced by the extensive atherosclerosis found in autopsies of Masai individuals,[68] and in ancient Inuit remains.[69]

10.11 ACCEPTABILITY

Clinicians who are new to the clinical use of plant-based diets may wonder if such diets are easy to follow and acceptable to patients. Clinical trials have addressed this issue directly. Using quantitative surveys, a plant-based diet was found to have an acceptability in individuals with type 2 diabetes that was comparable to that of a conventional portion-controlled diet.[70] Similar findings have been reported in individuals with cardiovascular disease,[71] young healthy women,[72] and older overweight individuals.[73] Randomized trials using plant-based diets have continued for several years, and cohort studies have included thousands of individuals following vegan diets for many years—or for life—showing that long-term adherence is indeed an approachable prospect.

The acceptability of vegan diets stems from several factors. They do not restrict carbohydrate or overall calorie intake, so they do not cause hunger or carbohydrate craving. Their predictable ability to reduce weight, blood sugar, lipids, and blood pressure and to ameliorate other physical issues (e.g., constipation and gastro-esophageal reflux) rewards continued adherence.[74] The popularity of plant-based diets for other reasons (environmental and animal welfare concerns) has engendered an increasing number of convenient products. In 2018, plant-based product sales increased by

20% over the previous year, with total sales exceeding \$3.3 billion.[75] These included increased sales of meat alternatives (24%) and plant-based versions of milks (9%), cheeses (43%), yogurts (55%), and creamers (131%). This increasing popularity has also meant a wide variety of resources for individuals seeking recipes, health information, and social support.

10.12   HOW TO BEGIN

A vegan diet is surprisingly easy to adopt and maintain. Patients are generally willing to try it, provided its rationale has been explained and a simple pathway is laid out for them[76]; many find it to be life-changing. Here is a simple and highly effective sequence for introducing a vegan diet in clinical practice or in research settings:

1. **Physician Validation**: The treating clinician should briefly educate the patient as to how a diet change leads to clinical improvements and what the recommended diet consists of, in general terms. A word from a physician on the role of a healthful diet in diabetes management plays both an educational role and a motivational role, in the same way as a doctor mentioning the need to quit smoking can have a measurable clinical effect.

   The clinician's role is very brief. As an analogy, in the case of a bacterial pneumonia, the physician simply lets the patient know that (1) the growth of bacteria in the lungs and the body's response to it are responsible for the patient's symptoms; (2) an antibiotic, in combination with the patient's immune defenses, will attack the infection; and (3) the antibiotic must be taken with a specific frequency and duration to be effective. In the case of dietary interventions for type 2 diabetes, the key points are (1) microscopic fat particles have built up inside the muscle and liver cells, making it harder for insulin to escort sugar into the cells; (2) eliminating animal products and minimizing oils will cause that built-up fat to diminish; and (3) blood sugars will then likely fall, making it necessary to monitor blood glucose and adjust insulin and oral hypoglycemic agents accordingly. This explanation typically takes 2–3 minutes.

2. **Dietetic Teaching**: The patient should be referred to a registered dietitian or, in the absence of a dietitian, to a nurse, health coach, or other nutrition expert who can work with the patient to draw up a menu of familiar foods that meet the treatment requirements. In many cases, these will be simply modifications of current favorites.

   It is important that the patient's spouse or other family member(s) be included in this session because family members can either support or interfere with the process of change. In a meeting lasting approximately 45 minutes, the patient will come up with an ample list of suitable foods. The need for vitamin B12 supplementation should also be discussed.

3. **Check out the Possibilities**: The dietitian then asks the patient to try out healthful vegan foods over the next 7 days. The idea is not to give up anything during this week. Instead, the patient simply tries out vegan breakfasts, lunches, dinners, and snacks to add to the growing list.

4. **Three-Week Test Drive**: In a return visit a week later, the patient is asked to adopt a fully vegan diet for a 3-week period. This is easy to do because it is a short time frame and the patient has already developed a list of suitable foods. At the end of 3 weeks, patients who have done this reasonably well notice not only significant physical changes, particularly weight loss and improved blood sugars, but also changes in tastes and attitudes and a new-found desire to explore healthful foods. The opportunity to break from the taste of unhealthful foods and to learn new tastes is often a dramatic experience for patients and their families.

It is important that clinicians avoid the temptation to water down the dietary recommendations. Clinicians who advise patients to "just do the best you can" tacitly encourage them to deviate from the recommended diet, in the same way that encouraging a smoker to just "try to cut down" is an invitation to not quit. Instead, patients should be encouraged to give the process of change 100%, to allow themselves to adjust to new tastes and forget old ones. If a patient has a slip, as some will, they will find that their progress slows markedly. In such cases, it is essential to avoid moralizing; rather, it is best to simply encourage patients to pick up where they left off.

In addition to this simple and effective structured sequence, some practices also provide in-office or online classes for patients and families, which are a cost-effective way to follow-up with many patients at once. Such sessions can provide tips for handling practical challenges, such as selecting restaurants (e.g., favoring those serving Italian, Asian, Latin American, or other "international" cuisines), dealing with travel (e.g., focusing on planning ahead), and talking with unhelpful family members. It goes without saying that clinicians working with patients on nutrition issues should adopt the same healthful diet themselves in order to be effective in answering questions and motivating patients.

Practices that do not yet work with registered dietitians should remedy that deficiency. Diabetes is an illness for which diet is always a central treatment consideration, and it should always be addressed as such.

10.13 MEDICATIONS

A few important considerations about medication should be mentioned:

Medications for Glycemic Control: Because vegan diets are highly effective for glucose management, patients taking insulin or other diabetes medications must be educated on how to handle hypoglycemia, must check their blood glucose levels appropriately, and must be in regular touch with their caregivers to reduce their medication regimens so as to avoid hypoglycemia, which can occur within days of a diet change.

Antihypertensive Medications: Because plant-based diets also reduce blood pressure, it is important to work with patients to anticipate hypotension and to reduce or stop antihypertensive medications as appropriate.

Anticoagulants: Some patients using warfarin are fearful of consuming vegetables because of their vitamin K content. However, warfarin use is not a contraindication for a vegetable-rich diet. The best course is to have an abundance of vegetables and to keep the amount of vegetables in the diet reasonably consistent from day to day so that the warfarin dose can be established. Newer anticoagulants allow clinicians to sidestep this issue.

10.14 PLANT-BASED DIETS IN THE COVID-19 ERA

Plant-based diets gained particular urgency with the emergence of COVID-19. When SARS-CoV-2 arose in China, it was soon clear that mortality was much higher among those with diabetes, particularly in those with elevated blood glucose concentrations.[77] Plant-based diets, of course, reduce the risk of diabetes and improve its management, in addition to improving management of weight problems, hypertension, and dyslipidemia, all of which are associated with COVID-19 vulnerability.

The COVID Symptom Study, including 592,571 participants of whom 31,815 developed COVID-19, reported in 2021 that dietary patterns highest in fruits, vegetables, and plant-based foods in general were associated with a 41% lower risk of severe COVID-19 and a 9% reduction of COVID-19 infection of any severity, compared with diets lowest in these foods.[78] Similarly, a 2021 case–control study of healthcare workers in six countries reported that individuals following largely plant-based diets had 73% lower odds of developing moderate-to-severe COVID-19 than those following other diets.[79]

10.15 RESOURCES

The 21-Day Vegan Kickstart is a free app designed to help individuals transition to vegan diets, providing menus, recipes, and cooking videos in English and Spanish.

The Nutrition Guide for Clinicians provides details on the use of dietary interventions for a wide variety of clinical conditions and is available online at no charge.

NutritionCME.org provides free continuing medical education on nutrition in medical practice.

REFERENCES

1. Yokoyama Y, Barnard ND, Levin SM, Watanabe M. Vegetarian diets and glycemic control in diabetes: a systematic review and meta-analysis. *Cardiovasc Diagn Ther.* 2014;4(5):373–82.
2. Tsilas CS, de Souza RJ, Mejia SB, et al. Relation of total sugars, fructose and sucrose with incident type 2 diabetes: a systematic review and meta-analysis of prospective cohort studies. *CMAJ.* 2017 May 23;189(20):711–720. doi: 10.1503/cmaj.160706
3. Shulman GI. Ectopic fat in insulin resistance, dyslipidemia, and cardiometabolic disease. *N Engl J Med.* 2014;371(12):1131–41. doi: 10.1056/NEJMra1011035

4. Petersen KF, Dufour S, Befroy D, Garcia R, Shulman GI. Impaired mitochondrial activity in the insulin-resistant offspring of patients with type 2 diabetes. *N Engl J Med.* 2004;350:664–71.

5. Meyer KA, Kushi LH, Jacobs DR Jr, Folsom AR. Dietary fat and incidence of type 2 diabetes in older Iowa women. *Diabetes Care.* 2001 Sep;24(9):1528–35. doi: 10.2337/diacare.24.9.1528

6. Thanopoulou AC, Karamanos BG, Angelico FV, et al. Dietary fat intake as risk factor for the development of diabetes: multinational, multicenter study of the Mediterranean Group for the Study of Diabetes (MGSD). *Diabetes Care.* 2003 Feb;26(2):302–7. doi: 10.2337/diacare.26.2.302

7. Bachmann OP, Dahl DB, Brechtel K, et al. Effects of intravenous and dietary lipid challenge on intramyocellular lipid content and the relation with insulin sensitivity in humans. *Diabetes.* 2001;50(11):2579–84.

8. Petersen KF, Dufour S, Morino K, Yoo PS, Cline GW, Shulman GI. Reversal of muscle insulin resistance by weight reduction in young, lean, insulin-resistant offspring of parents with type 2 diabetes. *Proc Natl Acad Sci U S A.* 2012;109(21):8236–40. doi:10.1073/pnas.1205675109

9. Goff LM, Bell JD, So PW, Dornhorst A, Frost GS. Veganism and its relationship with insulin resistance and intramyocellular lipid. *Eur J Clin Nutr.* 2005;59:291–98.

10. Kahleova H, Petersen KF, Shulman GI, et al. Effect of a low-fat vegan diet on body weight, insulin sensitivity, postprandial metabolism, and intramyocellular and hepatocellular lipids in overweight adults: a randomized clinical trial. *JAMA Netw Open.* 2020 Nov 2;3(11):e2025454. doi: 10.1001/jamanetworkopen.2020.25454

11. Tonstad S, Butler T, Yan R, Fraser GE. Type of vegetarian diet, body weight and prevalence of type 2 diabetes. *Diabetes Care.* 2009;32:791–6.

12. Tonstad S, Stewart K, Oda K, Batech M, Herring RP, Fraser GE. Vegetarian diets and incidence of diabetes in the Adventist Health Study-2. *Nutr Metab Cardiovasc Dis.* 2013 Apr;23(4):292–9. doi: 10.1016/j.numecd.2011.07.004

13. Pan A, Sun Q, Bernstein AM, Manson JE, Willett WC, Hu FB. Changes in red meat consumption and subsequent risk of type 2 diabetes mellitus: three cohorts of US men and women. *JAMA Intern Med.* 2013;173:1328–35.

14. InterAct Consortium, Bendinelli B, Palli D, Masala G, et al. Association between dietary meat consumption and incident type 2 diabetes: the EPIC-InterAct study. *Diabetologia.* 2013;56:47–59.

15. Chiu TH, Huang HY, Chiu YF, et al. Taiwanese vegetarians and omnivores: dietary composition, prevalence of diabetes and IFG. *PLoS One.* 2014 Feb 11;9(2):e88547. doi: 10.1371/journal.pone.0088547

16. Chiu THT, Pan WH, Lin MN, Lin CL. Vegetarian diet, change in dietary patterns, and diabetes risk: a prospective study. *Nutr Diabetes.* 2018;8(1):12. doi: 10.1038/s41387-018-0022-4

17. Barnard RJ, Jung T, Inkeles SB. Diet and exercise in the treatment of NIDDM: the need for early emphasis. *Diabetes Care.* 1994;17:1469–72.

18. Barnard ND, Cohen J, Jenkins DJ, et al. A low-fat, vegan diet improves glycemic control and cardiovascular risk factors in a randomized clinical trial in individuals with type 2 diabetes. *Diabetes Care.* 2006;29:1777–83.

19. Barnard ND, Cohen J, Jenkins DJ, et al. A low-fat vegan diet and a conventional diabetes diet in the treatment of type 2 diabetes: a randomized, controlled, 74-week clinical trial. *Am J Clin Nutr.* 2009;89(suppl):1588S–96S.

20. Crane MG, Sample C. Regression of diabetic neuropathy with total vegetarian (vegan) diet. *J Nutr Med.* 1994;4:431–9.

21. Bunner AE, Wells CL, Gonzales J, Agarwal U, Bayat E, Barnard ND. A dietary intervention for chronic diabetic neuropathy pain: a randomized controlled pilot study. *Nutr Diabetes*. 2015 May 26;5:e158. doi: 10.1038/nutd.2015.8.
22. Anderson JW, Zeigler JA, Deakins DA, et al. Metabolic effects of high-carbohydrate, high-fiber diets for insulin-dependent diabetic individuals. *Am J Clin Nutr*. 1991;54(5):936–43.
23. Riccardi G, Rivellese AA, Giacco R. Role of glycemic index and glycemic load in the healthy state, in prediabetes, and in diabetes. *Am J Clin Nutr*. 2008;87(1):269S–74S.
24. Kahleova H, Carlsen B, Berrien-Lopez R, Barnard ND. Plant-based diets for type 1 diabetes. *J Diab Metab*. 2020;11:847. doi: 10.35248/2155-6156.20.11.847
25. Reece EA, Leguizamon G, Wiznitzer A. Gestational diabetes: the need for a common ground. *Lancet*. 2009;373(9677):1789–97. doi: 10.1016/S0140-6736(09)60515-8 5.
26. American Diabetes Association. Gestational diabetes mellitus. *Diabetes Care*. 2004 Jan;27(suppl 1):s88–s90. doi: 10.2337/diacare.27.2007.S88
27. Santos S, Voerman E, Amiano P, et al. Impact of maternal body mass index and gestational weight gain on pregnancy complications: an individual participant data metaanalysis of European North American and Australian cohorts. *BJOG*. 2019;126 (8):984–95. doi: 10.1111/1471-0528.15661
28. Kesary Y, Avital K, Hiersch L. Maternal plant-based diet during gestation and pregnancy outcomes. *Arch Gynecol Obstet*. 2020 Oct;302(4):887–98. doi: 10.1007/s00404-020-05689-x.
29. Hassani Zadeh S, Bofetta P, Hosseinzadeh M. Dietary patterns and risk of gestational diabetes mellitus: a systematic review and meta-analysis of cohort studies. *Clin Nutr ESPEN*. 2020;36:1–9. doi: 10.1016/j.clnesp.2020.02.009
30. Quan W, Zeng M, Jiao Y, et al. Western dietary patterns, foods, and risk of gestational diabetes mellitus: a systematic review and meta-analysis of prospective cohort studies. *Adv Nutr*. 2021;12(4):1353–64. doi: 10.1093/advances/nmaa184.
31. Simões-Wüst AP, Moltó-Puigmartí C, van Dongen MCJM, Thijs C. Organic food use, meat intake, and prevalence of gestational diabetes: KOALA birth cohort study. *Eur J Nutr*. 2021 Jun 5. doi: 10.1007/s00394-021-02601-4.
32. Zhang C, Liu S, Solomon CG, Hu FB. Dietary fiber intake, dietary glycemic load, and the risk for gestational diabetes mellitus. *Diabetes Care*. 2006;29:2223–30.
33. Longo-Mbenza B, Kadima-Tshimanga B, Buassa-bu-Tsumbu B, M'Buyamba K Jr. Diets rich in vegetables and physical activity are associated with a decreased risk of pregnancy induced hypertension among rural women from Kimpese, DR Congo. *Niger J Med* 2008;17(1):45–9.
34. Carter JP, Furman T, Hutcheson HR. Preeclampsia and reproductive performance in a community of vegans. *South Med J*. 1987;80:692–7.
35. Spencer EA, et al. Diet and body mass index in 38,000 EPIC-Oxford meat-eaters, fish-eaters, vegetarians, and vegans. *Int J Obesity*. 2003;27:728–34.
36. Barnard ND, Scialli AR, Turner-McGrievy G, Lanou AJ, Glass J. The effects of a low-fat, plant-based dietary intervention on body weight, metabolism, and insulin sensitivity. *Am J Med*. 2005;118(9):991–97.
37. Turner-McGrievy GM, Barnard ND, Scialli AR. A two-year randomized weight loss trial comparing a vegan diet to a more moderate low-fat diet. *Obesity*. 2007;15: 2276–281.
38. Barnard ND, Levin SM, Yokoyama Y. A systematic review and meta-analysis of changes in body weight in clinical trials of vegetarian diets. *J Acad Nutr Diet*. 2015;115(6): 954–69.
39. Huang RY, Huang CC, Hu FB, Chavarro JE. Vegetarian diets and weight reduction: ameta-analysis of randomized controlled trials. *J Gen Intern Med*. 2015;31(1):109–116.

40. Anderson AS, Haynie KR, McMillan RP, et al. Early skeletal muscle adaptations to short-term high-fat diet in humans before changes in insulin sensitivity. *Obesity.* 2015;23:720–24.
41. Sparks LM, Xie H, Koza RA, et al. A high-fat diet coordinately downregulates genes required for mitochondrial oxidative phosphorylation in skeletal muscle. *Diabetes.* 2005;54:1926–33.
42. Neelakantan N, Seah JYH, van Dam RM. The effect of coconut oil consumption on cardiovascular risk factors: a systematic review and metaanalysis of clinical trials. *Circulation.* 2020;141:803–14. doi: 10.1161/CIRCULATIONAHA.119.043052
43. Food and Nutrition Board, Institute of Medicine. *Dietary Reference Intakes for Energy, Carbohydrate, Fiber, Fat, Fatty Acids, Cholesterol, Protein, and Amino Acids.* Washington, DC: National Academies Press; 2002/2005.
44. Hegsted M. Serum-cholesterol response to dietary cholesterol: a re-evaluation. *Am J Clin Nutr.* 1986;44:299–305.
45. Hopkins PN. Effects of dietary cholesterol on serum cholesterol: a meta-analysis and review. *Am J Clin Nutr.* 1992;55:1060–70.
46. Berger S, Raman G, Vishwanathan R, Jacques PF, Johnson EJ. Dietary cholesterol and cardiovascular disease: a systematic review and meta-analysis. *Am J Clin Nutr.* 2015;102(2):276–94.
47. Weggemans RM, Zock PL, Meyboom S, Funke H, Katan MB. Dietary cholesterol from eggs increases the ratio of total cholesterol to high-density lipoprotein cholesterol in humans: a meta-analysis. *Am J Clin Nutr.* 2001;73(5): 885–91.
48. Rouhani MH, Rashidi-Pourfard N, Salehi-Abargouei A, Karimi M, Haghiatdoost F. Effects of egg consumption on blood lipids: a systematic review and meta-analysis of randomized clinical trials. *J Am Coll Nutr.* 2018;37(2):99–110.
49. Vincent MJ, Allen B, Palacios OM, Haber LT, Maki KC. Meta-regression analysis of the effects of dietary cholesterol intake on LDL and HDL cholesterol. *Am J Clin Nutr.* 2019;109:7–16.
50. Barnard ND, Long MB, Ferguson JM, Flores R, Kahleova H. Industry funding and cholesterol research: a systematic review. *Am J Lifestyle Med.* 2019;15(2):165–72.
51. Wang F, Zheng J, Yang B, Jiang J, Fu Y, Li D. Effects of vegetarian diets on blood lipids: a systematic review and meta-analysis of randomized controlled trials. *J Am Heart Assoc.* 2015;4:e002408.
52. Jenkins DJ, Kendall CW, Marchie A, et al. Direct comparison of a dietary portfolio of cholesterol-lowering foods with a statin in hypercholesterolemic participants. *Am J Clin Nutr.* 2005;81:380–7.
53. Chobanian AV, Bakris GL, Black HR, et al. The seventh report of the joint national committee on prevention, detection, evaluation, and treatment of high blood pressure: the JNC 7 report. *JAMA.* May 21 2003;289(19):2560–72.
54. Yokoyama Y, Nishimura K, Barnard ND, et al. Vegetarian diets and blood pressure: a meta-analysis. *JAMA Intern Med.* 2014;174(4):577–87.
55. Rizzo NS, Jaceldo-Siegl K, Sabate J, Fraser GE. Nutrient profiles of vegetarian and nonvegetarian dietary patterns. *J Acad Nutr Diet.* 2013 Dec;113(12):1610–9.
56. Ernst E, Pietsch L, Matrai A, Eisenberg J. Blood rheology in vegetarians. *Br J Nutr.* 1986;56(3):555–60.
57. Sacks FM, Obarzanek E, Windhauser MM, et al. Rationale and design of the Dietary Approaches to Stop Hypertension trial (DASH). A multicenter controlled-feeding study of dietary patterns to lower blood pressure. *Ann Epidemiol.* 1995;5(2):108–18.
58. Estruch R, Ros E, Salas-Salvadó J, et al. Primary prevention of cardiovascular disease with a mediterranean diet supplemented with extra-virgin olive oil or nuts. *N Engl J Med.* 2018 21;378(25):e34.

59. Martínez-González MA, Sánchez-Tainta A, Corella D, et al. A provegetarian food pattern and reduction in total mortality in the Prevención con Dieta Mediterránea (PREDIMED) study. *Am J Clin Nutr.* 2014 Jul;100(Suppl 1):320S–8S.

60. Barnard ND, Alwarith J, Rembert E, et al. A Mediterranean Diet and low-fat vegan diet to improve body weight and cardiometabolic risk factors: a randomized, cross-over trial. *J Am Coll Nutr.* 2021 Feb;41:127–39.

61. Turner-McGrievy GM, Barnard ND, Cohen J, Jenkins DJA, Gloede L, Green AA. Changes in nutrient intake and dietary quality among participants with type 2 diabetes following a low-fat vegan diet or a conventional diabetes diet for 22 weeks. *J Am Diet Assoc.* 2008;108:1636–45.

62. Melina V, Craig W, Levin S. Position of the academy of nutrition and dietetics: vegetarian diets. *J Acad Nutr Diet.* 2016 Dec;116(12):1970–80. doi: 10.1016/j.jand.2016.09.025

63. Bastide NM, Pierre FH, Corpet DE. Heme iron from meat and risk of colorectal cancer: a meta-analysis and a review of the mechanisms involved. *Cancer Prev Res.* 2011; 4(2):177–84.

64. Ayton S, Wang Y, Diouf I, et al. Brain iron is associated with accelerated cognitive decline in people with Alzheimer pathology. *Mol Psychiatry.* 2019 Feb 18. doi: 10.1038/s41380-019-0375-7

65. Allen LH. How common is vitamin B12 deficiency? *Am J Clin Nutr.* 2009;89:693S–6.

66. Scott RS, Ungar PS, Bergstrom TS, Brown CA, Grine FE, Teaford MF, Walker A. Dental microwear texture analysis shows within-species diet variability in fossil hominins. *Nature.* 2005 Aug 4;436(7051):693–5.

67. Hardy K, Brand-Miller J, Brown KD, Thomas MG, Copeland L. The importance of dietary carbohydrate in human evolution. *Q Rev Biol.* 2015 Sep;90(3):251–68. doi: 10.1086/682587

68. Mann GV. The Masai, milk and the yogurt factor: an alternative explanation. *Atherosclerosis.* 1978;29:265.

69. Wann LS, Narula J, Blankstein R, Thompson RC, Frohlich B, Finch CE, Thomas GS. Atherosclerosis in 16th-century greenlandic inuit mummies. *JAMA Network Open.* 2019;2(12):e1918270. doi: 10.1001/jamanetworkopen.2019.18270.

70. Barnard ND, Gloede L, Cohen J, Jenkins DJA, Turner-McGrievy G, Green AA, Ferdowsian H. A low-fat vegan diet elicits greater macronutrient changes, but is comparable in adherence and acceptability, compared with a more conventional diabetes diet among individuals with type 2 diabetes. *J Am Diet Assoc.* 2009;109:263–72.

71. Barnard ND, Scherwitz LW, Ornish D. Adherence and acceptability of a low-fat, vegetarian diet among patients with cardiac disease. *J Cardiopulm Rehab.* 1992;12:423–31.

72. Barnard ND, Scialli AR, Bertron P, Hurlock D, Edmonds K. Acceptability of a therapeutic low-fat, vegan diet in premenopausal women. *J Nutr Educ.* 2000;32:314–9.

73. Barnard ND, Scialli AR, Turner-McGrievy GM, Lanou AJ. Acceptability of a very-low-fat, vegan diet compares favorably to a more moderate low-fat diet in a randomized, controlled trial. *J Cardiopulm Rehab.* 2004;24:229–35.

74. Barnard ND, Gloede L, Cohen J, et al. A low-fat vegan diet elicits greater macronutrient changes, but is comparable in adherence and acceptability, compared with a more conventional diabetes diet among individuals with type 2 diabetes. *J Am Diet Assoc.* 2009;109:263–72.

75. Retail Sales Data 2018. *Plant Based Foods Association.* 2020. https://plantbasedfoods. org/consumer-access/nielsen-data-release–2018/

76. Lee V, McKay T, Ardern CI. Awareness and perception of plant-based diets for the treatment and management of type 2 diabetes in a community education clinic: a pilot study. *J Nutr Metab.* 2015;2015:236234. doi: 10.1155/2015/236234

77. Zhu L, She ZG, Cheng X, et al. Association of blood glucose control and outcomes in patients with COVID-19 and pre-existing type 2 diabetes. *Cell Metab.* 2020;31:1–10.

78. Merino J, Joshi AD, Nguyen LH. Diet quality and risk and severity of COVID-19: a prospective cohort study. *medRxiv.* 2021. doi: 10.1101/2021.06.24.21259283
79. Kim H, Rebholz CM, Hegde S, et al. Plant-based diets, pescatarian diets and COVID-19 severity: a population-based case–control study in six countries. *BMJ Nutr Prev Health.* 2021;4:257. doi: 10.1136/bmjnph-2021-000272

11 Physical Activity

Andrea Delgado Nieves and Michael A. Via
Icahn School of Medicine at Mount Sinai

Jeffrey I. Mechanick
Kravis Center for Cardiovascular Health at Mount Sinai Heart
Icahn School of Medicine at Mount Sinai

CONTENTS

11.1 INTRODUCTION

Various terms will need to be defined to place physical activity (PA) in proper context. Physical activity is defined as any bodily movement produced by skeletal muscles that results in an increased metabolic rate over resting energy expenditure.[1,2] Exercise is defined as a form of leisure-time physical activity that is structured with respect to specific intent/format, repetitiveness, duration, and ultimate goal to improve health.[2] When prescribed by a physician or exercise specialist, the regimen specifies mode, intensity, frequency, and duration of such activity. Sports are a form of exercise but

DOI: 10.1201/9781003206637-11

227

with an intent that can but does not need to be health promotion *per se* (e.g., competition, fun, entertainment, and socialization). Health can be defined in terms of three parts: (1) achieving evidence-based metrics that are associated with decreased chronic disease risk (e.g., body mass index [BMI; weight/height-squared], hemoglobin A1c [A1C], land low-density lipoprotein cholesterol [LDL-C]), (2) decreased symptom burden that is associated with increased quality of life; and (3) happiness.

Chronic disease is any pathophysiological state persisting >3 months, progressing through defined stages, resulting from one or more drivers (key mechanistic causal events), and modulated by social determinants of health and transcultural factors.[3,4] Lifestyle medicine is the nonpharmacological and/or nonprocedural management of chronic disease.[3,4] Lastly, cardiometabolic risk is interpreted using the three-dimensional cardiometabolic-based chronic disease (CMBCD) model whereby primary drivers (genetics, environment, and behavior creating a unique lifestyle) lead to secondary, metabolic drivers (abnormal adiposity, dysglycemia, hypertension, dyslipidemia, and other metabolic syndrome traits) over four stages with their respective preventive care modalities ((1) risk [e.g., insulin resistance] and primordial prevention; (2) predisease [e.g., prediabetes or overweight] and primary prevention; (3) disease [e.g., type 2 diabetes {T2D} or obesity]; and (4) complications [e.g., cardiovascular disease {CVD}]),[3,4] In short, PA should be implemented as early as possible in the CMBCD model to successfully prevent CVD risk and events.[3,4]

Total energy expenditure in humans can be divided into three components: basal metabolic rate, thermic effect of food, and the energy expenditure of activity (activity thermogenesis).[7] Basal metabolic rate is the energy expended when an individual is at complete rest. Thermic effect of food is defined as the increase in energy expenditure associated with digestion, absorption, and storage of food and accounts for approximately 10% of the total daily energy expenditure. Activity thermogenesis is the thermogenesis that accompanies physical activities, which in turn can be divided into exercise and non-exercise activity thermogenesis. Non-exercise activity thermogenesis includes activities of daily living, fidgeting, spontaneous muscle contraction, and maintaining posture when non-recumbent.

Physical activity is an integral part of human life, which influences development and overall health.[1] This general concept includes leisure-time PA, exercise, sport, transportation, occupational work, and chores. In numerous studies, PA has been shown to promote cardiometabolic wellness, improve cognitive performance, and aid in the prevention and treatment of a variety of health conditions, including CVD, T2D, and other disorders of insulin resistance.[1] The human species evolved a physiology dependent on habitual PA to meet environmental demands and requirements. In contrast, the absence of regular PA, which is common in modern societies, leads to detrimental metabolic physiology, insulin resistance, T2D, and CMBCD.[1]

11.2   RECOMMENDED PHYSICAL ACTIVITY

The Physical Activity Guidelines for Americans (PAGA), released in 2008 by the U.S. Department of Health and Human Services, recommend that adults participate in at least 150 minutes/week of moderate-intensity physical activity, 75 minutes/week of vigorous-intensity physical activity, or a combination of moderate and vigorous physical activity.[8] Like many general recommendations, this represents a standard minimum that may be adjusted to the individual patient.[8]

Activity may be gauged by the amount of energy utilized as a metabolic equivalent (MET), which is defined as the total energy cost of an activity as a multiple of resting metabolic rate.[9] In practice, this may be estimated through indirect calorimetry by oxygen consumed during PA. Moderate-intensity activities are defined as those with an energy expenditure of 3–5.9 METs. Some examples of moderate PA include brisk walking, dancing, gardening, housework, traditional hunting and gathering, general building tasks, and carrying/moving moderate loads (<20 kg). Activities are considered as vigorous intensity if they induce an expenditure of six or more METs and include running, walking/climbing up a hill, fast cycling, aerobics, competitive sports, heavy shoveling, and carrying/moving heavy loads (>20 kg).[9] Use of the MET concept provides a convenient method to describe functional capacity or exercise tolerance of an individual. Additionally, the MET descriptor can be used to define specific PAs in which a person may participate safely, without exceeding a prescribed intensity level.[9]

11.3 PHYSICAL INACTIVITY

Contrary to recommendations and guidelines that state adults should participate in at least 140 minutes/week of moderate-intensity physical activity, 75 minutes/week of vigorous-intensity exercise, or a combination of both, physical inactivity is defined as performing insufficient amounts of moderate- and vigorous-intensity activity.[10,11] Global estimates show that one in four adults and more than three-quarters of adolescents do not meet the recommendations for aerobic exercise as outlined in the 2010 Global Recommendations on Physical Activity for Health.[12] This puts more than 1.4 billion adults at risk of developing or exacerbating diseases associated with inactivity.[12]

In Westernized cultures, physical inactivity has significantly higher prevalence. The highest levels of inactivity were found in high-income Western countries, high-income Asia-Pacific countries, as well as in Latin America and the Caribbean.[12] In these areas, the prevalence of physical inactivity is nearly double compared with that of low-income countries.[12] A review of published studies demonstrates that 36.8% (95% CI 34.6–38.4) of the population of high-income Western countries meets criteria for physical inactivity.[12] Similarly, data collected in the U.S. in the 2017 National Health Interview Survey (NHIS) indicate that only 53.8% of adults met the PA guidelines for aerobic exercise, with less than a quarter (23.7%) meeting both aerobic and muscle-strengthening activities.[12] The high levels of frank physical inactivity or diminished PA noted among wealthier nations is attributed to the transition toward more sedentary occupations, choices of leisure-time sedentary behaviors (e.g., increased screen time: computers, video games, and television), and personal motorized transportation.[12] Risk factors leading to less PA participation, lower intensity of PA, and shorter duration of PA include higher income categories, living in lower- to middle-income countries (LMIC; mainly due to unhealthy built environments), unemployment, and lack of health insurance.[13,14] In general, people in low socioeconomic classes or with less education, even in high-income countries, are more likely to be economically disadvantaged and are at greater risk of being affected by chronic diseases, both contributing to physical inactivity.[15]

11.4 PHYSIOLOGICAL MECHANISMS

The seemingly simple act of PA has numerous complex physiological effects within metabolically active tissues and organs that serve as the basis for the observed health benefits. Some examples include improvement in glucose metabolism, skeletal muscle function, ventilator muscle strength, bone stability, locomotor coordination, psychological well-being, and other organ functions.[17]

11.4.1 GLUCOSE METABOLISM

Physical activity has effects at a cellular level in healthy individuals, as well as patients with dysglycemia-based chronic disease (DBCD): stage 1—insulin resistance, stage 2—prediabetes, stage 3—T2D, and stage 4—T2D with vascular complications.[16] Glucose utilization during PA is similar in both patients with T2D and those without, suggesting that non-insulin dependent mechanisms may have significant impacts in DBCD stages 1 and 2.[17] During exercise, many adaptive changes in skeletal muscle in patients with T2D decrease insulin resistance.[17] Therefore, since skeletal muscle is responsible for the majority of glucose uptake in the postprandial state, PA can profoundly affect glycemia and reduce the risk of downstream diabetic complications in DBCD stage 4.[17]

In the acute state, both insulin and exercise increase skeletal muscle glucose uptake by translocation of glucose transporter 4 (GLUT-4) to the plasma membrane.[18] However, different molecular pathways are invoked. Insulin causes phosphorylation of the insulin receptor with subsequent signal cascade.[19] In contrast, exercise activates pathways including the AMP-activated protein kinase (AMPK) and the calcium/calmodulin-dependent protein kinases pathways.[20] Further downstream, the pathways for insulin signal transduction and for exercise converge to enable GLUT-4 mobilization to the cellular surface. Some of the molecules involved in this common pathway are AS160, TBC1D1, and Rab proteins, which are involved in many membrane trafficking events, including vesicle budding, tethering, and fusion. This leads to cell surface translocation of GLUT-4.[21] In addition to the well-established roles of Rab proteins, there is evidence that the Rho family GTPase Rac1 is involved in both insulin- and exercise-stimulated GLUT-4 translocation.[21]

11.4.2 LIPID METABOLISM

The lipid profile is altered by PA. Exercise consumes carbohydrates and fat as energy sources.[22] The four major sources of energy during exercise can be found in: plasma glucose, free fatty acids (FFA) derived from adipose tissue lipolysis or hydrolysis of triacylglycerol in very low-density lipoproteins (VLDL), muscle glycogen, and intramyocellular triacylglycerols (IMTGs) within skeletal muscle fibers.[22] Fatty acid (FA) oxidation rate is the result of processes including triglyceride lipolysis, fatty acid transport from plasma to muscle sarcoplasm, availability and hydrolysis rate of intra-muscular triglycerides, and transport of FAs through the mitochondrial membrane.[22] Cardiac muscle, skeletal muscle, kidney, and liver tissues increase FFA uptake for energy substrate during exercise.[23] Preferential FA oxidation is maximized during moderate-intensity exercise, while glucose consumption is seen mostly during high-intensity training, though there is a shift back to lipid sources during periods of prolonged exercise.[23]

The majority of the FFA used during exercise is released from lipid stores in adipose tissue and skeletal muscle. Circulating lipoproteins are mobilized to replenish these stores. Consequently, resistance exercise causes a significant decrease in triglycerides and cholesterol within chylomicrons.[22] Aerobic and/or resistance exercise also decrease total cholesterol and LDL-C and increase high-density lipoprotein cholesterol (HDL-C).[22] The metabolism of lipids includes lipolysis, transport from the blood to cytosol of muscle, and FA transport to the mitochondria of muscles for oxidation and adenosine 5′-triphosphate (ATP) generation.[22] After chronic endurance training, plasma FA oxidation decreases and there is increased dependence on IMTGs as a fuelsource.[22] Exercise drives these processes through muscle contraction and hormonal mechanisms. Major endocrine mechanisms include epinephrine mediated hormone-sensitive lipase (HSL) and perilipin 1 activation, which in turn increases lipolysis.[22] Within mitochondria, there is an increase in the activities of β-oxidation enzymes, the tricarboxylic acid cycle, and the electron transport chain during exercise.[22] Rapid glycolysis during high-intensity exercise provides mitochondria with excess acetyl-coenzyme A (CoA) to form acetyl carnitine, which drives FA oxidation.[22]

11.4.3 Skeletal Muscle

Physical activity has effects on signaling cascades in several tissues including skeletal muscle.[24] Through muscular contraction and release of calcium from the sarcoplasmic reticulum, increased cytosolic calcium concentration leads to activation of signaling cascades that influence myocyte glucose uptake. Increased concentration of calcium/calmodulin complexes activate the calcium/calmodulin-dependent protein kinases, leading to enhanced expression of GLUT-4.[24] Activation of the calcium/calmodulin signaling pathways is enhanced by both increased intensity and duration of exercise.[24] Another key pathway in glucose uptake-related signaling is through activation of mammalian target of rapamycin (mTOR).[24] Muscle contraction stimulates mTOR signaling, leading to protein synthesis and myocyte hypertrophy.[24] Additional tissue allows for greater glucose uptake. Exercise-induced activation of mTOR signaling in endurance and resistance training appears to be time-dependent with continuous increase that persists after termination of PA.[24]

Inflammatory states can contribute to insulin resistance and muscle wasting.[25] The nuclear factor-κB (NFκB) inflammatory pathway is activated within skeletal muscles of patients with T2D.[25] The toll-like receptors (TLR) are the major drivers for this and are activated through inflammatory signaling including cytokines such as interleukin (IL)-6, tumor necrosis factor (TNF)-α, and IL-15.[26] Chronic exercise can lead to reduced TLR expression.[26] In addition, acute and chronic exercise can reduce activation of the NFκB pathway independent of exercise modality, age, and training status.[25] Acute PA increases IL-6 expression in skeletal muscle but suppresses IL-6 in adipose tissue. However, with chronic exercise, there is a decrease in plasma IL-6 concentration. The transient rise in IL-6 during acute exercise appears to be responsible for producing anti-inflammatory mediators such as IL-10 or IL-1 receptor antagonist.[25] These anti-inflammatory cytokines inhibit the secretion of proinflammatory cytokines TNF-α and IL-1β, suppress the secretion of the acute phase reactant c-reactive protein (CRP), downregulate monocyte TLR expression, and inhibit the NFκB pathway.[24]

The nucleotide-binding oligomerization domain (NOD)-like receptors (NLRs) represent another class of signal molecules that initiate inflammatory processes and affect glucose uptake-related signaling.[5] NLRs activate the inflammasome pathway, which in turn, activates proinflammatory cytokines such as IL-1β. Moreover, IL-1β has been shown to stimulate inflammatory processes leading to cell damage and apoptosis, particularly in pancreatic β-cells, and is suggested to drive progression of DBCD, that is insulin resistance to prediabetes/T2D.[5] Multiple animal studies have shown how chronic endurance and resistance training decreases the activity of the NLR/inflammasome pathway, specifically by decreased expression of IL-18 expression. However, this is yet to be studied in humans.[24]

The C-jun N-terminal kinase (JNK)/mitogen-activated protein kinase (MAPK) pathway is suppressed by exercise, which serves to modulate exercise dependent effects on glucose uptake and inflammatory response.[27] JNK/MAPK activity leads to systemic inflammation through TNF-α and IL-6 release and can also impair insulin receptor signaling, leading to insulin resistance.[28] In the acute setting, intense exercise can lead to stimulation of JNK signaling in skeletal muscle while long-term exercise reduces JNK phosphorylation, diminishing MAPK signaling and improving insulin sensitivity in adipose and hepatic tissue.[29]

Skeletal muscle mitochondrial dysfunction has also been associated with insulin resistance.[30] Patients with T2D demonstrate smaller, damaged, or dysfunctional mitochondria, and decreased expression of peroxisome proliferator-activated receptor-γ coactivator-1α, a marker of mitochondrial biogenesis.[30] Chronic exercise improves mitochondrial function and biogenesis within skeletal muscle.[30] A 12-week combined progressive training program (three times per week and 45 minutes per session, including aerobic and strength exercises) in people with T2D restored mitochondrial content and function to levels similar to those of controls without diabetes.[31]

11.4.4 Adipose Tissue

Adipose tissue is specialized for storage of energy in the form of triacylglycerols. It also releases peptides and factors that act in endocrine and paracrine fashion. PA can lead to a loss of adiposity or fat mass.[32] However, studies support that exercise has no preferential effect on visceral adipose tissue (VAT) or subcutaneous adipose tissue (SCAT).[32] In theory, PA-induced reduction in adiposity could be explained by either reduction in adipocyte size and/or number. Clinical studies demonstrate regular exercise reduces subcutaneous abdominal adipocyte size, with little to no change in adipocyte number.[33]

VAT accumulation is associated with low-grade systemic inflammation and contributes to insulin resistance. White adipose tissue (WAT), especially when located within VAT, secretes adipokines that regulate energy metabolism. These include the cytokines TNF-α, IL-6, adiponectin, leptin, omentin-1, and visfatin, among others.[34] Dysregulated production of adipokines affects insulin sensitivity, hypothalamic metabolic regulation, and systemically on glucose homeostasis.[33] PA reduces proinflammatory cytokine release within adipose tissue and diminishes inflammatory responses mediated by leukocytes.[32] The chronic effects of PA on cytokine levels are beneficial regardless of mode or intensity, with lower TNF-α, CRP, and IL-6 and higher anti-inflammatory modulators such as IL-4 and IL-10.

Exercise also induces increased production of adiponectin, a prominent adipokine with insulin sensitizing properties.[35] In macrophages, adiponectin reduces NFκB activation and thus inhibits TNF-α activity.[36] Adiponectin also improves pancreatic β-cell mass,[37] enhances GLUT-4 translocation in myocytes,[38] reduces hepatic glucose release,[39] reduces circulating triglycerides through increased lipoprotein lipase activity,[40] and improves vascular endothelial function through nitric oxide (NO) signaling.[41]

Levels of other adipokines are generally diminished by exercise. Leptin is an adipokine that regulates hypothalamic pathways of metabolic control and satiation, as well as skeletal muscle metabolism.[42] Studies have reported no changes or decreases in leptin levels in response to exercise.[42] An exercise-induced decrease in leptin levels is mediated through increased energy expenditure, increasing catecholamine concentrations, oxidative stress, testosterone levels, and reduction in fat mass.

Resistin is part of the newly described family of secretory proteins termed "resistin-like molecules," which are up-regulated in obesity and contribute to insulin resistance. During exercise, resistin concentrations are decreased in response to released catecholamines.[43] VAT-derived serpin (vaspin) is a member of the serine protease inhibitor family that is associated with fat mass expansion, impaired insulin sensitivity, fitness levels, and blood leptin concentrations.[44] There is no evidence of an association between PA and vaspin levels in patients with obesity. However, there are data that suggest that PA may lower vaspin levels by decreasing insulin resistance.[44] Omentin-1 is an adipokine that plays a role in improving insulin sensitivity.[45] It does so by stimulating glucose uptake in adipocytes by activating protein kinase B. Exercise training increases basal level of omentin-1 in individuals with obesity; however, the mechanism by which this is achieved is poorly understood. Retinol-binding protein (RBP)-4 is an adipokine secreted by the liver, skeletal muscles, and WAT, which is involved in increasing insulin resistance by inhibiting insulin signaling in muscles and increasing hepatic glucose output. Resistance training can decrease RBP-4 levels in persons with T2D in an intensity-dependent manner. Apelin is a peptide secreted by adipocytes which increases blood pressure and cardiac contractility.[45] In skeletal muscle, apelin enhances insulin sensitivity and glucose uptake. There are no studies regarding the effects of acute exercise on apelin levels, and there are a limited number of studies on the effects of chronic exercise showing mixed outcomes. Visfatin is another newly identified adipocytokine that possesses insulin-like metabolic effects that can improve insulin sensitivity.[45] Chronic exercise has been observed to decrease visfatin levels in individuals with obesity via negative energy balance and correlates with exercise duration. Monocyte chemoat-tractant protein (MCP)-1 is an adipokine released by adipose tissue and is increased by obesity-associated low-grade inflammation. Chronic aerobic exercise training has been seen to decrease MCP-1 levels likely by remodeling adipose tissue and decreasing inflammatory macrophages.

11.4.5 Cardiovascular System

Biochemical mechanisms involved in mediating exercise-induced cardiovascular effects can be classified into cardiac and vascular effects.[46]

11.4.5.1 Cardiac Effects

Cardiac level effects of PA in an individual with normal LV function can be divided into three categories: prevention of aging-related pathologies; prevention of impaired systolic and/or diastolic cardiac function associated with short-term challenges [e.g., ischemia/reperfusion (I/R)]; and adaptation resulting in myocardial hypertrophy (athlete's heart).[46] Regular exercise prevents cardiac pathologies associated with aging via: delayed accumulation of reactive oxygen species (ROS)-mediated cell damage by improving antioxidative protection; overexpression of heat shock proteins in cardiomyocytes to protect against ischemic damage and to increase cell survival; and protection against cardiomyocyte apoptosis by modulating proapop-totic and antiapoptotic genes.[46] Cardiac hypertrophy resulting from exercise training is mediated by increased cardiac insulin-like growth factor-1 (IGF-1) expression and activation of phophoinositide-3 kinase (PI3K).[46] In addition, downregulation of cardiac-specific microRNAs is also involved in exercise-induced cardiac hypertrophy.[43] Exercise-induced protection against ischemia-reperfusion damage is achieved by improved antioxidative protection, changes in mitochondrial metabolism and protein expression, increased expression of sarcolemmal/mitochondrial K_{ATP} channels, and attenuation of I/R-induced calpain activation.[46] Lastly, regular exercise attenuates the deleterious elevation of endothelial and myofibroblasts oxidative stress and reduces expression of pro-calcific genes, both of which contribute to aortic valve degeneration and sclerosis.[47]

11.4.5.2 Vascular Endothelium

Exercise-induced vascular effects depend on the level of the arterial vascular bed.[46] Four basic mechanisms have been identified to regulate vascular tone in response to local metabolic demand in the vascular territories: endothelium-mediated flow-induced vasodilation, myogenic control, metabolic vasodilation, and sympathetic control.[48] The relative contribution of these mechanisms to vasodilation is different in the various microdomains of the vascular tree. Endothelium-dependent vasodilation is most relevant in small conduit and resistance arteries. Metabolic control is dominant in small resistance arteries, in which the myogenic response to increased perfusion pressure is most pronounced. At the level of large arterial conduit vessels, endurance training is effective in attenuating the paradoxical arterial vasoconstriction in epicardial conduit vessels and increases average peak flow velocity. In addition, endurance training improves endothelium-dependent, flow-mediated dilation in conduit arteries.[49]

Along the arterial tree, arteries are exposed to two main forces: radial strain and laminar shear tress. As a result of pulsatile continuous blood flow, laminar shear stress is a survival signal for endothelial cells. At a molecular level, laminar shear stress affects multiple signaling pathways, including the PI3K, extracellular signal-regulated kinase 5, and NO pathways.[50] Exercise has been shown to increase the expression of endothelial NO synthase, which leads to higher NO production, and dilation of vascular smooth muscle cells. In addition, exercise induces vascular expression of antioxidative enzymes, reduces the expression of ROS generating enzymes, and decreases the expression of angiotensin II receptors.[50] During exercise, endothelial progenitor cells are mobilized from the bone marrow and contribute to the integrity of the endothelial cell layer. In terms of arterial resistance vessels, larger and medium-sized vasodilation is primarily mediated by the endothelium, whereas smaller arterioles are subject to metabolic and myogenic control. Metabolic control of resistance vessel dilation is based on the presence of an oxygen/metabolic sensor coupled to vascular smooth muscle cells.[48] Some molecules that induce vascular dilatation through these sensors include adenosine, carbon dioxide, and erythrocyte ATP release.[50] Exercise training increases resistance vessel sensitivity and maximal responsiveness to adenosine. In terms of myogenic control for smaller arterioles, exercise induces myogenic vasoconstriction to increase tissue perfusion pressure via mechanisms of L-type voltage-gated calcium channel activation and protein kinase C in smooth muscle.[48] Finally, several studies have shown that exercise training increases vascular endothelial growth factor transcription in skeletal muscle leading to increased vascularization.[51]

11.4.6 Hepatic Metabolism

Exercise is an effective strategy for mitigating the harmful effects of fructose consumption, especially on hepatic function.[52] High consumption of fructose has been related to the development of obesity. Fructose-rich beverages lead to increased body weight gain, elevated systolic blood pressure, hyperglycemia, hyperinsulinemia, and increased serum triglyceride concentrations.[52] In humans, high fructose consumption is related to high levels of fasting insulin, uric acid, and central adiposity[52]. Fructose consumption also increases serum triglyceride levels, decreases mobilization and oxidation of lipids, and increases leptin levels[52]. Consequently, dietary fructose has been shown to raise liver lipid accumulation.[52] Fructose is absorbed into the bloodstream by GLUT-5 receptors, and into hepatocytes by GLUT-2 receptors.[53] Inside hepatocytes, fructose is converted to fructose 1-phosphate, which acts as substrate for pathways leading to increased gluconeogenesis and hyperglycemia. Intracellular fructose also increases inflammatory processes and produces uric acid via AMP pathways. Fructose metabolism induces generation of triglycerides via peroxisome proliferator-activated receptor-gamma coactivator 1-β protein within the hepatocyte leading to nonalcoholic fatty liver disease, hypercholesterolemia, and dyslipidemia.[53] Resulting lipids may also travel to adipose tissue to generate hypertrophy, to the skeletal muscle triggering insulin resistance, or to the pancreas, which inhibits the secretion of insulin. Fructose consumption activates the formation of ROS and increases the expression of inflammatory proteins in hepatocytes leading to tissue damage and inflammation.[53]

Strength training decreases insulin levels, improves insulin sensitivity, and decreases in intra-abdominal adipose tissue. Combined aerobic exercise and strength training improves several deleterious effects of fructose consumption.[52] When performed on alternate days, aerobic exercise and strength training was able to improve glucose tolerance, insulin sensitivity[52], HDL-C levels, and hepatic TG accumulation.[52] In addition, decreased activation of NF-κB and decreased systemic inflammation.[52]

Sedentary individuals with obesity have an increased risk of developing nonalcoholic fatty liver disease (NAFLD).[54] NAFLD can progress into nonalcoholic steatohepatitis (NASH), which can place patients at risk of developing end-stage liver disease and consequently hepatocellular carcinoma (HCC). Diet and lifestyle modification leading to 10% weight loss or more has been proven to achieve resolution of NASH in > 90% of patients. Several studies have shown vigorous-intensity exercise to decrease the risk of developing NASH.[55] In addition, a study comparing doses and intensities of exercise regimens found significant reduction in liver fat even with low intensity and low volume intensity exercise. Studies comparing aerobic vs resistance training have shown similar benefits on hepatic fat content.[54] However, other studies suggest aerobic exercise had greater reduction in hepatic fat content than resistance exercise.[54] Moreover, a decrease in hepatic fat content has been achieved because of exercise, even in the absence of overall weight loss.[55] All of these findings suggest that PA has a beneficial impact on hepatic fat content irrespective of exercise regimen, frequency or intensity[56]. Therefore, exercise training should be encouraged and can be tailored in patients with NAFLD by individual preference for long-term adherence.

In the 2022 clinical practice guidelines on NAFLD by the American Association of Clinical Endocrinology and American Association for the Study of Liver Diseases, PA is recommended to optimize body composition and cardiometabolic health in adults (recommendation 3.2.3) and children (recommendation 4.3.1).

The beneficial effects of physical activity on NAFLD are achieved through several molecular mechanisms. Improvement in insulin resistance reduces the flux of free fatty acids to the liver.[55] Resistance and high-intensity aerobic exercise have both been shown to decrease the expression of sterol regulatory element-binding protein (SREBP)-1c, a transcription factor involved in lipogenesis that is overexpressed in NAFLD and NASH[54]. Expression of other hepatocyte proteins associated with lipid accumulation is decreased by exercise, including fatty acid synthase, stearoyl-CoA desaturase 1, and acetyl-CoA carboxylase.[54]

The liver can neutralize immunologically active FFA by four major pathways: esterification of FFA into triglycerides, sequestration into lipid droplets, excretion in very-low-density lipoprotein, and fatty acid oxidation in hepatocyte mitochondria.[57] A 7-day aerobic exercise course was found to have a significant increase in fatty acid oxidation in patients with NAFLD.[54] Running, as a standard cardiovascular exercise, improves liver mitochondrial function and increases the activity of carnitine palmitoyltransferase, an enzyme necessary for FA transport for oxidation.[58] Activity of peroxisome proliferator-activated receptor-α, which regulates the expression of multiple genes responsible for mitochondrial fatty acid oxidation, is also increased with exercise.[54] Activation of AMPK-regulated pathways represents another mechanism whereby exercise increases hepatic fatty acid oxidation.

Indirectly, exercise reduces ROS formation, which can cause FFA overabundance and mitochondrial damage in patients with NASH.[59] Hepatocyte damage induced by ROS and the toxic consequences of FFA can activate localized inflammation, leading to an increase in circulating cytokines and transaminase levels.[59] In patients with NASH, various exercise regimens have been shown to decrease levels of liver transaminases, serum cytokines, and other inflammatory markers, including IL-6, IL-8, TNF-α, ferritin, and CRP.[59]

In rats, a study of treadmill running regimen reduced markers of fibrosis and decreased activation of hepatic stellate cells, which is thought to be the cause of fibrosis in NASH.[60] In addition, in a mouse model of NASH that progresses to HCC, exercise-induced AMPK decreased mTOR activity, which attenuated hepatocyte proliferation and tumor formation.[61] Treadmill training not only decreased the risk of developing cancer, but also had a reduction in tumor reduction of primary liver cancer. Among patients with advanced cases of NASH, liver fibrosis can develop, with risk for progression to liver cancer.

11.4.7 CENTRAL NERVOUS SYSTEM EFFECTS

11.4.7.1 Hypothalamus

The hypothalamus is an important region for regulatory control of energy balance, feeding behavior, and body weight.[62] Leptin and melanocortin pathways are involved in the regulation of energy balance and glucose homeostasis in the arcuate nucleus of the hypothalamus, which receives input from several peripheral hormones that reflect energy stores and nutrient availability, including leptin, insulin, and ghrelin.[62] Within the arcuate nucleus, two neuronal cell groups comprise the melanocortin system: the anorexigenic pro-opiomelanocortin (POMC) neurons and orexigenic neuropeptide Y (NPY)/agouti-related peptide (AgRP) neurons. The AgRP population drives rapid feeding responses while the POMC population alters chronic feeding behavior.[62] In addition, activation of AgRP neurons results in swift modifications of body substrate utilization to carbohydrate metabolism, decreased fat usage, and decreased energy expenditure. In contrast, POMC neurons, via leptin receptors,[63] raise energy expenditure, decrease adiposity, and improve insulin sensitivity and glucose metabolism.[63] Exercise activates arcuate nuclei POMC and inhibits NPY/AgRP neurons.[62] Additionally, exercise increases leptin sensitivity within the arcuate nucleus. In aggregate, these central mechanisms act to reduce the risk of prediabetes, T2D, and T2D complications, especially CVD.

11.4.7.2 Psychological Effects

Exercise impacts mental health. Studies that include participants with anxiety disorders, major depression, dysthymic disorder, or depressive disorder demonstrate improved anxiety scores and reduced depression scores with either aerobic or non-aerobic exercises.[64] Several physiological mechanisms have been proposed to explain these mental health effects, including elevated plasma levels of endorphins and endocannabinoids after exercise.[64] An increase in body temperature after exercise has also been implicated in mood elevation and reduction in anxiety symptoms.[64] In specific areas such as the brainstem, an increase in temperature can decrease muscular tension and lead to a feeling of overall relaxation.

PA is also associated with increased neuronal mitochondriogenesis. Mitochondria play a key role in synaptic strength and cellular resilience of neuronal circuits within the brain and neuroplasticity of grey matter.[65] Poor mental health has been linked to poor neuroplasticity which may result in an inability to respond and adapt to stress. Exercise activates mTOR in brain regions that are involved with cognition and emotional behaviors.[64] This can improve mental health states by reducing the effects of stress, anxiety, and depression through cognitive and emotional function. Exercise has also been observed to increase serotonergic and adrenergic levels in the brain, acting similarly to serotonin reuptake inhibitor medications used for anxiety and depression.[64]

11.4.7.3 Sleep

There is strong evidence that regular PA can improve sleep.[66] Studies have shown improvement in non-rapid eye movement sleep, slow wave sleep, stage 2 sleep, and total sleep time, as well as reduced wake time after sleep onset.[66] Exercise programs improve sleep quality, latency, duration, efficiency, and total sleep time.[66] In addition, PA has been shown to decrease the use of sleep medications.[66] Moderate rather than vigorous-intensity exercise appears more beneficial in terms of sleep outcomes, though both show improvement in sleep measures. Compared to a single exercise activity, a combination of different types of exercise (e.g., aerobic, strength, and yoga) is more effective for improved sleep.[67,68]

11.4.8 Stem Cell Regeneration

In addition to organ and tissue effects of PA, there is growing evidence that exercise training activates mobilization of bone marrow progenitor cells to facilitate regeneration of metabolically active tissues.[2] These include endothelial progenitor cells promoting vascular regeneration, neural progenitor cells in ischemic stroke recovery, and cardiac progenitor cells to induce physiological cardiac hypertrophy.[2] Moreover, PA diminishes cellular quiescence within skeletal muscle and other tissues, a phenomenon of aging that is accelerated by insulin resistance.[5] This may also contribute to activity-induced improvements in metabolic function.

11.5 PRESCRIPTION OF ACTIVITY

Most interventions also recommend 30–40 minutes of moderate physical activity on all or most days of the week with variable emphasis on high-intensity and resistance training exercise. These recommendations are based on large clinical trial data and are summarized in Table 11.1. The Finnish Diabetes Prevention Study[6] published in 2000 aimed to assess the efficacy of an intensive diet–exercise program in preventing or delaying T2D in individuals with impaired glucose tolerance. This trial also evaluated the effect of the program on atherosclerotic vascular diseases and the incidence of cardiovascular events.[6] The main measure in the intervention group was individual dietary advice aimed at reducing weight and intake of saturated fat,

TABLE 11.1

Clinical Trial Data Demonstrating Beneficial Effects of Physical Activity on Cardiometabolic Parameters[a]

Name of Trial (Reference)	Type of Prevention	N	Intervention	Key Results
Finnish Diabetes Prevention Study[73]	Primary	522	Individualized dietary counseling plus circuit-type resistance training sessions	Intervention group had greater weight reduction and improvements on glycemia and lipemia
Diabetes Prevention Program[69]	Primary	3,234	Lifestyle modification program with at least 150 minutes of exercise a week	Intervention group had reduction of 58% incidence of diabetes
Look AHEAD trial[4]	Secondary	5,145	Intensive lifestyle intervention	Intervention group had greater reductions in weight loss, A1C, and cardiovascular risk factors (except LDL-C), and had greater initial improvements in exercise capacity
Stewart, 2004[98]	Primary	62	Six months of exercise in subjects with or at high risk for metabolic syndrome	Exercise group improved peak $\dot{V}O_2$, muscle strength, and lean body mass; reductions in total and abdominal fat related to improved CVD risk
Kartzmarzyk, 2003[99]	Primary	333	Twenty weeks of supervised aerobic exercise training	30.5% of patients were no longer classified as having metabolic syndrome after exercise training
Balducci, 2008[100]	Primary	234	Twice weekly aerobic and resistance training for 1 year	Exercise group improved fitness, A1C, and CVD risk profile

Abbreviations: A1C, hemoglobin A1c; CVD, cardiovascular disease; LDL-C, low-density lipoprotein cholesterol; $\dot{V}O_2$, maximal oxygen consumption.

[a] These selected clinical trials serve as examples that constitute the evidence base supporting the incorporation of different types of physical activity for specific cardiometabolic targets based on individualization of risk.

as well as increasing intake of dietary fiber. Additionally, the intervention subjects were individually guided to increase their level of PA, including aerobic exercise and resistance training. In contrast, the control group received general information about the benefits of weight reduction, PA, and healthy diet in the prevention of T2D. Results showed greater weight reduction (−4.6 kg) at 1 year in the intervention group compared with the control group (−0.9 kg). Additionally, at 1 year, the intervention group showed significantly greater reductions in post-challenge 2 hours glucose, fasting insulin, and 2 hours insulin, as well as blood pressure (systolic and diastolic) and serum triglycerides. These results show that a lifestyle intervention including regular PA can postpone the onset of T2D for many years.

Similarly, the Diabetes Prevention Program aimed to determine whether lifestyle intervention or pharmacological therapy (i.e., metformin) would prevent or delay the onset of T2D in individuals with impaired glucose tolerance (a descriptor for DBCD stage 2, or prediabetes; identifying patients at high risk for progression to DBCD stage 3, or T2D).[69–71] The two major prespecified lifestyle endpoints of the Diabetes Prevention Program were a minimum of 7% weight loss/weight maintenance and a minimum of 150 minutes of physical activity similar in intensity to brisk walking. Study groups included an intensive lifestyle intervention focusing on a healthy diet and exercise ($N = 1,079$), and two blinded medication treatment groups—metformin ($N = 1,073$) or placebo ($N = 1,082$)—combined with standard diet and exercise recommendations.[72] There were a total of 3,234 participants in the study, and the main finding was that intensive lifestyle intervention resulted in a 58% reduction in the incidence rate of T2D ($p < 0.001$).

The impact of PA on CVD has also been evaluated in several studies. The Look AHEAD trial assessed the effects of an intensive lifestyle intervention (ILI) that included PA but focused on cardiovascular morbidity, mortality, and other complications in 5,145 overweight/obese adults with T2D. Results showed clinically meaningful weight loss (5%) at year 8 in 50% of patients with T2D with lifestyle intervention that included regular PA.[8,73] While there was a differential effect on weight loss and fitness between the two groups, there was no effect on cardiovascular outcomes.[8,73] CVD events were less than half the projected rate in the control group.[8,73] Thus, there was a very low overall rate of events in both groups, which could explain the non-significant effects on CVD found in the study.[8,73] However, there were many other health benefits that occurred with ILI, including improved biomarkers of glucose and lipid control, less sleep apnea, lower liver fat, less depression, less urinary incontinence, less severe kidney disease, improved sexual dysfunction, reduced need of diabetes medications, maintenance of physical mobility, and improved quality of life.[8,73] PA was more specifically investigated in terms of CVD prevention and decreasing risk factors associated to CVD.[8,73] A 2008 randomized controlled trial aimed to compare the effects of fat loss induced by reduced energy intake (calorie restriction) or by increased energy expenditure (exercise) on several cardiovascular risk factors in healthy normal-weight and overweight middle-aged men and women.[74] Results provided evidence that calorie restriction and exercise-induced negative energy balance improve the CVD risk profile to a similar extent. Twelve months of these intervention programs resulted in an approximate 25% reduction in body fat mass in both groups. These results were accompanied by reductions in most of the major CVD risk factors, including plasma LDL-C concentration, total cholesterol/HDL-C ratio, CRP concentrations, and insulin resistance using the homeostatic model assessment, that were similar in the two groups. A second randomized controlled trial aimed to determine the effect of two behavioral programs, aerobic exercise training and stress management training, with routine medical care on psychosocial functioning and markers of cardiovascular risk.[75] The exercise intervention included usual medical care plus supervised aerobic exercise training for 35 minutes, three times per week for 16 weeks, vs. usual medical care alone. Results showed that exercise and stress management were associated with lower mean left ventricular wall motion abnormalities rating scores, flow-mediated dilation improvements, and baroreflex sensitivities, each versus usual care.

PA is an effective lifestyle medicine therapy for patients at risk for CVD (primary prevention) as well as patients with known CVD (secondary prevention).[76] However, patients with established CVD should follow exercise recommendations with varying levels of supervision and forms of exercise depending on the severity of the disease. Exercise therapy is a central part of cardiac rehabilitation, which is a complex intervention that may involve a variety of therapies, including exercise, risk factor education, behavior change, psychological support, and strategies that are aimed at targeting traditional risk factors for cardiovascular disease.[77] Patients who have been studied to benefit from these interventions as secondary prevention for CVD include individuals with known CAD or angina pectoris defined by angiography, previous myocardial infarction with coronary artery bypass graft (CABG) or percutaneous transluminal coronary angioplasty (PTCA), hypertension, and HF across a range of disease severities.[77,78] Adverse responses to acute exercise are infrequent, and the benefits of regular exercise are substantial. In patients with established CVD, regular exercise improves vascular function, may produce regression of atherosclerotic plaque, and reduces the risk factors associated with CVD, including lipidemia, obesity, insulin resistance/hyperglycemia, and hypertension.[76] Regular PA improves functional capacity and reduces myocardial oxygen demand.[76] Previous meta-analyses of the effects of exercise-based cardiac rehabilitation for CHD patients reported a statistically significant reduction in total and cardiac mortality, ranging from 20% to 32%, in patients receiving exercise therapy compared with usual medical care.[79–82] However, the revised Cochrane review in 2011 showed no difference between exercise-based cardiac rehabilitation and usual care groups in the risk of recurrent myocardial infarction or revascularization at any duration of follow-up.[77] This was majorly attributed to the population of the studies being predominantly male, middle-aged and low risk.[77]

The Physical Activity Readiness Questionnaire (PAR-Q) is a screening tool completed by people who plan to undergo a fitness assessment or to become much more physically active when initiating PA participation that is beyond a person's habitual daily activity level or when beginning a structured PA exercise program. Questions assess if patient has a known heart condition, if there is any chest pain or dizziness during PA, bone/joint problems exacerbated by PA, does patient take any medications for hypertension or heart disease. If a person provides a positive response to any question on the PAR-Q, he or she is directed to consult with his or her physician for clearance to engage in either unrestricted or restricted PA. The Physical Activity Readiness Medical Evaluation (PARmed-X) is a screening tool developed for use by physicians to assist in addressing the medical concerns related to PA participation that were identified by the PAR-Q.[83] It addresses the patient's medical conditions with its relative and absolute contraindications to physical activity. Absolute contraindications for exercise participation for patients with established CVD include unstable angina pectoris, aortic aneurysm, severe aortic stenosis, acute myocardial infarction, active myocarditis, uncontrolled ventricular tachycardia, multifocal premature ventricular contractions, a 2 kg or more increase in body mass over 1–3 days. Evidence indicates that those who are medically stable, who are involved with PA, and who have adequate physical ability can participate in PA of lower to moderate risk. Patients at higher risk can exercise in medically supervised programs.

A study conducted in 2019 analyzed the association between self-reported exercise and mortality in patients with stable CHD.[72] The study provided a questionnaire which evaluated the hours spent each week on mild, moderate, and vigorous exercise. Associations between volume of habitual exercise in metabolic equivalents of task hours/week and outcomes for 3.7 years were evaluated. It was concluded that in patients with stable CVD, more physical activity was associated with lower mortality. The largest benefits occurred between sedentary patient groups and between those with highest mortality risk.[84] Meta-analysis of randomized controlled trials shows that exercise training significantly improves survival time in patients with chronic heart failure due to left ventricular systolic dysfunction.[85] One explanation, applicable to patients with ischemic causes, is that exercise training improves myocardial perfusion by alleviating endothelial dysfunction and therefore dilating coronary vessels and by stimulating new vessel formation by way of intermittent ischemia.[85] Ventricular remodeling has been shown to be attenuated by exercise training.[85] The HF-ACTION randomized controlled trial evaluated the efficacy and safety of exercise training among patients with heart failure with reduced ejection fraction and included patients with ICD or biventricular pacemaker; exercise training was associated with modest significant reductions for both all-cause mortality or hospitalization and cardiovascular mortality or heart failure hospitalization.[86] In atrial fibrillation (AF), cohort studies have shown that meeting the 150 min of moderate-intensity physical activity guidelines was associated with lower risk of all-cause mortality, cardiovascular-related mortality, cardiovascular morbidity, and stroke compared with those not meeting the guidelines and those who were inactive and 170–240 minutes per week of moderate-intensity exercise and was consistently associated with a lower risk of mortality, stroke, and heart failure in patients with AF.[87] In addition, cardiac rehabilitation is associated with significant improvements in autonomic markers of neural regulation of the SA node, including heart rate variability and the gain of the overall spontaneous baroreflex, which can be affected after a major ischemic heart disease event.[88] These improvements may further explain the reduction in morbidity and mortality noted after formal cardiac rehabilitation and exercise training program.[88]

11.5.1 Prolonged Healthspan

Healthspan is the period of life free of major chronic clinical diseases and disability.[89] The main concept is that life can be divided roughly into two phases: a period of relatively healthy aging (healthspan) and a period of age-associated disease and disability. Although medical advances have resulted in increased mean lifespan, it is argued that most of this increase is the result of surviving longer with age-associated disease and disability, rather than by increasing healthspan.[90] Greater occupational and recreational PA, as well as higher levels of regular structured PA, are associated with better preservation of function with advancing age. Data from cross-sectional analyses indicate that the age at which decreases in key functions, such as cardio-respiratory fitness and muscle strength, reach levels associated with frailty can be delayed by up to 30 years in exercise-trained compared with inactive healthy adults.[91] This finding has been corroborated in a longitudinal study that demonstrates post-ponement in disability development and increased survival with advancing age in a population of runners compared with healthy community controls.[92]

Overall, regular PA improves not only healthspan, but also lifespan among individuals.[93] A prospective study aimed to examine PA recommendations in relation to mortality.

PA was assessed with two questionnaires which inquired about structured moderate (at least 30 minutes on most days of the week) or vigorous (at least 20 minutes 3 times per week) intensity exercise during the previous year. Meeting either of these benchmarks of activity was associated with 27% decrease in mortality compared with inactive individuals.[94] An exercise volume with a caloric expenditure of approximately 1,000 kcal per week appears to convey significant reduction in mortality risk.[95] A subsequent study evaluated the association between lower levels of PA and mortality. Findings indicated that PA is associated with decreased mortality rate, even among those who are active one or two days a week.[96, 97] Similarly, it has been shown that the same volume of higher intensity PA is associated with decreased mortality compared with lighter physical activity.[9]

Disclosures:
Jeffrey I. Mechanick received honoraria from Abbott Nutrition for lectures and serves on the Advisory Boards for Aveta.Life and Twin Health.

REFERENCES

1. Alberti KG, Zimmet P, Shaw J. International Diabetes Federation: a consensus on type 2 diabetes prevention. *Diabet Med* 2007; 24(5): 451–63.
2. Leitzmann MF, Park Y, Blair A, et al. Physical activity recommendations and decreased risk of mortality. *Arch Intern Med* 2007; 167(22): 2453–60.
3. Mechanick JI, Farkouh ME, Newman JD, Garvey WT. Cardiometabolic-based chronic disease, adiposity and dysglycemia drivers: JACC state-of-the-art review. *J Am Coll Cardiol* 2020; 75(5): 525–38.
4. Mechanick JI, Farkouh ME, Newman JD, Garvey WT. Cardiometabolic-based chronic disease, addressing knowledge and clinical practice gaps: JACC state-of-the-art review. *J Am Coll Cardiol* 2020; 75(5): 539–55.
5. Ding S, Xu S, Ma Y, Liu G, Jang H, Fang J. Modulatory mechanisms of the NLRP3 inflammasomes in diabetes. *Biomolecules* 2019; 9(12): 850.
6. Hamer M, Stamatakis E. Physical activity and mortality in men and women with diagnosed cardiovascular disease. *Eur J Cardiovasc Prev Rehabil* 2009; 16(2): 156–60.
7. Levine JA. Measurement of energy expenditure. *Public Health Nutr* 2005; 8(7A): 1123–32.
8. Look ARG. Eight-year weight losses with an intensive lifestyle intervention: the look AHEAD study. *Obesity* 2014; 22(1): 5–13.
9. Shiroma EJ, Lee IM, Schepps MA, Kamada M, Harris TB. Physical activity patterns and mortality: the weekend warrior and activity bouts. *Med Sci Sports Exerc* 2019; 51 (1): 35–40.

10. Ahmad LA, Crandall JP. Type 2 diabetes prevention: a review. *Clin Diabetes* 2010; 28 (2): 53–9.

11. Meex RC, Schrauwen-Hinderling VB, Moonen-Kornips E, et al. Restoration of muscle mitochondrial function and metabolic flexibility in type 2 diabetes by exercise training is paralleled by increased myocellular fat storage and improved insulin sensitivity. *Diabetes* 2010; 59(3): 572–9.

12. Bull FC, Al-Ansari SS, Biddle S, et al. World Health Organization 2020 guidelines on physical activity and sedentary behaviour. *Br J Sports Med* 2020; 54(24): 1451–62.

13. Ranasinghe PD, Pokhrel S, Anokye NK. Economics of physical activity in low-income and middle-income countries: a systematic review. *BMJ Open* 2021; 11(1): e037784.

14. Elshahat S, O'Rorke M, Adlakha D. Built environment correlates of physical activity in low-and middle-income countries: a systematic review. *PLoS One* 2020; 15(3): e0230454.

15. Haskell W, Bouchard C, Blair S. *Physical Activity and Health.* Champaign: Human Kinetics; 2007.

16. Mechanick JI, Garber AJ, Grunberger G, Handelsman Y, Garvey WT. Dysglycemia-based chronic disease: an American Association of Clinical Endocrinologists position statement. *Endocr Pract* 2018; 24(11): 995–1011.

17. Martin IK, Katz A, Wahren J. Splanchnic and muscle metabolism during exercise in NIDDM patients. *Am J Physiol* 1995; 269(3 Pt 1): E583–90.

18. Stanford KI, Goodyear LJ. Exercise and type 2 diabetes: molecular mechanisms regulating glucose uptake in skeletal muscle. *Adv Physiol Educ* 2014; 38(4): 308–14.

19. Posner BI. Insulin signalling: the inside story. *Can J Diabetes* 2017; 41(1): 108–13.

20. Combes A, Dekerle J, Webborn N, Watt P, Bougault V, Daussin FN. Exercise-induced metabolic fluctuations influence AMPK, p38-MAPK and CaMKII phosphorylation in human skeletal muscle. *Physiol Rep* 2015; 3(9): e12462.

21. Kido K, Ato S, Yokokawa T, Makanae Y, Sato K, Fujita S. Acute resistance exercise-induced IGF1 expression and subsequent GLUT4 translocation. *Physiol Rep* 2016; 4(16): e12907.

22. Muscella A, Stefàno E, Lunetti P, Capobianco L, Marsigliante S. The regulation of fat metabolism during aerobic exercise. *Biomolecules* 2020; 10(12): 1699.

23. Ranallo RF, Rhodes EC. Lipid metabolism during exercise. *Sports Med* 1998; 26(1): 29–42.

24. Röhling M, Herder C, Stemper T, Müssig K. Influence of acute and chronic exercise on glucose uptake. *J Diabetes Res* 2016; 2016: 2868652.

25. Hopps E, Canino B, Caimi G. Effects of exercise on inflammation markers in type 2 diabetic subjects. *Acta Diabetol* 2011; 48(3): 183–9.

26. Park JW, Kim KH, Choi JK, Park TS, Song KD, Cho BW. Regulation of toll-like receptors expression in muscle cells by exercise-induced stress. *Anim Biosci* 2021; 34(10): 1590–9.

27. Aronson D, Boppart MD, Dufresne SD, Fielding RA, Goodyear LJ. Exercise stimulates c-Jun NH2 kinase activity and c-Jun transcriptional activity in human skeletal muscle. *Biochem Biophys Res Commun* 1998; 251(1): 106–10.

28. Chen L, Chen R, Wang H, Liang F. Mechanisms linking inflammation to insulin resistance. *Int J Endocrinol* 2015; 2015: 508409.

29. Passos E, Pereira CD, Goncalves IO, et al. Role of physical exercise on hepatic insulin, glucocorticoid and inflammatory signaling pathways in an animal model of non-alcoholic steatohepatitis. *Life Sci* 2015; 123: 51–60.

30. Booth FW, Zwetsloot KA. Basic concepts about genes, inactivity and aging. *Scand J Med Sci Sports* 2010; 20(1): 1–4.

31. Stewart RAH, Held C, Hadziosmanovic N, et al. Physical activity and mortality in patients with stable coronary heart disease. *J Am Coll Cardiol* 2017; 70(14): 1689–700.

32. Thompson D, Karpe F, Lafontan M, Frayn K. Physical activity and exercise in the regulation of human adipose tissue physiology. *Physiol Rev* 2012; 92: 157–91.

33. Sahl RE, Andersen PR, Gronbaek K, et al. Repeated excessive exercise attenuates the anti-inflammatory effects of exercise in older men. *Front Physiol* 2017; 8: 407.

34. Mechanick JI, Zhao S, Garvey WT. The adipokine-cardiovascular-lifestyle network: translation to clinical practice. *J Am Coll Cardiol* 2016; 68(16): 1785–803.

35. Garcia-Hermoso A, Ceballos-Ceballos RJ, Poblete-Aro CE, Hackney AC, Mota J, Ramirez-Velez R. Exercise, adipokines and pediatric obesity: a meta-analysis of randomized controlled trials. *Int J Obes* 2017; 41(4): 475–82.

36. Yanai H, Yoshida H. Beneficial effects of adiponectin on glucose and lipid metabolism and atherosclerotic progression: mechanisms and perspectives. *Int J Mol Sci* 2019; 20(5).

37. Tao C, Sifuentes A, Holland WL. Regulation of glucose and lipid homeostasis by adiponectin: effects on hepatocytes, pancreatic beta cells and adipocytes. *Best Pract Res Clin Endocrinol Metab* 2014; 28(1): 43–58.

38. Shklyaev S, Aslanidi G, Tennant M, et al. Sustained peripheral expression of transgene adiponectin offsets the development of diet-induced obesity in rats. *Proc Natl Acad Sci U S A* 2003; 100(24): 14217–22.

39. Combs TP, Berg AH, Obici S, Scherer PE, Rossetti L. Endogenous glucose production is inhibited by the adipose-derived protein Acrp30. *J Clin Invest* 2001; 108(12): 1875–81.

40. Qiao L, Zou C, van der Westhuyzen DR, Shao J. Adiponectin reduces plasma triglyceride by increasing VLDL triglyceride catabolism. *Diabetes* 2008; 57(7): 1824–33.

41. Ouedraogo R, Wu X, Xu SQ, et al. Adiponectin suppression of high-glucose-induced reactive oxygen species in vascular endothelial cells: evidence for involvement of a cAMP signaling pathway. *Diabetes* 2006; 55(6): 1840–6.

42. Peng J, Yin L, Wang X. Central and peripheral leptin resistance in obesity and improvements of exercise. *Horm Behav* 2021; 133: 105006.

43. Cobbold C. Type 2 diabetes mellitus risk and exercise: is resistin involved? *J Sports Med Phys Fitness* 2018; 59(2): 290–7.

44. Kurowska P, Mlyczynska E, Dawid M, et al. Review: vaspin (SERPINA12) expression and function in endocrine cells. *Cells* 2021; 10(7): 1710.

45. Recinella L, Orlando G, Ferrante C, Chiavaroli A, Brunetti L, Leone S. Adipokines: new potential therapeutic target for obesity and metabolic, rheumatic, and cardiovascular diseases. *Front Physiol* 2020; 11: 578966.

46. Saeidi A, Haghighi MM, Kolahdouzi S, et al. The effects of physical activity on adipokines in individuals with overweight/obesity across the lifespan: a narrative review. *Obes Rev* 2021; 22(1): e13090.

47. Gielen S, Schuler G, Adams V. Cardiovascular effects of exercise training: molecular mechanisms. *Circulation* 2010; 122(12): 1221–38.

48. Schuttler D, Clauss S, Weckbach LT, Brunner S. Molecular mechanisms of cardiac remodeling and regeneration in physical exercise. *Cells* 2019; 8(10): 1128.

49. Kozakova M, Palombo C. Vascular ageing and aerobic exercise. *Int J Environ Res Public Health* 2021; 18(20): 10666.

50. Qiu S, Cai X, Yin H, et al. Exercise training and endothelial function in patients with type 2 diabetes: a meta-analysis. *Cardiovasc Diabetol* 2018; 17(1): 64.

51. Adams V, Reich B, Uhlemann M, Niebauer J. Molecular effects of exercise training in patients with cardiovascular disease: focus on skeletal muscle, endothelium, and myocardium. *Am J Physiol Heart Circ Physiol* 2017; 313(1): H72–H88.

52. Hoier B, Hellsten Y. Exercise-induced capillary growth in human skeletal muscle and the dynamics of VEGF. *Microcirculation* 2014; 21(4): 301–14.

53. Pereira RM, Botezelli JD, da Cruz Rodrigues KC, et al. Fructose consumption in the development of obesity and the effects of different protocols of physical exercise on the hepatic metabolism. *Nutrients* 2017; 9(4): 405.

54. Herman MA, Birnbaum MJ. Molecular aspects of fructose metabolism and metabolic disease. *Cell Metab* 2021; 33(12): 2329–54.

55. van der Windt DJ, Sud V, Zhang H, Tsung A, Huang H. The effects of physical exercise on fatty liver disease. *Gene Expr* 2018; 18(2): 89.

56. Semmler G, Datz C, Reiberger T, Trauner M. Diet and exercise in NAFLD/NASH: beyond the obvious. *Liver Int* 2021; 41(10): 2249–68.

57. Cusi K, Isaacs S, Barb D, et al. American Association of Clinical Endocrinology clinical practice guideline for the diagnosis and management of nonalcoholic fatty liver disease in primary care and endocrinology clinical settings: co-sponsored by the American Association for the Study of Liver Diseases (AASLD). *Endocr Pract* 2022; 28(5): 528–62.

58. Engin A. Non-alcoholic fatty liver disease. *Adv Exp Med Biol* 2017; 960: 443–67.

59. Gonçalves IO, Oliveira PJ, Ascensao A, Magalhães J. Exercise as a therapeutic tool to prevent mitochondrial degeneration in nonalcoholic steatohepatitis. *Eur J Clin Invest* 2013; 43(11): 1184–94.

60. Farzanegi P, Dana A, Ebrahimpoor Z, Asadi M, Azarbayjani MA. Mechanisms of beneficial effects of exercise training on non-alcoholic fatty liver disease (NAFLD): roles of oxidative stress and inflammation. *Eur J Sport Sci* 2019; 19(7): 994–1003.

61. Albano E, Mottaran E, Vidali M, et al. Immune response towards lipid peroxidation products as a predictor of progression of non-alcoholic fatty liver disease to advanced fibrosis. *Gut* 2005; 54(7): 987–93.

62. Piguet A-C, Saran U, Simillion C, et al. Regular exercise decreases liver tumors development in hepatocyte-specific PTEN-deficient mice independently of steatosis. *J Hepatol* 2015; 62(6): 1296–303.

63. Lieu L, Chau D, Afrin S, et al. Effects of metabolic state on the regulation of melanocortin circuits. *Physiol Behav* 2020; 224: 113039.

64. Mechanick JI, Zhao S, Garvey WT. Leptin, an adipokine with central importance in the global obesity problem. *Global Heart* 2018; 13(2): 113–27.

65. Mikkelsen K, Stojanovska L, Polenakovic M, Bosevski M, Apostolopoulos V. Exercise and mental health. *Maturitas* 2017; 106: 48–56.

66. Raefsky SM, Mattson MP. Adaptive responses of neuronal mitochondria to bioenergetic challenges: roles in neuroplasticity and disease resistance. *Free Radic Biol Med* 2017; 102: 203–16.

67. Vanderlinden J, Boen F, Van Uffelen J. Effects of physical activity programs on sleep outcomes in older adults: a systematic review. *Int J Behav Nutr Phys Act* 2020; 17(1): 1–15.

68. Bonardi JMT, Lima LG, Campos GO, et al. Effect of different types of exercise on sleep quality of elderly subjects. *Sleep Med* 2016; 25: 122–9.

69. Blumenthal JA, Sherwood A, Babyak MA, et al. Effects of exercise and stress management training on markers of cardiovascular risk in patients with ischemic heart disease: a randomized controlled trial. *JAMA* 2005; 293(13): 1626–34.

70. Brett JO, Arjona M, Ikeda M, et al. Exercise rejuvenates quiescent skeletal muscle stem cells in old mice through restoration of Cyclin D1. *Nat Med* 2020; 2(4): 307–17.

71. Group DPPR. The Diabetes Prevention Program (DPP) description of lifestyle intervention. *Diabetes Care* 2002; 25(12): 2165–71.

72. Knowler WC, Barrett-Connor E, Fowler SE, et al. Reduction in the incidence of type 2 diabetes with lifestyle intervention or metformin. *N Engl J Med* 2002; 346(6): 393–403.

73. Jeong S-W, Kim S-H, Kang S-H, et al. Mortality reduction with physical activity in patients with and without cardiovascular disease. *Eur Heart J* 2019; 40(43): 3547–55.

74. Pi-Sunyer X. The look AHEAD trial: a review and discussion of its outcomes. *Curr Nutr Rep* 2014; 3(4): 387–91.

75. Fontana L, Villareal DT, Weiss EP, et al. Calorie restriction or exercise: effects on coronary heart disease risk factors. A randomized, controlled trial. *Am J Physiol Endocrinol Metab* 2007; 293(1): E197–202.

76. Kokkinos P. Physical activity, health benefits, and mortality risk. *ISRN Cardiol* 2012; 2012: 718789.

77. Laaksonen DE, Lindstrom J, Lakka TA, et al. Physical activity in the prevention of type 2 diabetes: the Finnish diabetes prevention study. *Diabetes* 2005; 54(1): 158–65.

78. Heran BS, Chen JM, Ebrahim S, et al. Exercise-based cardiac rehabilitation for coronary heart disease. *Cochrane Database Syst Rev* 2011; 7: CD001800.

79. Hansen D, Niebauer J, Cornelissen V, et al. Exercise prescription in patients with different combinations of cardiovascular disease risk factors: a consensus statement from the EXPERT working group. *Sports Med* 2018; 48(8): 1781–97.

80. Oldridge NB, Guyatt GH, Fischer ME, Rimm AA. Cardiac rehabilitation after myocardial infarction. Combined experience of randomized clinical trials. *JAMA* 1988; 260(7): 945–50.

81. Jolliffe JA, Rees K, Taylor RS, Thompson D, Oldridge N, Ebrahim S. Exercise-based rehabilitation for coronary heart disease. *Cochrane Database Syst Rev* 2001; 1: CD001800.

82. Clark AM, Hartling L, Vandermeer B, McAlister FA. Meta-analysis: secondary prevention programs for patients with coronary artery disease. *Ann Intern Med* 2005; 143 (9): 659–72.

83. O'Connor GT, Buring JE, Yusuf S, et al. An overview of randomized trials of rehabilitation with exercise after myocardial infarction. *Circulation* 1989; 80(2): 234–44.

84. Warburton DE, Gledhill N, Jamnik VK, et al. Evidence-based risk assessment and recommendations for physical activity clearance: consensus document 2011. *Appl Physiol Nutr Metab* 2011; 36(Suppl 1): S266–98.

85. Saint-Maurice PF, Troiano RP, Berrigan D, Kraus WE, Matthews CE. Volume of light versus moderate-to-vigorous physical activity: similar benefits for all-cause mortality? *J Am Heart Assoc* 2018; 7(7): e008815.

86. Piepoli MF, Davos C, Francis DP, Coats AJ, ExTra MC. Exercise training meta-analysis of trials in patients with chronic heart failure (ExTraMATCH). *BMJ* 2004; 328(7433): 189.

87. O'Connor CM, Whellan DJ, Lee KL, et al. Efficacy and safety of exercise training in patients with chronic heart failure: HF-ACTION randomized controlled trial. *JAMA* 2009; 301(14): 1439–50.

88. Buckley BJ, Risom SS, Boidin M, Lip GY, Thijssen DH. Atrial fibrillation specific exercise rehabilitation: are we there yet? *J Pers Med* 2022; 12(4): 610.

89. Lucini D, Milani RV, Costantino G, Lavie CJ, Porta A, Pagani M. Effects of cardiac rehabilitation and exercise training on autonomic regulation in patients with coronary artery disease. *Am Heart J* 2002; 143(6): 977–83.

90. Tucker JM, Welk GJ, Beyler NK. Physical activity in U.S.: adults compliance with the physical activity guidelines for Americans. *Am J Prev Med* 2011; 40(4): 454–61.

91. Nilsson MI, Bourgeois JM, Nederveen JP, et al. Correction: lifelong aerobic exercise protects against inflammaging and cancer. *PLoS One* 2020; 15(5): e0233401.

92. van der Ploeg HP, Hillsdon M. Is sedentary behaviour just physical inactivity by another name? *Int J Behav Nutr Phys Act* 2017; 14(1): 1–8.

93. Chakravarty EF, Hubert HB, Lingala VB, Fries JF. Reduced disability and mortality among aging runners: a 21-year longitudinal study. *Arch Int Med* 2008; 168(15): 1638–46.

94. Mytton OT, Tainio M, Ogilvie D, Panter J, Cobiac L, Woodcock J. The modelled impact of increases in physical activity: the effect of both increased survival and reduced incidence of disease. *Eur J Epidemiol* 2017; 32(3): 235–50.

95. Neufer PD, Bamman MM, Muoio DM, et al. Understanding the cellular and molecular mechanisms of physical activity-induced health benefits. *Cell Metab* 2015; 22(1): 4–11.

96. Ozemek C, Lavie CJ, Rognmo Ø. Global physical activity levels-need for intervention. *Prog Cardiovasc Dis* 2019; 62(2): 102–7.

97. Seals DR, Justice JN, LaRocca TJ. Physiological geroscience: targeting function to increase healthspan and achieve optimal longevity. *J Physiol* 2016; 594(8): 2001–24.

98. Stewart KJ, Bacher AC, Turner K, et al. Exercise and risk factors associated with metabolic syndrome in older adults. *Am J Prev Med* 2005; 28(1): 9–18.

99. Katzmarzyk PT, Leon AS, Wilmore JH, et al. Targeting the metabolic syndrome with exercise: evidence from the HERITAGE Family Study. *Med Sci Sports Exerc* 2003; 35(10): 1703–9.

100. Balducci S, Zanuso S, Massarini M, et al. The Italian Diabetes and Exercise Study (IDES): design and methods for a prospective Italian multicentre trial of intensive lifestyle intervention in people with type 2 diabetes and the metabolic syndrome. *Nutr Metab Cardiovasc Dis* 2008; 18(9): 585–95.

12 Psychological Stress, Behavioral Modification, and Cardiometabolic Health

Amanda Bonano-Carambot and Michael A. Via
Icahn School of Medicine at Mount Sinai

Jeffrey I. Mechanick
Kravis Center for Cardiovascular Health at Mount Sinai Heart
Icahn School of Medicine at Mount Sinai

CONTENTS

DOI: 10.1201/9781003206637-12

12.1 INTRODUCTION

Successful adaptation to varying stressors – factors in our environment or from within our bodies that lead to harm – is a necessary part of health and is regarded as the "stress response" or more simply "stress." Cardiometabolic health is one of the most important topics of interest when discussing general medical well-being. There are many clinically significant risk factors that promote a spectrum of metabolic derangements leading to cardiovascular disease (CVD) and require structured approaches. More specifically, the union of metabolic drivers and CVD constitutes a framework to better contextualize cardiometabolic risks; this has been interpreted in a comprehensive cardiometabolic-based chronic disease (CMBCD) model (1,2). Drivers are causative factors and are considered as primary (genetic, environmental, and behavioral, which together create a personal lifestyle) and secondary/metabolic (abnormal adiposity, dysglycemia, hypertension, dyslipidemia, and other metabolic syndrome traits), which lead to a resultant CVD phenotype (1,2). As part of the behavioral primary driver, which is modifiable, psychological stress is highly involved in the development of CMBCD but unfortunately is given short shrift in clinical trials (research gap), medical training (knowledge gap), and routine clinical practice (practice gap).

To provide additional perspective, a stressor can be defined as a stimulus that produces a disturbance in homeostasis (e.g., the regulation of pH, heart rate, and temperature, characterized as "resistance to change"). Our body's response to this imbalance is to begin the process of allostasis (e.g., set-point alterations to optimize blood pressure control or adrenal activation for specific scenarios, and characterized as "stability through change"). In this way, many different behavioral, emotional, and biological changes are implemented together to adapt and subsequently endure the stressor. Allostasis is a complex process, allostatic load is the physiological cost of adaptation, and allostatic overload occurs when that cost cannot be repaid, or resources cannot be sufficiently replenished. Once a stressor is no longer present, the stress response should downregulate to restore equilibrium and start replenishing lost stores (e.g., nitrogen, calcium, glycogen, and fat), though there may be little evolutionary precedent for this in cases of severe stress since prior to the technological age, many such episodes resulted in death. In fact, impaired downregulation of the stress response can lead to "stress-vulnerability" in different psychiatric conditions (3). However, there may have been evolutionary pressure to target "revised" nadir levels to reduce the activation energy for subsequent stress responses with repeated exposures to the same or similar stressors (4,5). In this anticipatory model to promote a survival advantage, the stressor is presumed to be transient and the response is non-cognitive, conferred by genetic programming (6). However, if the stress response is sustained, repetitive, or otherwise disproportionate to innate responses, then pathophysiology can result (Table 12.1) (7). Ultimately, this challenges the body's ability and systemic limits to remain in a healthy state, with a new unhealthy phenotype emerging (e.g., chronic critical illness) (8) characterized by organ dysfunction, increased burden of disease, and decreased quality of life (7).

Stress can also interfere with normal cognitive processes, such as decision-making, behavioral self-regulation, and cognitive-emotional regulation (9), which can lead to unhealthy tendencies and behaviors. This includes having difficulty engaging and adhering to routine physical activity and a healthy diet. In terms of physical activity, stress can trigger sedentary behavior (10). The effect of stress on nutrition is interesting because the spectrum of reported effects is broad. Some sources report that stress is linked to increased cravings, gravitation toward calorie-dense, fatty, and sugary foods, and overeating in the form of increased portions or frequent snacking (11). Conversely, other sources report that stress can give rise to different eating patterns such as loss of appetite for prolonged periods of time with associated sudden urges to binge eat non-recommended foods (9). These actions generate subsequent feelings of guilt and regret (9). If these behavioral patterns remain unaddressed, they can predispose patients to an increased risk of weight gain, insulin resistance, and CMBCD. Mitigating the adverse effects of stress and associated unhealthy behaviors can assist in the efforts of combating CMBCD progression.

12.2   THE PSYCHOLOGICAL STRESS RESPONSE

12.2.1   INSULIN RESISTANCE

Dysglycemia-based chronic disease (DBCD) is another driver-based chronic disease model that configures insulin resistance, prediabetes, T2D, and vascular complications along a spectrum corresponding to natural history and encouraging early preventive measures (12). Several cross-sectional studies have investigated the relationship between the exposure to high allostatic load and development of insulin resistance, T2D, and CMBCD. For instance, in a cohort of 1,116 adults evaluated for allostatic load, the highest septile had odds ratios (ORs) of 5.7 for abdominal obesity, 6.2 for hypertension, 7.9 for T2D, and 4.3 for CVD (13). Another study showed an association of increased allostatic load and hypertension (14).

Allostatic stress can impact insulin sensitivity, which results in hyperinsulinemia with potential progression to chronic hyperglycemia and T2D. This mainly occurs through activation and upregulation of three pathways: the hypothalamic pituitary adrenal (HPA) axis, the sympathetic nervous system (SNS), and systemic inflammatory processes (15). Insulin resistance is a critical intermediating event in the development and progression of CMBCD, occupying the intersection point between abnormal adiposity and dysglycemia, and leading to dyslipidemia, hypertension, and atherosclerosis. Insulin resistance is defined as an impaired biologic response to insulin stimulation by target tissues (primarily liver, skeletal muscle, and adipose tissue) due to multiple pathophysiologic factors, including disrupted regulatory signaling, excess body fat, and epigenetic and genetic factors.

The functional physiology of the HPA axis consists of three main components: (1) hypothalamic transduction of information regarding "cognitive" (involving the cerebral cortex) and "non-cognitive" (primarily mediated by cytokines and suprahypothalamic neural pathways) stress that represent allostatic regulation and culminate in release of corticotropin-releasing hormone (CRH); (2) stimulation of pituitary proopiomelanocortin gene expression by CRH and other factors, and release of, among other peptides, adrenocorticotropic hormone (ACTH); and (3) stimulation of cortisol from the adrenal cortex by ACTH. Cortisol exerts pleiotropic effects on: energetics involving glucose, fatty acids, nitrogen stores, and insulin resistance; hemodynamics

TABLE 12.1

Mechanisms of the Stress Response Promoting Insulin Resistance, Adiposity, and Cardiometabolic-Based Chronic Disease

Hypothalamus-pituitary-adrenal axis activation
- Elevated cortisol activity (23)
- Disruption of circadian rhythms (29)

Autonomic dysfunction
- Activated sympathetic nervous system (32)
- Endothelial dysfunction (33)
- Elevated catecholamine activity (34)

Systemic inflammation
- Increased proinflammatory cytokine release (10)
- Macrophage and T-cell activation (20)
- Endothelial dysfunction (21)
- Adipose dysfunction (21)

involving systemic vascular resistance and blood pressure; and the immune system, depending on the chronicity of the stress response (acute – a blunted inflammatory response; chronic—a hyperactive/dysfunctional response that can promote tissue destruction) (16).

Allostatic activation of the SNS results in the release of catecholamines (primarily norepinephrine and epinephrine) produced by the adrenal medulla and peripheral nervous system. In general, norepinephrine exerts its actions locally in the periphery while epinephrine acts systemically. Catecholamine signaling plays a central role in increasing the heart rate, releasing proinflammatory cytokines and, alongside cortisol, elevating blood pressure and mobilizing energy stores in the form of lipids, as well as glucose via insulin resistance resulting in stress hyperglycemia (4,17).

In the setting of an acute stressor, a transient upregulation of tonic neuroendocrine pathways to appropriate and beneficial responses (i.e., "fight or flight") is normally observed. However, if the stressors are exaggerated, persistent, and/or repetitive, the chronic stress response may be associated with progression of insulin resistance (8,18). Rodent models of chronic stress based on learned helplessness, chronic restraint, water deprivation, and prolonged corticosterone exposure demonstrate insulin resistance and dyslipidemia (19–21). In primate studies, young bonnet macaques that were exposed to alternating easy (low stress) to difficult (high stress) accessibility of food over a 4 months time period were observed to have greater body weight and waist circumference, compared with controls (22).

Inflammation is another main contributor to the allostatic load that drives the development of insulin resistance, especially in patients with obesity. At first glance, one may appreciate the potential for confounding factors to play a role in this association given that inflammation promotes obesity, which can itself lead to insulin resistance. However, most studies support that inflammation plays a causal role in the development of insulin resistance (23). In order to comprehend how inflammatory pathways affect the body's normal response to insulin, it should be known that the insulin receptor is a tyrosine kinase that has the ability to auto-phosphorylate and intracellularly activate insulin receptor substrates and associated downstream pathways with the end goal of promoting glucose entry into target cells and an anabolic cellular state.

Inflammatory cells, mainly macrophages and T-cells (23), promote insulin resistance via multiple pathways. Once the inflammatory response begins, there is an increase in the production and release of major proinflammatory cytokines, including tumor necrosis factor (TNF)-α, interleukin (IL)-1β and interferon (INF)-γ. These, in turn, activate intracellular pathways that impair insulin signaling and induce insulin resistance (23,24). A main contributor to this process is the IκB kinase/nuclear factor κB enzyme complex, which acts by serine phosphorylation of insulin receptor substrate 1 or the insulin receptor itself, resulting in decreased tyrosine phosphorylation, insulin receptor activation, and downstream signaling, and ultimately fostering adipose tissue activation and insulin resistance (23,25). Other pathways that act similarly, via phosphorylation of insulin receptor substrates, are the c-Jun N-terminal kinases (target serine and threonine (24)) and mitogen-activated protein kinases (target serine (24)) pathways. The Janus kinase signal transducer and activation of transcription 1 and 3 pathways are also thought to contribute to insulin resistance by suppressing insulin receptor tyrosine kinase activity thereby interrupting receptor function and interaction with insulin receptor substrates (24). These effects of inflammation can impact the body's physiology both locally via autocrine/paracrine effects on adipocyte signaling and systemically by acting on other important tissues such as the skeletal muscles and liver (24).

12.2.2 Cortisol

Cortisol secretion follows a circadian rhythm, with high levels in the morning that decline throughout the day to nadir levels between approximately midnight and 4:00 am. On awakening, cortisol levels are elevated. During the 30–45 minutes following awakening, the cortisol awakening response unfolds and cortisol levels steadily increase until peak levels are achieved. This cycle is affected by sleep patterns, daily activities, and stress.

In settings of chronic stress exposure, prolonged increased levels of cortisol can lead to changes in glucose homeostasis (26). Hypercortisolism impairs insulin signaling and glucose uptake in skeletal muscles and activates gluconeogenesis directly leading to hyperglycemia. Lipolysis pathways are also activated, increasing circulating free fatty acids that accumulate in the liver. This promotes hepatocyte insulin resistance and diminishes hepatocyte glucose uptake, which further promotes hyperglycemia (27). In addition, chronic hypercortisolism drives abdominal and visceral adiposity, contributing further to insulin resistance (26,28). Epidemiological studies have demonstrated that chronic activation of the HPA axis leads to a dysregulated output of cortisol that is associated with increased central fat accumulation (29–31), abnormal function of pancreatic β-cells, hepatic gluconeogenesis, and insulin sensitivity (15).

Stress disrupts the circadian pattern of cortisol secretion leading to a rise in evening cortisol levels that is more pronounced in patients with either prediabetes or T2D. Patients with prediabetes also demonstrate a flattening of the downward slope (i.e., a slower decrease) in cortisol levels from the morning peak levels (32). In the Whitehall II prospective cohort study (32), which evaluated diurnal cortisol levels among 3,508 individuals, higher evening cortisol levels predicted new onset T2D (OR 1.18 [CI 1.01–1.37]) over 9 years of follow-up.

Hypercortisolism also drives insulin resistance through immune system activation of proinflammatory pathways. Under cortisol stimulation, visceral adipose tissue releases C-reactive protein, IL-6, IL-1β, TNF-α, and acute phase proteins (33). Glutathione pathways are diminished, leading to increased reactive oxygen species (33). Additionally, cortisol alters adipokine signaling, including increased leptin and decreased adiponectin (33). Both the released inflammatory mediators and the respective changes in adipokine signaling diminish the systemic response to insulin, as well as impairing pancreatic β-cell function leading to mistimed insulin release. These alterations induced by cortisol in the setting of chronic stress significantly contribute to dysregulation of glucose and energy metabolism, which drives the development of insulin resistance, prediabetes, and progression to T2D (15,34).

12.2.3 AUTONOMIC DYSFUNCTION

In addition to cortisol activity, stress-related autonomic dysregulation also contributes to insulin resistance through neuronal and humoral pathways. The SNS is activated both acutely and chronically in response to stress, directly stimulating vasoconstriction, elevating blood pressure, and promoting gluconeogenesis (35). Sympathetic activity may diminish endothelial nitric oxide synthase (eNOS) activity, further contributing to vasoconstriction and hypertension (36). Conversely, reduced eNOS activity may potentiate greater SNS signaling, amplifying the effect of stress (36). Increased plasma levels of epinephrine and norepinephrine, released through sympathetic stimulation, act to increase heart rate, blood pressure, and glycemia through glycogen breakdown and gluconeogenesis. Norepinephrine stimulates α1 and α2 receptors, which induce peripheral vasoconstriction leading to increased blood pressure. Through β1 stimulation, norepinephrine promotes sinus node activity, leading to increased chronotropy and inotropy. In contrast, low levels of epinephrine exert a dose-dependent effect on β1 and β2 adrenergic receptors, which promote lipolysis and hepatic/muscle glycogenolysis (37). Moreover, high levels of epinephrine activate α adrenergic receptors leading to vasoconstriction (37). Epidemiological studies associate chronic stress with insulin resistance, sympathetic activation (elevated resting heart rate and/or diminished heart rate variability), and cardiac dysfunction (30,31,38). These findings are also associated with the development of abdominal obesity, metabolic syndrome, and T2D (30,31,38). In one study, resting heart rate was shown to have a dose-response relationship with the incidence of T2D, in which every ten beats per minute increase in resting heart rate was associated with a 19% increased risk for developing T2D (39).

12.3 THE ROLE OF MOOD DISORDERS AND EMOTIONAL STRESS ON DEVELOPING CARDIOMETABOLIC DISEASE

12.3.1 DEPRESSION

Depression and emotional distress can be significant sources of stress for an individual and are associated with insulin resistance, T2D, and cardiometabolic risk.

Depression is characterized by symptoms of sleep disturbance, decreased interest/pleasure (anhedonia), guilt, feelings of worthlessness, decreased energy, difficulty concentrating, appetite changes, psychomotor changes, and suicidal ideations. Depression can induce amplification of the HPA axis and sympathetic activity, which potentiates the risk of CMBCD development and/or progression. Moreover, patients with clinical depression tend to exhibit behaviors that further increase this risk, including inactivity, food consumption (especially energy-dense/processed foods), and disrupted sleep (40,41).

Current views on the relationship of depression and DBCD suggest a bidirectional causality: mechanisms of depression can impel DBCD progression; and advancing DBCD stages, especially stage 4 (complications), may contribute to depressive symptoms (40). Depression is more common among patients with versus without chronic conditions, such as T2D (42–45). Specifically, the risk for incident depression is increased by 25% among patients with T2D when compared to those without (46–48). In addition, patients with T2D who do not meet the full criteria for diagnosis of clinical depression still commonly demonstrate increased prevalence of depressive symptoms, including hopelessness and the loss of pleasure (49,50).

Depression affects T2D disease management. In addition to enhanced HPA tone, sympathetic activity, and behavior choice, untreated depressive symptoms may hinder a patient's ability to self-manage and achieve glycemic targets (9). In cohort studies, elevated depressive symptom scores were associated with reduced levels of glycemic control (51,52), adherence (53), and self-care behaviors serving to increase complication risk and diminish the quality of life among patients with T2D (54,55).

12.3.2 ANXIETY

Anxiety is another a mood disorder that is more common among patients with T2D (56,57). An approximate 20% increase in the prevalence of anxiety is demonstrated in this population (58). HPA axis and sympathetic activity are enhanced by anxiety (59), and patients with anxiety also are less likely to make healthy behavior choices (58).

Specific to patients with T2D, anxiety may be rooted in the fear of experiencing a hypoglycemic episode or the possibility requiring additional glucose-lowering treatments in the future, both eventually leading to poor adherence and glycemic control (60). In this fashion, diabetes-related distress is an important stressor that refers to the unique burden of living with and managing T2D (51). In fact, 44.6% of patients with type 1 or 2 diabetes endorsed having distress relating to their diabetes. Furthermore, those identified as having a low-stress resiliency, meaning they are unable to maintain psychological well-being when faced with adversity, were observed to have hemoglobin A1c (A1C) levels 0.7% higher than the high and moderate resilience groups over a 1-year follow-up period (61).

12.3.3 PERSONALITY TRAITS

In addition to mood disorders, personality traits, such as anger and hostility, have also been identified as sources of stress related to T2D. Several studies have demonstrated this association, including the Multi-Ethnic Study of Atherosclerosis (62).

In this trial, 6,814 patients with diverse backgrounds (28% African American, 22% Latino, 12% Asian, and 39% Caucasian) were enrolled and anger was assessed by the Spielberger Anger Scale. Patients that fell within the highest anger levels had a 50% increase in incidence of T2D over 11 years. A second cohort trial of 32,586 men (mean age 31 years) demonstrated a 53% increase in incidence of T2D among those who report the highest levels of emotional stress over 6.3 years (63). After adjustment for known risks (e.g., body mass index [BMI] and physical activity), the observed incidence of T2D was increased by 114% within the high stress group (62,63).

12.3.4 Environmental Distress

Similar to internal stressors, external factors, such as one's environment, can also cause significant distress. Among these, work-related stress is one of the most common exposures that have been studied. A meta-analysis showed that job strain, defined as high job demand with low control at work, is associated with increased risk of T2D (64). Financial and socioeconomic factors are other categories of stressors that disproportionally affect patients with lower socioeconomic status and confer risk of obesity, T2D, and CVD (64). Additionally, the related stress of long working hours, defined as work >55 hours per week, is associated with an increased risk of developing T2D (64). Although stress is commonly perceived as a struggle of adulthood, early childhood stress can also have a meaningful impact on a person's development, as well as to their cardiometabolic risk. Studies show that adverse childhood experiences such as neglect and physical abuse demonstrate an increased associated risk of developing T2D in adulthood (OR 1.32 [CI 1.16–1.51]) (65).

12.4 THE STRESS RESPONSE AND MICROVASCULAR AND MACROVASCULAR COMPLICATIONS

Psychological stress exacerbates mechanistic drivers of each DBCD stage. Depression represents one of the most studied psychiatric factors in the context of T2D complications (15). Observational trials that include patients with both T2D and major depressive disorder demonstrate a 15%–20% increased risk of retinopathy and of chronic kidney disease (66–70). Development of foot ulcers in patients with T2D was increased by 30%–40% among those with depression (66–69). With regard to macrovascular disease, a 40% increase risk of cardiovascular complications and a 30%–50% increase risk of all-cause mortality were noted among patients with T2D and depressive symptoms, compared to those without depression (68,71–77). As a contributor to these already high risks, psychological stress adds considerable potential for severe complications warranting further evaluation and interventions (78).

12.5 LIFESTYLE INTERVENTION

Clinicians should be proactive in identifying patients who are exposed to psychological stressors, which may independently disrupt motivation to work toward a healthier lifestyle, and hinder potential for success (15). In a Danish study that followed initially healthy adults with a 10-year-follow-up period, perceived stress was linked with physical inactivity, unsuccessful smoking cessation, and alcohol reduction attempts; both the stress and failed interventions were detrimental to cardiometabolic health (79).

In general, the application of lifestyle interventions among patients with prediabetes, T2D, or cardiovascular complications improve clinical outcomes by controlling disease progression and delaying the need for pharmacological intervention (Table 12.2) (80). However, special considerations for patients facing psychological stress should be made. Many lifestyle interventions that benefit patients with insulin resistance, prediabetes, and T2D also improve mood disorders and stress. Achievable goal setting in each lifestyle intervention should be foremost; in fact, targets seen as unreachable can serve as psychological stressors and exacerbate rather than improve emotional distress and T2D (81).

12.5.1 PHYSICAL ACTIVITY

Increased physical activity is beneficial for patients with abnormal adiposity, insulin resistance, prediabetes, T2D, and CVD, as well as those with chronic psychological stress such as depression (82). Current recommendations for those diagnosed with prediabetes and T2D are to increase physical activity to weekly targets. This includes aerobic exercise of moderate intensity for 150 minutes per week spread over 3 days or more with no more than two consecutive days in between sessions (81). If vigorous resistance training is preferred, it should be performed at least every 2–3 days per week (81). The evidence-based initial weight loss goal is to achieve and maintain ≥5% loss of initial body weight for most patients who are overweight or obese, and ready to achieve weight loss (83,84). Depressive symptoms improve with this pattern of increased physical activity, and these may be reasonable targets among patients with psychological stress and T2D (82,85).

TABLE 12.2
Clinical Approaches to Psychologic Stress

Physical activity
- 150 minutes per week, spread over 2–3 non-consecutive days (78)

Sleep hygiene
- Increased physical activity, as above (78)
- Cyclic meditation (83)
- Involvement of multiple disciplines (e.g., psychiatry, social work, and sleep medicine) (79)

Dietary pattern
- Incorporation of a Mediterranean diet (89)

Stress reduction techniques
- Cognitive behavioral therapy (92)
- Consideration for pharmacological therapy of mood disorders (93)
- Involvement of multiple disciplines (e.g., psychiatry) (94)
- Group cardiac rehabilitation in patients with cardiovascular disease (95,96)

12.5.2 SLEEP HYGIENE

Sleep disturbances, which can exacerbate insulin resistance, are common among patients facing psychological stress and are often included in diagnostic criteria for common stress conditions. Methods and treatments of the stressor may help improve sleep quality. In one small study of patients with T2D and depressive symptoms, cyclic meditation improved scores in sleep quality by 7%, and depression symptoms by 26% after 4 weeks (86). However, this intervention may not achieve broad or longer-term success, and a multidisciplinary approach is often best to improve markers of clinical outcomes (82).

12.5.3 DIETARY PATTERNS

Improvement in dietary patterns can improve both T2D and depression (87–90). In a 2-year study that included patients with T2D and depression, a low carbohydrate diet improved depressive symptoms by 18% (91). In the Prevención con Dieta Mediterránea (PREDIMED Study) trial, a 41% decrease in incident depression was noted among the Mediterranean diet group that was supplemented with nuts (92).

12.5.4 STRESS REDUCTION

Although it may seem straightforward — that is, simply controlling stressors – stress modification has proven challenging and not consistently associated with improvement of glycemic control (15). In one study of 107 Latino patients with T2D, a program of eight stress management sessions given by a community health worker over 12 weeks improved depression and anxiety symptoms by 30%, though no improvements in glucose levels were noted (93). The practice of mindfulness similarly has not had consistent beneficial effects when employed in patients with depression and T2D (94). Other psychological interventions, such as cognitive behavioral therapy and psychodynamic supportive therapies, also yield mixed findings, though there is some evidence to suggest possible benefit (95). In contrast to non-pharmacological therapy, medication therapies, such as use of serotonin reuptake inhibitors or tricyclic antidepressants, to treat depression in patients with T2D demonstrate notable improvement in glycemic control. An approximate 0.4% reduction in A1C (CI −0.6 to −0.1) and association with short-term (OR of 2.88, CI 1.44–4.32) and medium-term (OR of 2.49, CI 1.44–4.32) remission of depression was observed in a Cochrane review of 19 published trials of these agents (96). At present, management of comorbid depression in the setting of chronic disease such as T2D should be through collaborative, multidisciplinary care (97).

In contrast to these studies, special populations such as patients with mood disorders and T2D who have developed CVD may benefit from non-pharmacological therapies. Cardiac rehabilitation group exercise programs demonstrate reduction in depressive symptoms, as well as reduction in onset of new cardiovascular events, likely due to the exercise and even the camaraderie of the group (98,99). This reiterates the large impact that coordinating tailored and individualized care regimens can have on patients' progress and successful achievement of their health goals.

12.6 CONNECTING THE PSYCHOLOGICAL STRESS RESPONSE WITH CARDIOVASCULAR DISEASE

The association of chronic stress and cardiovascular risk is well established (100). Activated mechanisms of the stress response that drive abnormal adiposity, insulin resistance, prediabetes, T2D, and hypertension also lead to increased risk of CVD. These include cytokine release and systemic inflammation that results in endothelial dysfunction, localized inflammation of arterial vessel walls, as well as infiltration of low-density lipoprotein particles and immune cells into the intimal layers of arteries (101). These processes promote coronary atherogenesis. In addition to these effects, stress-activation of the SNS diminishes heart rate variability, accelerates intracardiac pressure development, and raises cardiac oxygen demand, contributing to cardiac dysfunction (101,102). Stress also enhances platelet activation and promotes a pro-thrombotic state, potentially leading to acute cardiovascular events after atherosclerotic plaques are disrupted via rupture or erosion (103,104).

Clinical evidence for atherosclerosis risk in the setting of chronic stress includes cohort studies that associate stress with progression of carotid intima media thickness (105). Similarly, high-stress exposures during at least 3 years in adolescence are associated with increased cardiovascular reactivity to laboratory stressors, and increased carotid intima media thickness (106). In sum, pathways leading to increased cardiovascular risk are exacerbated through increased exposure to chronic stress (107).

Several techniques in stress reduction show benefits for mitigating cardiovascular risk factors. In an analysis of 17 studies that evaluate relaxation techniques (either Tai Chi or yoga), an 80% reduction in perceived stress was observed, with consequent improvement in heart rate variability (108). A study that examined the utility of a mindfulness-based program in patients with hypertension demonstrated reduced systolic blood pressure by 5 mm Hg after 8 weeks (109). This finding is in line with a published meta-analysis of meditation stress management techniques applied to patients with hypertension that demonstrated a systolic blood pressure reduction of 13.5 mm Hg and diastolic blood pressure reduction of 3.4 mm Hg (110). While these findings are suggestive, presently there is insufficient evidence to support stress reduction methods specifically for the prevention of cardiovascular events, as studies with these endpoints have not been conducted (111–113). However, a reduction in cardiac risk factors and an overall improvement in quality of life may guide the use of relaxation techniques, mindfulness-based techniques, or meditation stress management practices in at-risk patients.

12.7 CONNECTING THE PSYCHOLOGICAL STRESS RESPONSE WITH ADIPOSITY-BASED CHRONIC DISEASE

Adiposity-based chronic disease (ABCD) describes a dysmetabolic state wherein abnormal fat amount (i.e., increased total fat with elevated BMI in the overweight/obese range), distribution (e.g., increased waist circumference or imaging that demonstrates increased ectopic fat stores), and/or function (e.g., reflected by abnormal adipokine secretory signatures) are associated (epidemiologically and mechanistically) with chronic disease (i.e., organ dysfunction or "complications") (114). Similar to the other driver-based chronic disease models – DBCD and CMBCD – ABCD consists of four stages: (1) risk (primary drivers); (2) predisease (e.g., overweight); (3) disease (e.g., obesity); and (4) complications (e.g., CVD) (114). To be clear, "obesity" is defined solely in terms of BMI and corresponds to ABCD stage 3. Holistically, the ABCD state is interpreted as a secondary, metabolic driver of CMBCD primarily through insulin resistance and inflammation (e.g., infiltration of inflammatory macrophages within adipose tissue, altered adipokine secretion, and consequent β-cell phenomena that lead to hyperglycemia) (114).

Stress can exacerbate ABCD partially through mobilization of energy stores such as lipids, increased systemic inflammation, and dysregulated metabolism that further drives insulin resistance. In an animal model study with female cynomolgus monkeys, those who were subordinate were more likely to be exposed to aggression and were observed to have increased visceral adipose tissue in comparison with subcutaneous adipose tissue, and higher incidence of atherosclerosis when housed in social groups and fed atherogenic diets (115). Similarly, in the Whitehall II study (116), humans who were subjected to higher levels of psychological stress (assessed by questionnaire) had an increased risk of central obesity, BMI, and dyslipidemia.

Behavior therapy, as a lifestyle intervention that uses techniques to change an individual patient's exercise habits and dietary choices, is a key intervention when treating patients with ABCD (117). This centers around stimulus control, self-correction of problems that arise, use of rewards (verbal or otherwise), modification of unrealistic goals, and relapse prevention. A meta-analysis of seven trials demonstrates an improvement in weight loss (8.5 kg vs 0.4 kg, $p < 0.05$) in the early stages of weight loss journeys when regular behavior sessions are incorporated (118). By this finding, the authors conclude that the most effective programs for weight loss include practices in behavior modification combined with dietary changes and increased physical activity.

12.8   EVIDENCE-BASED METHODS OF BEHAVIORAL MODIFICATION

Behavior change is fundamental to lifestyle medicine in order to achieve optimization of cardiometabolic health. At times, this can be a difficult goal to reach given that the power of lifestyle intervention rests on both knowledge and successful execution. If implemented appropriately, lifestyle changes have the potential to delay T2D onset by an average of about 4 years, to reduce overall T2D incidence by 34% over 10 years (119), as well as to reduce cardiovascular and microvascular complications (120,121).

This great potential can be attained by patients that are willing and motivated to implement change. The high prevalence of insulin resistance and its sequelae suggests that even seemingly healthy patients may benefit from evaluation of lifestyle habits in order to maintain health and prevent disease. If cardiometabolic risk factors, such as stress, obesity, prediabetes, T2D, and CVD, are identified, engagement should be promoted as soon as risk is known. Unfortunately, this process can be difficult as some patients may express that they are not mentally or physically ready to make changes. At that point, it becomes the physician's duty to routinely reassess the patient's interest and confidence in their ability to work toward healthy lifestyle changes in subsequent encounters. Ideally, this should be addressed at every visit after diagnosis of prediabetes or T2D, since early engagement may benefit most from early intensive lifestyle intervention (81,121).

As with any change, significant behavioral and lifestyle modifications entail going through a set of stages prior to achieving and maintaining a change. The five-stage model for change includes precontemplation, contemplation, preparation, action, and maintenance (81). In the precontemplation stage, there is no perceivable problem to be solved and there is no interest in finding a solution, even though there are behaviors that may be negatively impacting a patient's health. Once there is awareness of a problem, the contemplation stage begins. Here, the person is mindful of the pros and cons associated with sustaining the unhealthy behaviors. However, at this point, pros seem to outweigh the cons, and thus, there is still a lack of intention to change behaviors. Once the preparation stage is reached, the problem is acknowledged, and cons appear to have a larger significance. At this point, patients typically are ready to consider the options that may aid in eliminating the problem – they are "activated for change." However, there is still no intention to actually implement a plan. However, once steps, big or small, are taken toward fixing the problem, the action phase is started. The maintenance stage is the final goal of this process and is achieved when new behaviors or actions can be continued for a prolonged period of time. At a given patient interaction, the goal may be simply to advance the patient to the next stage (81).

Rarely does meaningful change occur as a linear process; typically, progression is marred with lapses and relapses. Lapses are momentary deviations to plan that are brief in nature and end when the patient realigns with set goals. If a patient is unable to re-align with goals in a reasonably short timeframe or returns to original behaviors, this is known as a relapse. This is an important subject to discuss when beginning the process of change. Some patients can feel guilty and ashamed to admit when they've had setbacks in their journey which can lead to lack of transparency and suboptimal opportunities to provide support. Setbacks, themselves, can serve as a source of distress that may compound barriers that exist. For this reason, it's imperative to normalize lapses and relapses to prevent patients from becoming discouraged and quitting the process altogether. Clinicians can help by advising patients that "slips" are a normal part of the process of change. Additionally, if a patient experiences a lapse or a relapse, clinicians should prime patients to realize that the takeaway point should be to learn from the mistake experienced and to develop creative solutions to handle similar situations in the future in order to, hopefully, avoid further setbacks.

To minimize the incidence of lapses or relapses, the process of tailoring a patient's plan of action should be collaborative and include changes that are perceived as clear, realistic, and sustainable by the patient (81). Goals can be either quantitative in nature (A1C less than 7% or a 5% weight loss when compared to values on diagnosis) or qualitative (e.g., food portion control or exercising a few times a week). When helping a patient to tailor their plan of action, clinicians must listen closely to the obstacles that the patient anticipates facing in this journey (81). For example, if a patient considers equipment-based exercise to be boring or finds gyms are intimidating for a beginner, the patient may be encouraged to consider creative and enjoyable ways of exercising. Examples include yard work, biking, dancing, virtual instructor-led classes, and collaboration with a physical trainer. If a patient expresses lack of motivation and sense of accountability when it comes to diet changes, options such as documenting behaviors in a journal, use of digital applications to keep track of habits, joining support groups, and seeking help from nutritionists may be suggested (81). More modern approaches are also being studied in order to find new ways to help patients who have difficulty adhering to an exercise regimen. Specifically, the role of smartphones and digital resources has garnered a particular interest in the research community. In fact, the utility of smartphones and applications centered on providing reminders or nudges, monitoring and personalized feedback was studied in a small sample of T2D patients that lead a sedentary lifestyle. In that study, patients were provided a smartphone-based pedometer and personal physical activity plan and were sent a short message to encourage physical activity with varying frequency (between once a day to once a week). These prompts were coupled to a reinforcement learning algorithm to help with personalization and identify which prompts were successful in engaging patients with physical activity. Results showed that patients increased the amount of activity and pace of walking and those who had personalized messages had a greater reduction in A1C and increased engagement (122). Strategies like this one could also be applied to other modifiable factors that influence CMBCD, such as weight control and blood pressure control, to assist in health optimization.

To further promote a successful and positive experience with change, clinicians should express interest in learning what external factors may hinder their progress. An important task to complete when assessing this is to recognize any negative influences that may be present (81). For example, one may ask about family members, friends, and colleagues that may have tendencies to minimize or belittle all the efforts, sacrifices, and progress made by the patient. In addition to this, patients should be screened for psychological factors such as anxiety and depression (107,123) that may potentially affect their energy and motivation. If negative influences are identified, it's important to help them develop skills to endure or avoid these exposures (81) and, if medical evaluation and treatment is necessary, refer them to the appropriate specialists. While negative influences can be impactful, it's also important to identify and attempt to reinforce their relationship with sources of positivity and support that could promote compliance and adherence to desired changes. Positive influences include people who validate a patient's hard work, provide words and actions of encouragement, and assist the patient if lapses occur without judgment or even join them in their journey toward change. Unfortunately, physicians and other healthcare professionals often overlook the importance of identifying additional sources of support (81). Taking the time to ask about accomplishments and offering praise when working toward or achieving milestones can be encouraging, motivating, and empowering for patients (81). For example, a great way to discuss this is by asking the patient to share what benefits they've noticed (e.g., looser fitting clothes, better endurance, and less sweating) and provide congratulations on shared achievements that are making them proud of their hard work. Another source of support are specialists, such as nutritionists and exercise trainers, that can help patients demystify the intricacies of developing a well-balanced, healthy diet, and a good exercise routine that can be challenging, while also avoiding injuries (81). In interventional studies, such as the Look AHEAD and Diabetes Prevention Program studies, patients were provided coaching on healthy eating, physical exercise, and behavior techniques, which resulted in weight loss, reduced need for glucose lowering medications, and reduced micro- and macrovascular complications of T2D (85,119).

Once a plan is created and target changes are identified, it is good practice to schedule frequent contacts to check in on the patient's process and assess their perception on the sustainability of the implemented modifications (81). Additionally, if their latest goals have been reached, it is appropriate to take this as an opportunity to celebrate and congratulate them on their achievements and discuss the next milestones of interest. It is crucial to recognize that, even though the timeline for achieving a sustained lifestyle change is variable, patients must be made aware of the importance of long-term consistency and discipline given that longer periods of intervention correlate with sustained weight loss and engagement of physical activity (81,120,123,124). Visits should be slowly tapered once a patient appears to be comfortable with assuming more responsibility and independence in the process of setting new goals or has exhibited noteworthy control of maintaining their goal lifestyle.

Disclosures:

Jeffrey I. Mechanick received honoraria from Abbott Nutrition for lectures and serves on the Advisory Boards for Aveta.Life and Twin Health.

REFERENCES

1. Mechanick, Jeffrey I., Michael E. Farkouh, Jonathan D. Newman, and W. Timothy Garvey. 2020. "Cardiometabolic-Based Chronic Disease, Adiposity and Dysglycemia Drivers: JACC State-of-the-Art Review." *Journal of the American College of Cardiology* 75 (5): 525–38. https://doi.org/10.1016/j.jacc.2019.11.044.
2. Mechanick, Jeffrey I., Michael E. Farkouh, Jonathan D. Newman, and W. Timothy Garvey. 2020a. "Cardiometabolic-Based Chronic Disease, Addressing Knowledge and Clinical Practice Gaps: JACC State-of-the-Art Review." *Journal of the American College of Cardiology* 75 (5): 539–55. https://doi.org/10.1016/j.jacc.2019.11.046.
3. van Oort, Jasper, Nils Kohn, J. N. Vrijsen, Rose Collard, F. A. Duyser, S. C. A. Brolsma, Guillen Fernandez, A. H. Schene, Indira Tendolkar, and P. F. van Eijndhoven. 2020. "Absence of Default Mode Downregulation in Response to a Mild Psychological Stressor Marks Stress-Vulnerability across Diverse Psychiatric Disorders." *NeuroImage. Clinical* 25 (102176): 102176. https://doi.org/10.1016/j.nicl.2020.102176.
4. Mechanick, Jeffrey I. 2006. "Metabolic Mechanisms of Stress Hyperglycemia." *JPEN. Journal of Parenteral and Enteral Nutrition* 30 (2): 157–63. https://doi.org/10.1177/0148607106030002157.
5. Stumvoll, Michael, P. Antonio Tataranni, Norbert Stefan, Barbora Vozarova, and Clifton Bogardus. 2003. "Glucose Allostasis." *Diabetes* 52 (4): 903–9. https://doi.org/10.2337/diabetes.52.4.903.
6. Deans, Carrie. 2021. "Biological Prescience: The Role of Anticipation in Organismal Processes." *Frontiers in Physiology* 12: 672457. https://doi.org/10.3389/fphys.2021.672457.
7. McEwen, Bruce S. 2017. "Neurobiological and Systemic Effects of Chronic Stress." *Chronic Stress* 1: 247054701769232. https://doi.org/10.1177/2470547017692328.

8. Schulman, Rifka C., and Jeffrey I. Mechanick. 2012. "Metabolic and Nutrition Support in the Chronic Critical Illness Syndrome." *Respiratory Care* 57 (6): 958–77. https://doi.org/10.4187/respcare.01620.

9. Wallace, Deshira D., Clare Barrington, Sandra Albrecht, Nisha Gottfredson, Lori Carter-Edwards, and Leslie A. Lytle. 2021. "The Role of Stress Responses on Engagement in Dietary and Physical Activity Behaviors among Latino Adults Living with Prediabetes." *Ethnicity & Health*, 1–15. https://doi.org/10.1080/13557858.2021.1880549.

10. Stults-Kolehmainen, Matthew A., and Rajita Sinha. 2014. "The Effects of Stress on Physical Activity and Exercise." *Sports Medicine* 44 (1): 81–121. https://doi.org/10.1007/s40279-013-0090-5.

11. Zellner, Debra A., Susan Loaiza, Zuleyma Gonzalez, Jaclyn Pita, Janira Morales, Deanna Pecora, and Amanda Wolf. 2006. "Food Selection Changes under Stress." *Physiology & Behavior* 87 (4): 789–93. https://doi.org/10.1016/j.physbeh.2006.01.014.

12. Mechanick, Jeffrey I., Alan J. Garber, George Grunberger, Yehuda Handelsman, and W. Timothy Garvey. 2018. "Dysglycemia-Based Chronic Disease: An American Association of Clinical Endocrinologists Position Statement." *Endocrine Practice: Official Journal of the American College of Endocrinology and the American Association of Clinical Endocrinologists* 24 (11): 995–1011. https://doi.org/10.4158/PS-2018-0139.

13. Mattei, Josiemer, Serkalem Demissie, Luis M. Falcon, Jose M. Ordovas, and Katherine Tucker. 2010. "Allostatic Load Is Associated with Chronic Conditions in the Boston Puerto Rican Health Study." *Social Science & Medicine (1982)* 70 (12): 1988–96. https://doi.org/10.1016/j.socscimed.2010.02.024.

14. Carlsson, A. C., A. Nixon Andreasson, and P. E. Wändell. 2011. "Poor Self-Rated Health Is Not Associated with a High Total Allostatic Load in Type 2 Diabetic Patients-but High Blood Pressure Is." *Diabetes & Metabolism* 37 (5): 446–51. https://doi.org/10.1016/j.diabet.2011.03.005.

15. Hackett, Ruth A., and Andrew Steptoe. 2017. "Type 2 Diabetes Mellitus and Psychological Stress — a Modifiable Risk Factor." *Nature Reviews. Endocrinology* 13 (9): 547–60. https://doi.org/10.1038/nrendo.2017.64.

16. Tsigos, Constantine, Ioannis Kyrou, Eva Kassi, and George P. Chrousos. 2020. "Stress: Endocrine Physiology and Pathophysiology." In *Endotext [Internet]*. Feingold K, editor. South Dartmouth, MA: MDText.com.

17. Paravati, Stephen, Alan Rosani, and Steven J. Warrington. 2021. "Physiology, Catecholamines." In *StatPearls [Internet]*. Hughes E and Rubio G, editors. Treasure Island, FL: StatPearls Publishing.

18. Van den Berghe, Greet, Francis de Zegher, and Roger Bouillon. 1998. "Clinical Review 95: Acute and Prolonged Critical Illness as Different Neuroendocrine Paradigms." *The Journal of Clinical Endocrinology and Metabolism* 83 (6): 1827–34. https://doi.org/10.1210/jcem.83.6.4763.

19. Karatsoreos, Ilia N., Sarah M. Bhagat, Nicole P. Bowles, Zachary M. Weil, Donald W. Pfaff, and Bruce S. McEwen. 2010. "Endocrine and Physiological Changes in Response to Chronic Corticosterone: A Potential Model of the Metabolic Syndrome in Mouse." *Endocrinology* 151 (5): 2117–27. https://doi.org/10.1210/en.2009-1436.

20. Fransson, Liselotte, Stephanie Franzén, Victoria Rosengren, Petra Wolbert, Åke Sjöholm, and Henrik Ortsäter. 2013. "β-Cell Adaptation in a Mouse Model of Glucocorticoid-Induced Metabolic Syndrome." *The Journal of Endocrinology* 219 (3): 231–41. https://doi.org/10.1530/JOE-13-0189.

21. Lopez, Joëlle, and Rosemary C. Bagot, 2021. "Defining Valid Chronic Stress Models for Depression with Female Rodents." *Biological Psychiatry* 90 (4): 226–35. https://doi.org/10.1016/j.biopsych.2021.03.010.

22. Kaufman, Daniel, Mary Ann Banerji, Igor Shorman, Eric L. P. Smith, Jeremy D. Coplan, Leonard A. Rosenblum, and John G. Kral. 2007. "Early-Life Stress and

the Development of Obesity and Insulin Resistance in Juvenile Bonnet Macaques." *Diabetes* 56 (5): 1382–86. https://doi.org/10.2337/db06-1409.

23. Wu, Huaizhu, and Christie M. Ballantyne. 2020. "Metabolic Inflammation and Insulin Resistance in Obesity." *Circulation Research* 126 (11): 1549–64. https://doi. org/10.1161/CIRCRESAHA.119.315896.

24. Rehman, Kanwal, and Muhammad Sajid Hamid Akash. 2016. "Mechanisms of Inflammatory Responses and Development of Insulin Resistance: How Are They Interlinked?" *Journal of Biomedical Science* 23 (1): 87. https://doi.org/10.1186/s12929-016-0303-y.

25. Shoelson, Steven E., Jongsoon Lee, and Allison B. Goldfine. 2006. "Inflammation and Insulin Resistance." *The Journal of Clinical Investigation* 116 (7): 1793–1801. https:// doi.org/10.1172/JCI29069.

26. Ortiz, Robin, Bjoern Kluwe, James B. Odei, Justin B. Echouffo Tcheugui, Mario Sims, Rita R. Kalyani, Alain G. Bertoni, Sherita H. Golden, and Joshua J. Joseph. 2019. "The Association of Morning Serum Cortisol with Glucose Metabolism and Diabetes: The Jackson Heart Study." *Psychoneuroendocrinology* 103: 25–32. https://doi.org/10.1016/j. psyneuen.2018.12.237.

27. Arnaldi, Giorgio, Valerio Mattia Scandali, Laura Trementino, Marina Cardinaletti, Gloria Appolloni, and Marco Boscaro. 2010. "Pathophysiology of Dyslipidemia in Cushing's Syndrome." *Neuroendocrinology* 92 (Suppl 1): 86–90. https://doi. org/10.1159/000314213.

28. Kamba, Aya, Makoto Daimon, Hiroshi Murakami, Hideyuki Otaka, Kota Matsuki, Eri Sato, Jutaro Tanabe, et al. 2016. "Association Between Higher Serum Cortisol Levels and Decreased Insulin Secretion in a General Population." *PloS One* 11 (11): e0166077. https://doi.org/10.1371/journal.pone.0166077.

29. McEwen, Bruce S. 2006. "Protective and Damaging Effects of Stress Mediators: Central Role of the Brain." *Dialogues in Clinical Neuroscience* 8 (4): 367–81. https:// doi.org/10.31887/dcns.2006.8.4/bmcewen.

30. Licht, Carmilla M. M., Sophie A. Vreeburg, Arianne K. B. van Reedt Dortland, Erik J. Giltay, Witte J. G. Hoogendijk, Roel H. DeRijk, Nicole Vogelzangs, Frans G. Zitman, Eco J. C. de Geus, and Brenda W. J. H. Penninx. 2010. "Increased Sympathetic and Decreased Parasympathetic Activity Rather than Changes in Hypothalamic-Pituitary-Adrenal Axis Activity Is Associated with Metabolic Abnormalities." *The Journal of Clinical Endocrinology and Metabolism* 95 (5): 2458–66. https://doi.org/10.1210/ jc.2009-2801.

31. Mancia, Giuseppe, Pascal Bousquet, Jean Luc Elghozi, Murray Esler, Guido Grassi, Stevo Julius, John Reid, and Peter A. Van Zwieten. 2007. "The Sympathetic Nervous System and the Metabolic Syndrome." *Journal of Hypertension* 25 (5): 909–20. https:// doi.org/10.1097/HJH.0b013e328048d004.

32. Hackett, Ruth A., Andrew Steptoe, and Meena Kumari. 2014. "Association of Diurnal Patterns in Salivary Cortisol with Type 2 Diabetes in the Whitehall II Study." *The Journal of Clinical Endocrinology and Metabolism* 99 (12): 4625–31. https://doi. org/10.1210/jc.2014-2459.

33. Siddiqui, Azaz, Nimesh G. Desai, Suman B. Sharma, Mohammad Aslam, Uday K. Sinha, and Sri V. Madhu. 2019. "Association of Oxidative Stress and Inflammatory Markers with Chronic Stress in Patients with Newly Diagnosed Type 2 Diabetes." *Diabetes/Metabolism Research and Reviews* 35 (5): e3147. https://doi.org/10.1002/ dmrr.3147.

34. Wang, Xia, Wei Bao, Jun Liu, Ying-Ying Ouyang, Di Wang, Shuang Rong, Xiao Xiao, et al. 2013. "Inflammatory Markers and Risk of Type 2 Diabetes: A Systematic Review and Meta-Analysis." *Diabetes Care* 36 (1): 166–75. https://doi.org/10.2337/dc12-0702.

35. DeLorey, Darren S. 2021. "Sympathetic Vasoconstriction in Skeletal Muscle: Modulatory Effects of Aging, Exercise Training, and Sex." *Applied Physiology Nutrition and Metabolism* 46 (12): 1437–47. https://doi.org/10.1139/apnm-2021-0399.
36. Liskova, S. 2021. "The Organ-Specific Nitric Oxide Synthase Activity in the Interaction with Sympathetic Nerve Activity: A Hypothesis." *Physiological Research* 70 (2): 169–75. https://doi.org/10.33549/physiolres.934676.
37. Motiejunaite, Justina, Laurence Amar, and Emmanuelle Vidal-Petiot. 2021. "Adrenergic Receptors and Cardiovascular Effects of Catecholamines." *Annales d'endocrinologie* 82 (3–4): 193–97. https://doi.org/10.1016/j.ando.2020.03.012.
38. Thayer, Julian F., and Esther Sternberg. 2006. "Beyond Heart Rate Variability: Vagal Regulation of Allostatic Systems." *Annals of the New York Academy of Sciences* 1088: 361–72.
39. Aune, D., B. Ó Hartaigh, and L. J. Vatten. 2015. "Resting Heart Rate and the Risk of Type 2 Diabetes: A Systematic Review and Dose--Response Meta-Analysis of Cohort Studies." *Nutrition, Metabolism, and Cardiovascular Diseases: NMCD* 25 (6): 526–34. https://doi.org/10.1016/j.numecd.2015.02.008.
40. Tabák, Adam G., Tasnime N. Akbaraly, G. David Batty, and Mika Kivimäki. 2014. "Depression and Type 2 Diabetes: A Causal Association?" *The Lancet. Diabetes & Endocrinology* 2 (3): 236–45. https://doi.org/10.1016/S2213-8587(13)70139-6.
41. Privitera, Gregory J., Quentin W. King-Shepard, Kayla N. Cuifolo, and P. Murali Doraiswamy. 2019. "Differential Food Intake and Food Choice by Depression and Body Mass Index Levels Following a Mood Manipulation in a Buffet-Style Setting." *Journal of Health Psychology* 24 (2): 199–208. https://doi.org/10.1177/1359105316650508.
42. Ali, S., M. A. Stone, J. L. Peters, M. J. Davies, and K. Khunti. 2006. "The Prevalence of Co-Morbid Depression in Adults with Type 2 Diabetes: A Systematic Review and Meta-Analysis: Review Article." *Diabetic Medicine: A Journal of the British Diabetic Association* 23 (11): 1165–73. https://doi.org/10.1111/j.1464-5491.2006.01943.x.
43. Anderson, Ryan J., Kenneth E. Freedland, Ray E. Clouse, and Patrick J. Lustman. 2001. "The Prevalence of Comorbid Depression in Adults with Diabetes: A Meta-Analysis." *Diabetes Care* 24 (6): 1069–78. https://doi.org/10.2337/diacare.24.6.1069.
44. Roy, Tapash, and Cathy E. Lloyd. 2012. "Epidemiology of Depression and Diabetes: A Systematic Review." *Journal of Affective Disorders* 142 (Suppl): S8–21. https://doi.org/10.1016/S0165-0327(12)70004-6.
45. Vancampfort, Davy, Alex J. Mitchell, Marc De Hert, Pascal Sienaert, Michel Probst, Roselien Buys, and Brendon Stubbs. 2015. "Type 2 Diabetes in Patients with Major Depressive Disorder: A Meta-Analysis of Prevalence Estimates and Predictors: Review: Depression and Diabetes." *Depression and Anxiety* 32 (10): 763–73. https://doi.org/10.1002/da.22387.
46. Mezuk, Briana, William W. Eaton, Sandra Albrecht, and Sherita Hill Golden. 2008. "Depression and Type 2 Diabetes over the Lifespan: A Meta-Analysis." *Diabetes Care* 31 (12): 2383–90. https://doi.org/10.2337/dc08-0985.
47. Rotella, F., and E. Mannucci. 2013. "Diabetes Mellitus as a Risk Factor for Depression. A Meta-Analysis of Longitudinal Studies." *Diabetes Research and Clinical Practice* 99 (2): 98–104. https://doi.org/10.1016/j.diabres.2012.11.022.
48. Nouwen, Arie, Kirsty Winkley, J. Twisk, C. E. Lloyd, Mark Peyrot, K. Ismail, F. Pouwer, and European Depression in Diabetes (EDID) Research Consortium. 2010. "Type 2 Diabetes Mellitus as a Risk Factor for the Onset of Depression: A Systematic Review and Meta-Analysis." *Diabetologia* 53 (12): 2480–86. https://doi.org/10.1007/s00125-010-1874-x.
49. Demakakos, Panayotes, Paola Zaninotto, and Arie Nouwen. 2014. "Is the Association between Depressive Symptoms and Glucose Metabolism Bidirectional? Evidence from the English Longitudinal Study of Ageing." *Psychosomatic Medicine* 76 (7): 555–61. https://doi.org/10.1097/PSY.0000000000000082.

50. Rotella, Francesco, and Edoardo Mannucci. 2013. "Depression as a Risk Factor for Diabetes: A Meta-Analysis of Longitudinal Studies." *The Journal of Clinical Psychiatry* 74 (1): 31–37. https://doi.org/10.4088/JCP.12r07922.

51. Fisher, Lawrence, Joseph T. Mullan, Patricia Arean, Russell E. Glasgow, Danielle Hessler, and Umesh Masharani. 2010. "Diabetes Distress but Not Clinical Depression or Depressive Symptoms Is Associated with Glycemic Control in Both Cross-Sectional and Longitudinal Analyses." *Diabetes Care* 33 (1): 23–28. https://doi.org/10.2337/dc09-238.

52. Aikens, James E. 2012. "Prospective Associations between Emotional Distress and Poor Outcomes in Type 2 Diabetes." *Diabetes Care* 35 (12): 2472–78. https://doi.org/10.2337/dc12-0181.

53. Gonzalez, Jeffrey S., Mark Peyrot, Lauren A. McCarl, Erin Marie Collins, Luis Serpa, Matthew J. Mimiaga, and Steven A. Safren. 2008. "Depression and Diabetes Treatment Nonadherence: A Meta-Analysis." *Diabetes Care* 31 (12): 2398–2403. https://doi.org/10.2337/dc08-1341.

54. Ali, Saima, Margaret Stone, Timothy Chas Skinner, Noelle Robertson, Melanie Davies, and Kamlesh Khunti. 2010. "The Association between Depression and Health-Related Quality of Life in People with Type 2 Diabetes: A Systematic Literature Review." *Diabetes/Metabolism Research and Reviews* 26 (2): 75–89. https://doi.org/10.1002/dmrr.1065.

55. Schram, Miranda T., Caroline A. Baan, and François Pouwer. 2009. "Depression and Quality of Life in Patients with Diabetes: A Systematic Review from the European Depression in Diabetes (EDID) Research Consortium." *Current Diabetes Reviews* 5 (2): 112–19. https://doi.org/10.2174/157339909788166828.

56. Grigsby, Allison B., Ryan J. Anderson, Kenneth E. Freedland, Ray E. Clouse, and Patrick J. Lustman. 2002. "Prevalence of Anxiety in Adults with Diabetes: A Systematic Review." *Journal of Psychosomatic Research* 53 (6): 1053–60.

57. Smith, Kimberley J., Mélanie Béland, Matthew Clyde, Geneviève Gariépy, Véronique Pagé, Ghislaine Badawi, Rémi Rabasa-Lhoret, and Norbert Schmitz. 2013. "Association of Diabetes with Anxiety: A Systematic Review and Meta-Analysis." *Journal of Psychosomatic Research* 74 (2): 89–99. https://doi.org/10.1016/j.jpsychores.2012.11.013.

58. Li, C., L. Barker, E. S. Ford, X. Zhang, T. W. Strine, and A. H. Mokdad. 2008. "Diabetes and Anxiety in US Adults: Findings from the 2006 Behavioral Risk Factor Surveillance System." *Diabetic Medicine: A Journal of the British Diabetic Association* 25 (7): 878–81. https://doi.org/10.1111/j.1464-5491.2008.02477.x.

59. Juruena, Mario F., Filip Eror, Anthony J. Cleare, and Allan H. Young. 2020. "The Role of Early Life Stress in HPA Axis and Anxiety." *Advances in Experimental Medicine and Biology* 1191: 141–53. https://doi.org/10.1007/978-981-32-9705-0_9.

60. Hajós, Tibor R. S., William H. Polonsky, Frans Pouwer, Linda Gonder-Frederick, and Frank J. Snoek. 2014. "Toward Defining a Cutoff Score for Elevated Fear of Hypoglycemia on the Hypoglycemia Fear Survey Worry Subscale in Patients with Type 2 Diabetes." *Diabetes Care* 37: 102–8.

61. Yi, Joyce P., Peter P. Vitaliano, Ronald E. Smith, Jean C. Yi, and Katie Weinger. 2008. "The Role of Resilience on Psychological Adjustment and Physical Health in Patients with Diabetes." *British Journal of Health Psychology* 13 (Pt 2): 311–25. https://doi.org/10.1348/135910707X186994.

62. Abraham, Sherley, Nina G. Shah, Ana Diez Roux, Felicia Hill-Briggs, Teresa Seeman, Moyses Szklo, Pamela J. Schreiner, and Sherita Hill Golden. 2015. "Trait Anger but Not Anxiety Predicts Incident Type 2 Diabetes: The Multi-Ethnic Study of Atherosclerosis (MESA)." *Psychoneuroendocrinology* 60: 105–13. https://doi.org/10.1016/j.psyneuen.2015.06.007.

63. Golden, Sherita Hill, Janice E. Williams, Daniel E. Ford, Hsin-Chieh Yeh, Catherine Paton Sanford, F. Javier Nieto, and Frederick L. Brancati. 2006. "Anger Temperament

Is Modestly Associated with the Risk of Type 2 Diabetes Mellitus: The Atheroslcerosis Risk in Communities Study." *Psychoneuroendocrinology* 31 (3): 325–32. https://doi.org/10.1016/j.psyneuen.2005.08.008.

64. Kivimäki, Mika, Marianna Virtanen, Ichiro Kawachi, Solja T. Nyberg, Lars Alfredsson, G. David Batty, Jakob B. Bjorner, et al. 2014. "Long Working Hours, Socioeconomic Status, and the Risk of Incident Type 2 Diabetes: A Meta-Analysis of Published and Unpublished Data from 222 120 Individuals." *The Lancet. Diabetes & Endocrinology* 3 (1): 27–34. https://doi.org/10.1016/S2213-8587(14)70178-0.

65. Huang, Hao, Peipei Yan, Zhilei Shan, Sijing Chen, Moying Li, Cheng Luo, Hui Gao, Liping Hao, and Liegang Liu. 2015. "Adverse Childhood Experiences and Risk of Type 2 Diabetes: A Systematic Review and Meta-Analysis." *Metabolism: Clinical and Experimental* 64 (11): 1408–18. https://doi.org/10.1016/j.metabol.2015.08.019.

66. Williams, Lisa H., Carolyn M. Rutter, Wayne J. Katon, Gayle E. Reiber, Paul Ciechanowski, Susan R. Heckbert, Elizabeth H. B. Lin, et al. 2010. "Depression and Incident Diabetic Foot Ulcers: A Prospective Cohort Study." *The American Journal of Medicine* 123 (8): 748–754.e3. https://doi.org/10.1016/j.amjmed.2010.01.023.

67. Sieu, Nida, Wayne Katon, Elizabeth H. B. Lin, Joan Russo, Evette Ludman, and Paul Ciechanowski. 2011. "Depression and Incident Diabetic Retinopathy: A Prospective Cohort Study." *General Hospital Psychiatry* 33 (5): 429–35. https://doi.org/10.1016/j.genhosppsych.2011.05.021.

68. Novak, Marta, Istvan Mucsi, Connie M. Rhee, Elani Streja, Jun L. Lu, Kamyar Kalantar-Zadeh, Miklos Z. Molnar, and Csaba P. Kovesdy. 2016. "Increased Risk of Incident Chronic Kidney Disease, Cardiovascular Disease, and Mortality in Patients with Diabetes with Comorbid Depression." *Diabetes Care* 39 (11): 1940–47. https://doi.org/10.2337/dc16-0048.

69. Gonzalez, J. S., L. Vileikyte, J. S. Ulbrecht, R. R. Rubin, A. P. Garrow, C. Delgado, P. R. Cavanagh, A. J. M. Boulton, and M. Peyrot. 2010. "Depression Predicts First but Not Recurrent Diabetic Foot Ulcers." *Diabetologia* 53 (10): 2241–48. https://doi.org/10.1007/s00125-010-1821-x.

70. Iversen, Marjolein M., Grethe S. Tell, Birgitte Espehaug, Kristian Midthjell, Marit Graue, Berit Rokne, Line Iden Berge, and Truls Østbye. 2015. "Is Depression a Risk Factor for Diabetic Foot Ulcers? 11-Years Follow-up of the Nord-Trøndelag Health Study (HUNT)." *Journal of Diabetes and Its Complications* 29 (1): 20–25. https://doi.org/10.1016/j.jdiacomp.2014.09.006.

71. Ting, Rose Z. W., Eric S. H. Lau, Risa Ozaki, Winnie W. Y. Lau, Alice P. S. Kong, Andrea O. Y. Luk, Chun-Chung Chow, et al. 2013. "High Risk for Cardiovascular Disease in Chinese Type 2 Diabetic Patients with Major Depression--a 7-Year Prospective Analysis of the Hong Kong Diabetes Registry." *Journal of Affective Disorders* 149 (1–3): 129–35. https://doi.org/10.1016/j.jad.2013.01.012.

72. Scherrer, Jeffrey F., Lauren D. Garfield, Timothy Chrusciel, Paul J. Hauptman, Robert M. Carney, Kenneth E. Freedland, Richard Owen, William R. True, and Patrick J. Lustman. 2011. "Increased Risk of Myocardial Infarction in Depressed Patients with Type 2 Diabetes." *Diabetes Care* 34 (8): 1729–34. https://doi.org/10.2337/dc11-0031.

73. Lin, Elizabeth H. B., Carolyn M. Rutter, Wayne Katon, Susan R. Heckbert, Paul Ciechanowski, Malia M. Oliver, Evette J. Ludman, et al. 2010. "Depression and Advanced Complications of Diabetes: A Prospective Cohort Study." *Diabetes Care* 33 (2): 264–69. https://doi.org/10.2337/dc09-1068.

74. Rådholm, Karin, A-B Wiréhn, J. Chalmers, and Carl Johan Östgren. 2015. "Use of Antidiabetic and Antidepressant Drugs Is Associated with Increased Risk of Myocardial Infarction: A Nationwide Register Study." *Diabetic Medicine: A Journal of the British Diabetic Association* 33 (2): 218–23. https://doi.org/10.1111/dme.12822.

75. Park, Mijung, Wayne J. Katon, and Fredric M. Wolf 2013. "Depression and Risk of Mortality in Individuals with Diabetes: A Meta- Analysis and Systematic Review." *General Hospital Psychiatry* 35: 217–25.

76. Van Dooren, Fleur E. P., Giesje Nefs, Miranda T. Schram, Frans R. J. Verhey, Johan Denollet, and François Pouwer. 2013. "Depression and Risk of Mortality in People with Diabetes Mellitus: A Systematic Review and Meta-Analysis." *PloS One* 8 (3): e57058. https://doi.org/10.1371/journal.pone.0057058.

77. Hofmann, Mareike, Birgit Köhler, Falk Leichsenring, and Johannes Kruse. 2013. "Depression as a Risk Factor for Mortality in Individuals with Diabetes: A Meta-Analysis of Prospective Studies." *PloS One* 8 (11): e79809. https://doi.org/10.1371/journal.pone.0079809.

78. Dalsgaard, Else-Marie, Mogens Vestergaard, Mette V. Skriver, Helle T. Maindal, Torsten Lauritzen, Knut Borch-Johnsen, Daniel Witte, and Annelli Sandbaek. 2014. "Psychological Distress, Cardiovascular Complications and Mortality among People with Screen-Detected Type 2 Diabetes: Follow-up of the ADDITION-Denmark Trial." *Diabetologia* 57 (4): 710–17. https://doi.org/10.1007/s00125-014-3165-4.

79. Rod, Naja Hulvej, M. Grønbaek, P. Schnohr, E. Prescott, and T. S. Kristensen. 2009. "Perceived Stress as a Risk Factor for Changes in Health Behaviour and Cardiac Risk Profile: A Longitudinal Study." *Journal of Internal Medicine* 266 (5): 467–75. https://doi.org/10.1111/j.1365-2796.2009.02124.x.

80. Rippe, James M. 2018. "Lifestyle Medicine: The Health Promoting Power of Daily Habits and Practices." *American Journal of Lifestyle Medicine* 12 (6): 499–512. https://doi.org/10.1177/1559827618785554.

81. Koenigsberg, Marlon Russell, and Jennifer Corliss. 2017. "Diabetes Self-Management: Facilitating Lifestyle Change." *American Family Physician* 96 (6): 62–70.

82. Moulton, Calum D., John C. Pickup, and Khalida Ismail. 2015. "The Link between Depression and Diabetes: The Search for Shared Mechanisms." *The Lancet. Diabetes & Endocrinology* 3 (6): 461–71. https://doi.org/10.1016/S2213-8587(15)00134-5.

83. American Diabetes Association. 2021. "Cardiovascular Disease and Risk Management: Standards of Medical Care in Diabetes-2021." *Diabetes Care* 44 (Suppl 1): S125–50. https://doi.org/10.2337/dc21-S010.

84. American Diabetes Association. 2021a. "Obesity Management for the Treatment of Type 2 Diabetes: Standards of Medical Care in Diabetes-2021." *Diabetes Care* 44 (Suppl 1): S100–110. https://doi.org/10.2337/dc21-S008.

85. Rubin, Richard R., Thomas A. Wadden, Judy L. Bahnson, George L. Blackburn, Frederick L. Brancati, George A. Bray, Mace Coday, et al. 2014. "Impact of Intensive Lifestyle Intervention on Depression and Health-Related Quality of Life in Type 2 Diabetes: The Look AHEAD Trial." *Diabetes Care* 37 (6): 1544–53. https://doi.org/10.2337/dc13-1928.

86. Varghese, Mathew P., Ragavendrasamy Balakrishnan, and Subramanya Pailoor. 2018. "Association between a Guided Meditation Practice, Sleep and Psychological Well-Being in Type 2 Diabetes Mellitus Patients." *Journal of Complementary & Integrative Medicine* 15 (4). https://doi.org/10.1515/jcim-2015-0026.

87. Breymeyer, Kara L., Johanna W. Lampe, Bonnie A. McGregor, and Marian L. Neuhouser. 2016. "Subjective Mood and Energy Levels of Healthy Weight and Overweight/Obese Healthy Adults on High-and Low-Glycemic Load Experimental Diets." *Appetite* 107: 253–59. https://doi.org/10.1016/j.appet.2016.08.008.

88. Harvey, Cliff J. D. C., Grant M. Schofield, Caryn Zinn, and Simon Thornley. 2019. "Effects of Differing Levels of Carbohydrate Restriction on Mood Achievement of Nutritional Ketosis, and Symptoms of Carbohydrate Withdrawal in Healthy Adults: A Randomized Clinical Trial." *Nutrition* 67–68: 100005. https://doi.org/10.1016/j.nutx.2019.100005.

89. Brinkworth, Grant D., Jonathan D. Buckley, Manny Noakes, Peter M. Clifton, and Carlene J. Wilson. 2009. "Long-Term Effects of a Very Low-Carbohydrate Diet and a Low-Fat Diet on Mood and Cognitive Function." *Archives of Internal Medicine* 169 (20): 1873–80. https://doi.org/10.1001/archinternmed.2009.329.

90. McClernon, F. Joseph, William S. Yancy Jr, Jacqueline A. Eberstein, Robert C. Atkins, and Eric C. Westman. 2007. "The Effects of a Low-Carbohydrate Ketogenic Diet and a Low-Fat Diet on Mood, Hunger, and Other Self-Reported Symptoms." *Obesity* 15 (1): 182–87. https://doi.org/10.1038/oby.2007.516.

91. Kakoschke, Naomi, Ian T. Zajac, Jeannie Tay, Natalie D. Luscombe-Marsh, Campbell H. Thompson, Manny Noakes, Jonathan D. Buckley, Gary Wittert, and Grant D. Brinkworth. 2021. "Effects of Very Low-Carbohydrate vs. High-Carbohydrate Weight Loss Diets on Psychological Health in Adults with Obesity and Type 2 Diabetes: A 2-Year Randomized Controlled Trial." *European Journal of Nutrition* 60 (8): 4251–62. https://doi.org/10.1007/s00394-021-02587-z.

92. Sánchez-Villegas, Almudena, Miguel Angel Martínez-González, Ramón Estruch, Jordi Salas-Salvadó, Dolores Corella, Maria Isabel Covas, Fernando Arós, et al. 2013. "Mediterranean Dietary Pattern and Depression: The PREDIMED Randomized Trial." *BMC Medicine* 11 (1): 208. https://doi.org/10.1186/1741-7015-11-208.

93. Wagner, Julie Ann, Angela Bermudez-Millan, Grace Damio, Sofia Segura-Perez, Jyoti Chhabra, Cunegundo Vergara, Richard Feinn, and Rafael Perez-Escamilla. 2016. "A Randomized, Controlled Trial of a Stress Management Intervention for Latinos with Type 2 Diabetes Delivered by Community Health Workers: Outcomes for Psychological Wellbeing, Glycemic Control, and Cortisol." *Diabetes Research and Clinical Practice* 120: 162–70. https://doi.org/10.1016/j.diabres.2016.07.022.

94. Noordali, Farhan, Jennifer Cumming, and Janice L. Thompson. 2017. "Effectiveness of Mindfulness-Based Interventions on Physiological and Psychological Complications in Adults with Diabetes: A Systematic Review." *Journal of Health Psychology* 22 (8): 965–83. https://doi.org/10.1177/1359105315620293.

95. Dickens, Chris, Andrea Cherrington, Isabel Adeyemi, Kate Roughley, Peter Bower, Charlotte Garrett, Christine Bundy, and Peter Coventry. 2013. "Characteristics of Psychological Interventions That Improve Depression in People with Coronary Heart Disease: A Systematic Review and Meta-Regression." *Psychosomatic Medicine* 75 (2): 211–21. https://doi.org/10.1097/PSY.0b013e31827ac009.

96. Baumeister, Harald, Nico Hutter, and Jürgen Bengel. 2012. "Psychological and Pharmacological Interventions for Depression in Patients with Diabetes Mellitus and Depression." *Cochrane Database of Systematic Reviews* 12: CD008381. https://doi.org/10.1002/14651858.CD008381.pub2.

97. National Institute for Health and Care Excellence. 2009. "Depression in Adults with a Chronic Physical Health Problem: Recognition and Management."

98. Taylor, C. Barr, N. Houston-Miller, David K. Ahn, W. Haskell, and R. F. DeBusk. 1986. "The Effects of Exercise Training Programs on Psychosocial Improvement in Uncomplicated Postmyocardial Infarction Patients." *Journal of Psychosomatic Research* 30 (5): 581–87. https://doi.org/10.1016/0022-3999(86)90031-0.

99. Gellis, Zvi D., and Christina Kang-Yi. 2012. "Meta-Analysis of the Effect of Cardiac Rehabilitation Interventions on Depression Outcomes in Adults 64 Years of Age and Older." *The American Journal of Cardiology* 110 (9): 1219–24. https://doi.org/10.1016/j.amjcard.2012.06.021.

100. Hare, David L., Samia R. Toukhsati, Peter Johansson, and Tiny Jaarsma. 2014. "Depression and Cardiovascular Disease: A Clinical Review." *European Heart Journal* 35 (21): 1365–72. https://doi.org/10.1093/eurheartj/eht462.

101. Hansson, Göran K., and Andreas Hermansson. 2011. "The Immune System in Atherosclerosis." *Nature Immunology* 12 (3): 204–12. https://doi.org/10.1038/ni.2001.

102. Gresham, Kenneth S., Ranganath Mamidi, Jiayang Li, Hyerin Kwak, and Julian E. Stelzer. 2017. "Sarcomeric Protein Modification during Adrenergic Stress Enhances Cross-Bridge Kinetics and Cardiac Output." *Journal of Applied Physiology* 122 (3): 520–30. https://doi.org/10.1152/japplphysiol.00306.2016.

103. Kaplan, J. R., Haiying Chen, and Stephen B. Manuck. 2009. "The Relationship between Social Status and Atherosclerosis in Male and Female Monkeys as Revealed by Meta-Analysis." *American Journal of Primatology* 71 (9): 732–41. https://doi.org/10.1002/ajp.20707.

104. Kaplan, Jay R., Stephen B. Manuck, Thomas B. Clarkson, Frances M. Lusso, David M. Taub, and Eric W. Miller. 1983. "Social Stress and Atherosclerosis in Normocholesterolemic Monkeys." *Science* 220 (4598): 733–35. https://doi.org/10.1126/science.6836311.

105. Hamer, Mark, Romano Endrighi, Shreenidhi M. Venuraju, Avijit Lahiri, and Andrew Steptoe. 2012. "Cortisol Responses to Mental Stress and the Progression of Coronary Artery Calcification in Healthy Men and Women." *PloS One* 7 (2): e31356. https://doi.org/10.1371/journal.pone.0031356.

106. Chida, Yoichi, and Andrew Steptoe. 2010. "Greater Cardiovascular Responses to Laboratory Mental Stress Are Associated with Poor Subsequent Cardiovascular Risk Status: A Meta-Analysis of Prospective Evidence: A Meta-Analysis of Prospective Evidence." *Hypertension* 55 (4): 1026–32. https://doi.org/10.1161/HYPERTENSION AHA.109.146621.

107. Steptoe, Andrew, and Mika Kivimäki. 2013. "Stress and Cardiovascular Disease: An Update on Current Knowledge." *Annual Review of Public Health* 34 (1): 337–54. https://doi.org/10.1146/annurev-publhealth-031912-114452.

108. Zou, Liye, Jeffer Eidi Sasaki, Gao-Xia Wei, Tao Huang, Albert S. Yeung, Octávio Barbosa Neto, Kevin W. Chen, and Stanley Sai-Chuen Hui. 2018. "Effects of Mind-Body Exercises (Tai Chi/Yoga) on Heart Rate Variability Parameters and Perceived Stress: A Systematic Review with Meta-Analysis of Randomized Controlled Trials." *Journal of Clinical Medicine* 7 (11): 404. https://doi.org/10.3390/jcm7110404.

109. Hughes, Joel W., David M. Fresco, Rodney Myerscough, Manfred H. M. van Dulmen, Linda E. Carlson, and Richard Josephson. 2013. "Randomized Controlled Trial of Mindfulness-Based Stress Reduction for Prehypertension." *Psychosomatic Medicine* 75 (8): 721–28. https://doi.org/10.1097/PSY.0b013e3182a3e4e5.

110. Goldstein, Carly M., Richard Josephson, Susan Xie, and Joel W. Hughes. 2012. "Current Perspectives on the Use of Meditation to Reduce Blood Pressure." *International Journal of Hypertension* 2012: 578397. https://doi.org/10.1155/2012/578397.

111. Hartley, Louise, Mariana Dyakova, Jennifer Holmes, Aileen Clarke, Myeong Soo Lee, Edzard Ernst, and Karen Rees. 2014. "Yoga for the Primary Prevention of Cardiovascular Disease." *Cochrane Database of Systematic Reviews* (5): CD010072. https://doi.org/10.1002/14651858.CD010072.pub2.

112. Hartley, Louise, Nadine Flowers, Myeong Soo Lee, Edzard Ernst, and Karen Rees. 2014. "Tai Chi for Primary Prevention of Cardiovascular Disease." *Cochrane Database of Systematic Reviews* (4): CD010366. https://doi.org/10.1002/14651858.CD010366. pub2.

113. Hartley, Louise, Myeong Soo Lee, Joey S. W. Kwong, Nadine Flowers, Daniel Todkill, Edzard Ernst, and Karen Rees. 2015. "Qigong for the Primary Prevention of Cardiovascular Disease." *Cochrane Database of Systematic Reviews* (6): CD010390. https://doi.org/10.1002/14651858.CD010390.pub2.

114. Mechanick, Jeffrey I., Daniel L. Hurley, and W. Timothy Garvey. 2017. "Adiposity-Based Chronic Disease as a New Diagnostic Term: The American Association of Clinical Endocrinologists and American College of Endocrinology Position Statement." *Endocrine Practice: Official Journal of the American College of Endocrinology and*

the American Association of Clinical Endocrinologists 23 (3): 372–78. https://doi.org/10.4158/EP161688.PS.

115. Shively, Carol A., Thomas C. Register, and Thomas B. Clarkson. 2009. "Social Stress, Visceral Obesity, and Coronary Artery Atherosclerosis: Product of a Primate Adaptation." *American Journal of Primatology* 71 (9): 742–51. https://doi.org/10.1002/ajp.20706.

116. Kubera, Britta, Claudine Leonhard, Andreas Rößler, and Achim Peters. 2017. "Stress-Related Changes in Body Form: Results from the Whitehall II Study." *Obesity* 25 (9): 1625–32. https://doi.org/10.1002/oby.21928.

117. Teixeira, Pedro J., and Marta M. Marques. 2017. "Health Behavior Change for Obesity Management." *Obesity Facts* 10 (6): 666–73. https://doi.org/10.1159/000484933.

118. Lang, Astrid, and Erika Sivarajan Froelicher. 2006. "Management of Overweight and Obesity in Adults: Behavioral Intervention for Long-Term Weight Loss and Maintenance." *European Journal of Cardiovascular Nursing: Journal of the Working Group on Cardiovascular Nursing of the European Society of Cardiology* 5 (2): 102–14. https://doi.org/10.1016/j.ejcnurse.2005.11.002.

119. Diabetes Prevention Research Group. 2015. "Long-Term Effects of Lifestyle Intervention or Metformin on Diabetes Development and Microvascular Complications over 15-Year Follow-up: The Diabetes Prevention Program Outcomes Study." *The Lancet. Diabetes & Endocrinology* 3 (11): 866–75. https://doi.org/10.1016/s2213-8587(15)00291-0.

120. Look AHEAD Research Group. 2014. "Eight-Year Weight Losses with an Intensive Lifestyle Intervention: The Look AHEAD Study: 8-Year Weight Losses in Look AHEAD." *Obesity* 22 (1): 5–13. https://doi.org/10.1002/oby.20662.

121. Gregg, Edward W., Haiying Chen, Lynne E. Wagenknecht, Jeanne M. Clark, Linda M. Delahanty, John Bantle, et al. 2012. "Association of an Intensive Lifestyle Intervention with Remission of Type 2 Diabetes." *JAMA: The Journal of the American Medical Association* 308 (23): 2489. https://doi.org/10.1001/jama.2012.67929.

122. Yom-Tov, Elad, Guy Feraru, Mark Kozdoba, Shie Mannor, Moshe Tennenholtz, and Irit Hochberg. 2017. "Encouraging Physical Activity in Patients with Diabetes: Intervention Using a Reinforcement Learning System." *Journal of Medical Internet Research* 19 (10): e338. https://doi.org/10.2196/jmir.7994.

123. American Diabetes Association. 2016. "Standards of Medical Care in Diabetes-2016 Abridged for Primary Care Providers." *Clinical Diabetes: A Publication of the American Diabetes Association* 34 (1): 3–21. https://doi.org/10.2337/diaclin.34.1.3.

124. Dutton, Gareth R., and Cora E. Lewis. 2015. "The Look AHEAD Trial: Implications for Lifestyle Intervention in Type 2 Diabetes Mellitus." *Progress in Cardiovascular Diseases* 58 (1): 69–75. https://doi.org/10.1016/j.pcad.2015.04.002.

13 Sleep Hygiene

Geetika Arora and Michael A. Via
Icahn School of Medicine at Mount Sinai

Jeffrey I. Mechanick
Kravis Center for Cardiovascular Health at Mount Sinai Heart
Icahn School of Medicine at Mount Sinai

CONTENTS

Type 2 diabetes (T2D) is a major health problem worldwide. Today, 9.3% of adults aged 20–79 years – a staggering 463 million people – are living with diabetes. The International Diabetes Federation estimates that there will be 578 million adults with T2D by 2030, and 700 million by 2045 [1]. The rising prevalence of obesity and insulin resistance contributes significantly to T2D and atherosclerotic complications. It is within this context that sleep disturbances have gained attention as they are emerging as novel risk factors for cardiometabolic disease development.

In contemporary society, adults are sleeping less, which influences cardiometabolic risk. The importance of sleep for metabolic function and specifically glucose homeostasis is widely accepted, as many studies have shown a correlation between sleep deprivation or poor sleep quality and an increased risk of T2D [2]. The rapid increase in the prevalence of obesity and T2D results from environmental, socioeconomic, behavioral, and demographic factors as they interact with individual genetic predisposition. Besides traditional lifestyle factors, such as dietary choices and sedentary habits, other behavioral and environmental factors could be contributing to the epidemic of obesity and T2D [2]. At the same time, people are sleeping less, and sleep disorders are on the rise. According to recent polls from the U.S. Centers for Disease Control and Prevention, approximately 29% of U.S. adults report sleeping less than 7 hours per night, and 50–70 million have chronic sleep and wakefulness disorders [3]. The average sleep debt (calculated as the difference between self-reported actual and preferred weekday sleep duration) has increased with average daily sleep decreasing from 9 hours to just above 7 hours among adults between 1960 and 2000 [4]. This sleep curtailment is in part self-imposed, as the pace and the opportunities of modern society place more demands on time for work and leisure activities, leaving less for sleep [2].

13.1 SLEEP AND GLUCOSE HOMEOSTASIS

Glucose tolerance varies in a circadian rhythm, as well as with the different stages of sleep [2]. Sleep has five stages: rapid eye movement (REM) sleep and stages 1, 2, 3, and 4 of non-REM sleep. The deeper stages of non-REM sleep, i.e., stages 3 and 4, are also known as slow-wave sleep and are thought to be the most restorative. Additionally, the onset of slow-wave sleep is temporally associated with transient metabolic, hormonal, and neurophysiologic changes, all of which can affect glucose homeostasis.

With slow-wave sleep, the brain uses less glucose [5], the pituitary gland releases more growth hormone and less corticotropin [6], the sympathetic nervous system is less active, and vagal tone is increased [7]. In the first part of the night, when slow-wave sleep predominates, brain glucose metabolism is slower and contributes to a two-thirds fall in systemic glucose utilization and higher blood glucose levels. These effects are reversed in the second part of the night, when REM sleep, stage 1 non-REM sleep, and awakenings are more likely. In view of these important changes in glucose metabolism during sleep, it is not surprising that getting less sleep or poorer sleep on a regular basis could affect overall glucose homeostasis [2]. Epidemiologic and laboratory/interventional evidence supports an association between either short sleep duration (<7 hours per night) or poor sleep quality and an increased risk of T2D [2].

A number of epidemiologic studies examined the relationships between sleep duration and sleep disturbances and T2D risk [8]. The Sleep Heart Study was a large, cross-sectional, community-based study of the cardiovascular consequences of sleep-disordered breathing [9]. The authors assessed the relationship between reported sleep duration and impaired glucose tolerance or T2D in more than 1,400 men and women who had no history of insomnia. After adjustment for age, sex, race, body habitus, and apnea-hypopnea index, the prevalence of impaired glucose tolerance (IGT) and T2D was higher in those who reported sleeping 6 hours or less per night. Compared with those sleeping 7–8 hours per night, subjects sleeping 5 hours or less and 6 hours per night had adjusted odds ratios for T2D of 2.51 (95% CI, 1.57–4.02) and 1.66 (95% CI, 1.15–2.39), respectively. Adjusted odds ratios for IGT were 1.33 (95% CI, 0.83–2.15) and 1.58 (95% CI, 1.15–2.18), respectively. The major limitations of the study were that it was cross-sectional in design, sleep duration was self-reported, the reasons for sleep curtailment were unknown, and possible confounding variables as physical activity, diet, and socioeconomic status were not measured.

In 1969, Kuhn et al. [10] performed the very first laboratory study of the effect of sleep deprivation on metabolism. In this study, 28 healthy young adults were kept awake for 72–126 hours by simple psychic and physical stimulation and glucose tolerance testing worsened to prediabetic levels. From a real-world standpoint, total sleep deprivation is uncommon in humans and inevitably followed by sleep recovery, with normalization of glucose metabolism. Nevertheless, people in modern society commonly experience recurrent partial sleep deprivation and this could be a contributing factor for abnormal glucose tolerance. For example, in a landmark series of laboratory studies of partial sleep deprivation in healthy, lean adults, Spiegel et al. [11], demonstrated that restricting sleep to 4 hours per night for six nights resulted in a 40% decrease in glucose tolerance, levels similar to those seen in older adults with impaired glucose tolerance. This metabolic change was paralleled by an increase in the activity of sympathetic nervous system, and both effects reversed with sleep recovery.

More recently, Nedeltcheva et al. [12] examined the effects of less-severe sleep curtailment (5.5 hours per night for 14 nights) in sedentary middle-aged men and women. This degree of bedtime restriction led to a decrease in glucose tolerance due to decreased insulin sensitivity in the absence of adequate β-cell compensation. Such recurrent bedtime restriction is closer to the short sleep duration experienced by many people in everyday life. In at-risk patients, sleep deprivation at this level may facilitate the development of insulin resistance, reduced glucose tolerance, and ultimately T2D.

Knutson et al. examined the association between self-reported sleep duration and sleep quality and hemoglobin A1c (A1C) levels in 161 African American patients with T2D [13]. In patients without diabetic complications, glycemic control correlated with perceived sleep debt: a perceived sleep debt of 3 hours per night predicted a A1C value 1.1 absolute percentage points higher than the median value. The analyses were controlled for age, sex, body mass index, insulin use, and the presence of major complications; the analyses excluded patients whose sleep was frequently disrupted by pain. The effect size was comparable to (but opposite) that of oral antidiabetic drugs. However, the direction of causality cannot be confirmed from this association since it is possible that poor glycemic control in patients with T2D could impair their ability to achieve sufficient sleep.

To date, some major prospective studies have also looked at the association between short sleep duration or sleep problems and the risk of developing T2D in adults. The Nurses' Health Study [14] followed 70,000 women who did not have diabetes. With a 10-year follow-up, nurses who slept 5 hours or less per 24 hours had a relative risk of T2D of 1.57, as compared to those who slept 7–8 hours per day, even after controlling for body mass index, shift work, hypertension, exercise, and depression. The first National Health and Nutrition Examination Survey (NHANES I) examined the effect of sleep duration on the risk of incidence of T2D in roughly 9,000 men and women over a period of 8–10 years [15]. The statistical model included body mass index and hypertension and adjusted for physical activity, depression, alcohol consumption, ethnicity, education, marital status, and age. It was found that those who slept 5 hours or less per night were significantly more likely to develop T2D than were those who slept 7 hours per night (odds ratio 1.47, 95% confidence interval [CI] 1.03–2.09). Kawakami et al. [16] followed 2,649 Japanese men for 8 years. Those who had difficulty going to sleep and staying asleep, which are both likely to result in shorter sleep duration, had higher age-adjusted risks of developing T2D, with hazard ratios of 2.98 and 2.23, respectively. Nilsson et al. [17] followed 6,599 nondiabetic Swedish men for an average of 15 years. Self-reported difficulty sleeping predicted the development of T2D with an odds ratio of 1.52 even after controlling for age, body mass index at screening, changes in body mass index at follow-up, baseline glucose level, follow-up time, physical activity, family history of T2D, smoking, social class, and alcohol intake. Interestingly, the authors found that the resting heart rate was higher at baseline in the men who later developed T2D. This finding could be interpreted as reflecting greater sympathetic nervous system activity, a putative mediator of the metabolic dysfunction associated with both short sleep duration and obstructive sleep apnea (OSA).

A meta-analysis of ten prospective studies, with 107,756 participants followed for a median of 9.5 years, representing all prospective studies published to date demonstrated a 28% increase in incidence of T2D with short sleep duration (defined as either ≤5 or <6 hours within different studies) [18]. Additionally, the risk of T2D was 48% higher among individuals with long sleep duration (>8 hours), 57% higher with difficulty going to sleep, and 84% higher with difficulty staying asleep [18].

One consideration when interpreting these results is that sleep duration was self-reported in these studies and was not directly measured. For instance, self-reported sleeping more than 8 hours per night may include significant time in bed trying to fall asleep and not actually sleeping. Another consideration is that the higher incidence of T2D in people who slept longer per day is due to undiagnosed OSA, which is associated with daytime sleepiness and possibly longer sleep time to compensate for inefficient sleep. Finally, depressive symptoms, unemployment, a low level of physical activity, and undiagnosed health conditions have all been associated with longer sleep duration and could affect the relationship with T2D risk.

In summary, the weight of scientific evidence using different methodologies and from different geographic locations have consistently indicated that short or poor sleep may increase the risk of developing T2D and suggest that such an association spans different countries, cultures, and ethnic groups.

13.2   MECHANISM OF SLEEP DEPRIVATION AND DISTURBANCE LEADING TO INCREASED INSULIN RESISTANCE

13.2.1   HORMONAL DYSREGULATION

The effects of sleep loss on glucose metabolism are likely multifactorial, involving several interacting pathways, especially in the brain. Decreased brain glucose utilization has been shown on positron emission tomography in sleep-deprived subjects [19]. Sleep deprivation is associated with disturbances in the secretion of the counter-regulatory pituitary hormone growth hormone (GH) [20]. Young, healthy volunteers (22 ± 1 year) who were allowed to sleep only 4 hours per night for six nights showed a change in pattern of GH release from a normal single pulse to a biphasic pattern [20]. In this study, a higher overall amount of GH was found in the sleep-deprived condition, which could contribute to higher glucose levels. The hypothalamic-pituitary-adrenal axis is also affected with sleep deprivation. Evening cortisol levels were significantly higher in young, healthy men who were allowed to sleep only 4 hours per night for six nights [11], as well as in young, healthy women who were allowed to sleep only 3 hours for one night [21]. A cross-sectional analysis that included 2,751 men and women also demonstrated that short sleep duration and sleep disturbances are independently associated with more cortisol secretion in the evening [22]. Elevated evening cortisol levels can lead to insulin resistance, weight gain, and the development of T2D [23].

13.2.2 INFLAMMATION

Levels of inflammatory cytokines, inflammation, or both increase as sleep duration decreases, which in turn, can also increase insulin resistance [24]. A number of cytokines have previously been found to be associated with sleep, including IL-1, tumor necrosis factor-α (TNF-α), and IL-6 [25]. In one study, following a night of total sleep deprivation, levels of the pro-inflammatory cytokine IL-6 in healthy adults were increased during the day and decreased during the following night. These changes were associated with greater somnolence and fatigue during the day and deeper sleep the night after deprivation [26]. When healthy adult men were subjected to partial or total sleep deprivation for 4 days, the latter (but not the former) was associated with significant increases in plasma concentrations of IL-6 and a receptor for the pro-inflammatory cytokine TNF-α, TNF-α R1 [27]. C-reactive protein has also recently been found to be elevated in individuals at risk for cardiovascular disease and T2D [28–30]. Increasing evidence suggests that CRP is an important marker of cardiovascular risk in both apparently healthy populations and those with established vascular disease, to the extent that clinical guidelines for risk associated with CRP levels have been established [30]. In an experimental study conducted by Kritikou et al. [31], 77 subjects with OSA and 39 controls were studied in the sleep laboratory for four nights. Measures of sleepiness (objective and subjective), performance, serial 24-hour blood samples for IL-6, tumor necrosis factor receptor (TNFR)-1, leptin and adiponectin, and single samples for high-sensitivity C-reactive protein (hsCRP), fasting glucose, and insulin levels were obtained. The study proved that apneic males were significantly sleepier and had significantly higher hsCRP, IL-6, leptin, and insulin resistance than controls. Also, OSA was associated with inflammation and insulin resistance, even in nonobese males leading to conclusion that sleep deprivation or disturbance-induced inflammatory state could be contributing to development of insulin resistance, T2D, and cardiovascular diseases.

13.2.3 SYMPATHETIC NERVOUS SYSTEM ACTIVITY

Patients who have been sleep-deprived have been shown to have higher sympathetic nervous system activity, lower parasympathetic activity, or both [32]. The sympathetic nervous system inhibits insulin release, while the parasympathetic system stimulates insulin release. Changes of sleep deprivation on both have the potential to increase glucose levels. Overactivity of the sympathetic nervous system can also result in insulin resistance. Reduced skeletal muscle blood flow resulting from neural vasoconstriction leading to reduced glucose uptake may possibly be the primary cause of the insulin resistance. Sympathetic nervous activation can also directly contribute to the lipid changes that are part of the metabolic syndrome. Metabolism of chylomicrons in the periphery and of chylomicron remnants by the liver is slowed by adrenergic vasoconstriction, which reduces regional blood flows and chylomicron clearance [33].

13.2.4 HYPERACTIVITY OF OREXIN SYSTEM

A primary mechanism linking sleep deprivation and weight gain is likely hyperactivity of the orexin system. Orexigenic neurons play a central role in wakefulness, and they also promote feeding [34]. Animal models demonstrate an overactive orexin system during sleep deprivation, possibly mediated by the increase in sympathetic activity [35]. Increased sympathetic activity also affects the levels of peripheral appetite hormones inhibiting leptin release [36] and stimulating ghrelin release [37]. Lower leptin levels and increased ghrelin levels act in concert to further activate orexin neurons (NPY Neuropeptide Y; AGRP agouti-related protein; MCH melanin concentrating hormone), resulting in increased food intake [38,39].

13.2.5 REDUCED ENERGY EXPENDITURE

Sleep loss, with its associated sleepiness and fatigue, may result in reduced energy expenditure, partly due to less exercise, but also due to less non-exercise activity thermogenesis [40]. In one study, resting metabolic rate diminished by 5% and thermic effect of digestion decreased by 20% after one night of sleep deprivation [41]. In many people with overweight/obesity, this cascade of negative events is likely to be accelerated by sleep-disordered breathing, a reported independent risk factor for insulin resistance [42,43].

13.2.6 REDUCTION IN MELATONIN PRODUCTION

Melatonin plays a major role in the regulation of the circadian temporal internal order. The anti-obesogenic and the weight-reducing effects of melatonin depend on several mechanisms and actions. Experimental evidence demonstrates that melatonin is necessary for the proper synthesis, secretion, and action of insulin, though high melatonin may impair insulin release [44]. Cell culture studies and animal models demonstrate a reduction in glucotoxicity-induced β-cell apoptosis with the administration of melatonin, and improvement of pancreatic endocrine remodeling in the presence of melatonin, suggesting melatonin may preserve β-cell function [45]. Melatonin also acts by regulating GLUT4 expression and/or triggering [46]. Activation of melatonin receptors enhance phosphorylation of the insulin receptor and its intracellular substrates mobilizing the insulin-signaling pathway through a G-coupled signal mechanism [44].

In general, melatonin acts as a powerful chronobiotic, responsible, in part, for the daily distribution of metabolic processes so that the activity/feeding phase of the day is associated with high insulin sensitivity, and the rest/fasting is synchronized to the insulin-resistant metabolic phase of the day. Furthermore, melatonin is responsible for the establishment of an adequate energy balance mainly by regulating energy flow to and from the stores and directly regulating the energy expenditure through the activation of brown adipose tissue and participating in the browning process of white adipose tissue. The reduction in melatonin production, as during aging, shift work, or illuminated environments during the night, induces insulin resistance, glucose intolerance, sleep disturbance, and metabolic circadian disorganization, characterizing a state of chronodisruption leading to obesity and increased risk of T2D [46].

Mounting evidence as a result of various studies suggests that insufficient sleep is also linked to obesity, hypertension, and cardiovascular disease, as well as mood disturbances [47–50]. As a result, in 2015, a Joint Consensus Statement of the American Academy of Sleep Medicine and Sleep Research Society recommended that adults should sleep seven or more hours per night on a regular basis to promote optimal health [51].

13.3   SLEEP ARCHITECTURE AND INSULIN RESISTANCE IN ADOLESCENTS

Over the past decades, sleep duration has been declining in the United States, with one-third of adults reporting insufficient sleep. Increasing social and work obligations, along with the availability of electronic media, likely contribute to sleep curtailment in modern society. Studies conducted in the U.S. have shown that high school–aged students and adolescents do not get enough sleep, and the average total sleep duration for adolescents has decreased to less than 8 hours [52].

Three types of circadian typology have been described in human beings: morning (larks), evening (owls), and intermediate. Each type shows individual preferences for activity realization during a specified period of the day [53]. The evening-type individuals showed worse quality of sleep when compared with the morning and intermediate types [54]. In a cross-sectional study conducted by Rawat et al. [55], 203 adolescent subjects were enrolled and divided into three groups: definite evening chronotype, intermediate chronotype, and definite morning chronotype. Sleep quality was measured by the Pittsburgh Sleep Quality Index (PSQI), and daytime sleepiness and chronotype were measured by the Epworth Sleepiness Score and Morningness-Eveningness Questionnaire Self-Assessment version, respectively. Results show that definite evening chronotypes had higher mean value of body mass index (BMI) (23.06 vs 22.50/21.89, p 0.029), higher 2-hour blood glucose levels following oral glucose tolerance testing (131.84 vs 124.61/126.6; $p < 0.001$), and increased insulin resistance (determined by using the homeostasis model of assessment for insulin resistance [HOMA-IR] 2.97 vs 2.76/2.19; p 0.038) compared with the other two chronotypes. Subjects of evening chronotype had significant positive correlation of 2-hour blood glucose levels and HOMA-IR values with poor sleep quality when compared with subjects of intermediate and morning chronotypes. This study highlighted that evening chronotype adolescents have unhealthy sleep habits and are at higher risk of future development of insulin resistance.

A disrupted circadian rhythm changes sleep–wake habits that lead to poor sleep quality. Poor sleep quality may be due to substance abuse, such as alcohol, and incongruity between intrinsic sleep–wake cycle and actual bedtime due of social factors [56]. Disrupted sleep–wake cycle and poor sleep quality can lead to alteration in glucose metabolism and the metabolic syndrome [57–59]. This stresses the importance of promoting awareness, as part of screening and counseling, regarding the importance of circadian typology, sleep hygiene, and the negative cost of challenging the internal clock [55].

13.4   SLEEP ARCHITECTURE AND INSULIN RESISTANCE IN NIGHT SHIFT WORKERS

Shift work is defined as a work schedule involving irregular or unusual hours, compared with those of a normal daytime work schedule. In the era of globalization, demands on individuals are continually increased. Shift working is a human resource management strategy aimed to maximize work productivity and to complete the customer's needs [60]. Epidemiological studies have shown that shift workers are at higher risk for development of obesity, insulin resistance, and associated metabolic conditions including T2D [61–63]. In a cross-sectional study comparing 137 healthcare shift workers (HCSW) with 135 healthcare non-shift workers (HCNSW), mean HOMA-IR index levels in HCSW were above the cut-off (normal range: 2.5) and significantly higher (2.8 vs 1.5; $p < 0.001$) compared with HCNSW [64].

Aberrantly timed eating behavior, known as eating out of circadian rhythm synchrony, also leads to increased cardiometabolic risk [65]. Intrinsic or endogenous clocks function as internal circadian timing systems, which control sleep/wake and feeding/fasting cycles, as well as many metabolic processes, including the timing of eating behaviors, and processes involved in glucose homeostasis. Rodent studies have shown that eating out of phase with the endogenous clock results in desynchronization between rhythms of the central and peripheral clock systems [66,67] and between rhythms of different tissue clocks (e.g., liver and muscle clocks) [68,69]. In western 24/7 society, a large portion of the population that includes shift workers and others with varying daily schedules are at risk for similar metabolic derangement as eating moments are distributed predominantly over late evening [70]. Specifically, clock gene mutations, exposure to artificial light–dark cycles, disturbed sleep, shift work, and social jet lag are factors that may contribute to circadian disruption and insulin resistance [71].

13.5   POSSIBLE MECHANISM OF INSULIN RESISTANCE IN SHIFT WORKERS

13.5.1   Clock Control of Insulin Sensitivity

Glucose homeostasis is maintained through a series of clock-controlled uptake and release processes among different organs, including the pancreas, liver, skeletal muscle, and adipose tissue. The suprachiasmatic nucleus (SCN) is responsible for the 24-hour rhythm in plasma glucose concentrations peaking at the start of the active period, independent of feeding conditions [72,73]. Furthermore, glucose transporters and glucagon receptors fluctuate with the circadian cycle, and synthesis of glucose via gluconeogenesis is highly rhythmically controlled [74]. The SCN also regulates the daily variation in glucose tolerance, which is highest at the beginning of the activity period, followed by a gradual reduction toward the end of the activity period [75]. The higher morning glucose tolerance is partly the result of increased β-cell responsiveness, accompanied by a tendency to improved insulin action and lower hepatic insulin extraction as compared to later in the day [75]. Skeletal muscle has a day-night rhythm in mitochondrial respiratory capacity [76], thereby contributing to the daily rhythm of carbohydrate and lipid oxidation. Besides the crucial role of the central brain clock in regulating glucose homeostasis, the timing of food intake is also an important determinant for glucose regulation, as feeding at "inappropriate" times of the day can cause hyperglycemia and evoke insulin release at a phase opposite to the phase of other physiological rhythms dictated by the SCN master clock, contributing to a net metabolic imbalance [72].

13.5.2 Problems in Glucose Homeostasis Arising from Misalignment/Shift Work

Temporary circadian misalignment introduced in a controlled laboratory setting, similar to what occurs during jet lag or chronically during shift work, results in decreased glucose tolerance and insulin sensitivity, lower leptin levels, higher mean arterial pressure, lower sleep efficiency, and a complete reversion of the cortisol profile. The abnormally high cortisol levels at the beginning of the sleep period have been proposed to contribute to the development of insulin resistance and hyperglycemia [77,78]. Circadian misalignment affected postprandial glucose more than fasting glucose levels, suggesting that misalignment affects fat/muscle metabolism or β-cell function more than hepatic gluconeogenesis [77]. During a short-term misalignment study, Wefers et al. [79] found that endogenous glucose production, measured with a two-step hyperinsulinemic-euglycemic clamp, was not affected. In contrast, circadian misalignment resulted in decreased muscle insulin sensitivity, indicating that the process of glucose uptake, rather than glucose production, is disturbed during misalignment [79].

In healthy rotational shift workers, higher postprandial glucose peaks, accompanied by a lower first-phase insulin response, were observed during a simulated night shift than during a simulated day shift [80]. This suggests increased insulin resistance occurs with the night shift and may contribute to the development of T2D. Shift-work conditions commonly cause people to consume meals at a time of day when the β-cell responses are reduced within the normal daily variation [81]. Notably, factors such as gastrointestinal absorption, hepatic glucose production suppression, and non–insulin-dependent glucose metabolic pathways also contribute to the circadian misalignment effects on glucose tolerance [82].

13.5.3 Desynchronization between Organs

In a study by Wehrens et al. [83], shifting mealtimes resulted in a phase change for plasma glucose (peripheral) rhythms, including a phase delay for the clock gene *PER2* in white adipose tissue. However, there were no rhythm changes for melatonin and cortisol (output parameters of the SCN), indicating misalignment between the SCN and peripheral rhythms [83]. By applying a constant routine protocol in which participants are kept in constant conditions without photic or timing cues after either 3 days of simulated night shifts or day shifts, Skene et al. [84] showed that traditional markers of SCN phase generation (melatonin, cortisol, and core clock gene *PER3* expression) remained relatively stable. This contrasts with 95% of the studied plasma metabolites (e.g., glutathione, proline, sarcosine, leucine, and isoleucine), which dissociated from the SCN rhythm and aligned with the shifted behavioral cycles of feeding/fasting and sleep/wake [84]. These changes in metabolite rhythms indicated peripheral (e.g., liver, pancreas, and digestive tract) clock dysfunction. This disruption in the circadian organization might represent a pathway through which shift work is associated with metabolic disease [84]. The observation that these altered rhythms persisted under constant routine conditions in the absence of any externally imposed rhythm suggests an after effect of nightshift work on metabolism, corroborating well-known long-term negative effects of shift work. To summarize, timing most of the calorie consumption to coincide with the time that the endocrine system is most responsive, during the daytime, seems most beneficial for cardiometabolic health.

13.6   RELATIONSHIP OF NOCTURNAL LIGHT EXPOSURE AND INSULIN RESISTANCE

The electric light ranks among the most influential of human inventions. The widespread use of electric lighting within a modern 24/7 lifestyle is accompanied by self-imposed changes to patterns of light-dark exposure, which may include limited daytime exposure to natural sunlight and increased nocturnal artificial light exposure [85]. These behavioral changes affect cardiometabolic health [86,87]. There are at least two potential mechanisms by which alterations in light-dark exposure may impact hunger and metabolism: one is via the circadian system and the other is via physiological arousal.

The strongest exogenous modulator of the central circadian clock is the pattern of light-dark exposure, with the circadian system most sensitive to blue wavelength light [88–90]. Not only does light-dark exposure change throughout the day, but the wavelengths of light also vary throughout the day with a relatively higher contribution of blue light during evenings [91]. Light exposure also impacts the level of physiological arousal leading to high cortisol levels, which reduces insulin sensitivity [92].

Recent studies in humans have examined the impact of light exposure on body weight and metabolism. Studies manipulating morning light exposure are typically associated with leaner body weight, lower body fat, and altered appetite outcomes. In a crossover, placebo-controlled, randomized clinical trial by Danilenko et al. [93], 34 women between 20 and 54 years of age who were overweight were given a 3-week in-home session of morning bright light treatment using a device of light-emitting diodes, and a 3-week placebo session by means of a deactivated ion generator, separated by an off-protocol period. With bright light treatment, fat mass and the percentage of fat, as well as appetite were significantly lower (average fat reduction 0.35 kg) than placebo [93]. In another randomized controlled study by Dunai et al. [94], 25 subjects with overweight/obesity were assigned to 6 weeks of moderate exercise with or without bright light treatment. In this study, the addition of bright light significantly reduced body fat. On the other hand, in a study conducted by Reid et al. [95], there was a strong association observed between later timing of habitual light exposure over 500 lux (MLiT500) and higher BMI. In another study, 19 healthy adults were randomized to 3 hours of blue-enriched light exposure for 1 day starting either 0.5 hours (morning group) or 10.5 hours (evening group) after waking [92]. In both the morning and evening groups, insulin total area and HOMA-IR were increased, and subjective sleepiness was reduced with blue-enriched light compared with dim light. The evening group, but not the morning group, had significantly higher glucose peak values during blue-enriched light exposure compared with dim light.

Taken together, these studies offer some causative relationships between types and timing of light exposure, independent of sleep timing/duration, with abnormal adiposity and insulin resistance, and by extension, cardiometabolic risk. Thus, environmental light exposure is a potentially modifiable cardiometabolic risk factor.

13.7 SCREEN TIME AND METABOLIC HEALTH

Sedentary behavior, and specifically screen-based sedentary behavior, has been a focus for health researchers, engineers, telecommunications companies, gamers, and the media for many years. In recent years, research in this area has proliferated at an exponential rate. On one side, arguments have been made that screen time is harmful to the healthy growth and development of children and youth. On the other side, modern technology has far surpassed any prediction of success and become a fixture of daily living, making life easier and providing opportunities never thought possible. Regardless, screens have become omnipresent in our society, and it is important to understand the risks and the benefits associated with their use. Excessive time spent in various sedentary behaviors can coexist in a lifestyle that includes sufficient levels of moderate- to vigorous-intensity physical activity, but research has shown that for optimal health benefits, individuals should be both physically active and limit their sedentary behaviors, especially screen time [96]. Various studies have shown that adults who spend an excessive amount of time in front of a television are at greater risk for insulin resistance, T2D, and cardiovascular risk [97,98]. However, in the era of tablets, smartphones, and laptops, the question arises if the same relationships are observed in children and adolescents?

To address this, Nightingale et al. [99] conducted The Child Heart and Health Study in England, a cross-sectional survey of heart health among 4495 children aged 9–10 years who attended 200 primary schools. Cardiometabolic risk factors, anthropometric measurements, and reported daily screen times were assessed. Compared with children who reported ≤1 hour of screen time daily, those who reported more than 3 hours had a 1.95 higher ponderal index (weight/height^3), 4.5% higher skinfold thickness, 3.3% higher fat mass index, 9.2% higher leptin level, and 10.5% higher insulin resistance [99]. Associations with insulin resistance remained after adjustment for adiposity, socioeconomic markers, and physical activity [99]. Similarly, the 2005 Korean National Health and Nutrition Examination Surveys (KNHANES) included cross-sectional data of 845 children and adolescents (10–18 years of age) that demonstrated an odds ratio for development of metabolic syndrome of 2.23 (95% CI, 1.02–4.86) in subjects with ≥35 hours screen time/week, compared to those with ≤16 hours screen time/week [100]. Strong graded associations between screen time, adiposity, and insulin resistance suggested that reducing screen time may facilitate early T2D prevention.

In addition to adverse effects of screen time on physical health, psychosocial health indicators can be affected by high levels of screen time. For instance, a recent systematic review reported a strong association between high duration of screen time and indicators of mental health, including hyperactivity/inattention problems, internalizing problems, lower psychological well-being, and perceived quality of life [101]. Similarly, a systematic review that focused on adolescent girls found that higher levels of screen time were associated with depression and poor social support [102].

The adverse effects of screen are not just limited to physical inactivity. For example, messages emanating from screens, such as advertisements for unhealthy foods, are important factors to take into consideration [103]. This can be coupled with more mindless eating in front of the screen device (distracting activity) and therefore overconsumption of food. Screen exposure is also associated with increased sleep disturbances [104]. For example, the blue light of screens has been shown to suppress melatonin secretion, which may delay sleep onset [105]. Many individuals are using screen devices within the hour before trying to fall asleep or using cell phones in bed, which interferes with the ability to fall asleep at nighttime. The adverse effects of screen time on cardiometabolic risk are manifold and both independent and dependent on sleep hygiene [106].

13.8   OBSTRUCTIVE SLEEP APNEA AND T2D

The most robust evidence relating sleep duration and quality on T2D risk derives from metabolic studies in patients with OSA. As an increasingly prevalent disorder, OSA is characterized by recurrent episodes of partial or complete upper airway obstruction with intermittent hypoxia and microarousals, resulting in low amounts of slow-wave sleep and overall decreased sleep quality [107]. OSA is common in patients with T2D, and clinical and epidemiological studies suggest that when left untreated, T2D risk or control can worsen [42,43,108].

The Sleep AHEAD (Action for Health in Diabetes) study revealed that more than 84% of patients with T2D and obesity had OSA (with an apnea-hypopnea index ≥5) [109]. In a study conducted in 60 patients with T2D, Aronsohn et al. [110], found that 46 (77%) had OSA. Additionally, greater severity of OSA was associated with worsened glycemic control. After controlling for age, sex, race, BMI, number of T2D medications, level of exercise, years since diagnosis of T2D, and total sleep time, the adjusted mean A1C was increased by 1.49% in patients with mild OSA ($p = .0028$),

1.93% in patients with moderate OSA ($p = .0033$), and 3.69% in patients with severe OSA ($p < .0001$), compared to patients without OSA.

A more recent prospective study of 544 patients without diabetes showed that the risk of developing T2D over an average of 2.7 years of follow-up was associated with severity of OSA: for each increased quartile of severity there was a 43% increase in the incidence of T2D [111]. Additionally, in patients with moderate-to-severe OSA, regular use of continuous positive airway pressure (CPAP) was associated with an attenuated risk [111]. Similarly, the Veterans Affairs' Metabolism Obstructed and Non-Obstructed Sleep (VAMANOS) trial included 928 patients with OSA but without diabetes. Over a 5-month period, incidence of T2D was inversely associated with adherence to CPAP usage [112]. Despite these findings, a meta-analysis of six randomized trials that included patients with both T2D and OSA, showed no benefit in A1C at 12 and 24 weeks among those treated with CPAP (Mean difference= −0.10; Confidence interval −0.25 to 0.04). Subgroup analysis by adherence to CPAP (>4 hours or < 4 hours) confirmed these results [113]. These studies indicate that treatment of OSA can significantly impact glucose metabolism among patients who have not yet developed T2D.

There are several mechanisms of how OSA leads to T2D. High levels of sympathetic nervous system activity, intermittent hypoxia, sleep fragmentation, and sleep loss in OSA may all lead to dysregulation of the hypothalamic-pituitary axis, endothelial dysfunction, and alterations in cytokine and adipokine release, each affecting glucose metabolism in this population. These metabolic abnormalities can be partially corrected by CPAP treatment, though this may be more pronounced in patients with prediabetes.

13.9   WHAT SHOULD CLINICIANS TELL PATIENTS?

In aggregate, the current evidence suggests that strategies to improve the duration and the quality of sleep should be considered as a potential intervention to prevent or delay the development of T2D and cardiometabolic risk (Table 13.1). While further studies are needed to better elucidate the mechanisms of the relationship between sleep loss and T2D risk and to affirm whether extending sleep and treating OSA decreases the risk of T2D, clinicians should recommend at least 7 hours of uninterrupted sleep per night as a goal in maintaining a healthy lifestyle for their patients. In addition, patients should also be advised to have dim light during nighttime, bright light during daytime, and avoiding screen use for at least 1 hour before bedtime. Lastly, clinicians should systematically evaluate the risk of OSA in patients who have T2D, especially with other cardiometabolic risk factors, and conversely, should assess for T2D in patients with known OSA.

Disclosures:
Jeffrey I. Mechanick received honoraria from Abbott Nutrition for lectures and serves on the Advisory Boards for Aveta.Life and Twin Health.

TABLE 13.1

Table Summarizing Studies Showing Evidence of Relationship between Sleep Disturbance and Risk of Development of T2D

Study	Type of Study	Sleep Hygiene Factor	Associated Cardiometabolic Effect	Recommendations	Comments
Kuhn et al. [10]	Experimental	Twenty-eight subjects kept awake for 72–126 hours by psychic and physical stimulation.	Glucose tolerance curve changed after 3–4 days to a prediabetic curve.		Such extreme sleep deprivation uncommon in real life.
Spiegel et al. [11]	Experimental	Eleven subjects with sleep restriction to 4 hours per night for six nights. Data compared with sleep recovery period (12 hours per night for six nights)	Glucose tolerance lower in sleep-debt condition than in fully rested condition ($p < 0.02$).	Sleep debt has a harmful impact on carbohydrate metabolism and endocrine function	
The Sleep Heart Study [9]	Cross-sectional study	The relation of sleep time to DM and IGT was examined in 1,400 men and women.	Compared with those sleeping 7–8 hours per night, subjects sleeping 5 hours or less and 6 hours per night had adjusted odds ratios for T2D of 2.51 (95% CI 1.57–4.02) and 1.66 (95% CI 1.15–2.39), respectively.	Voluntary sleep restriction may contribute to the large public health burden of T2D.	Sleep duration was self-reported, the reasons for sleep curtailment were unknown, and possible confounding variables were not measured.
Nedeltcheva et al. [12]	Randomized crossover study	Eleven participants: two 14-day periods of controlled exposure to sedentary living with 5.5- or 8.5-hour bedtimes.	Recurrent sleep restriction resulted in reduced oral glucose tolerance (2-hour glucose value, 144 ± 25 vs. 132 ± 36 mg/dL; $p < 0.01$) and insulin sensitivity [3.3 ± 1.1 vs. 4.0 ± 1.6; $p < 0.03$].	Bedtime restriction may facilitate the development of insulin resistance and reduced glucose tolerance.	Such recurrent bedtime restriction is closer to real-life experiences.
Knutson et al. [13]	Cross-sectional study	One hundred sixty-one participants were assessed for A1C levels and sleep quality using PSQI.	The predicted increase in A1C level for a perceived sleep debt of 3 hours per night was 1.1% above median.	Optimizing sleep duration and quality should be tested as an intervention to improve glucose control in patients with T2D.	The direction of causality cannot be confirmed.

(Continued)

TABLE 13.1 (Continued)
Table Summarizing Studies Showing Evidence of Relationship between Sleep Disturbance and Risk of Development of T2D

Study	Type of Study	Sleep Hygiene Factor	Associated Cardiometabolic Effect	Recommendations	Comments
The Nurses' Health Study [14]	Prospective (Cohort) study	Seventy thousand twenty-six women without diabetes were followed for 10 years for diagnosis of T2D.	Long and short sleep durations were associated with an increased risk of T2D diagnosis. The relative risks for short (slept ≤5 hours per day) and long (slept ≥9 hours per day) sleepers were 1.57 (95% CI 1.28–1.92) and 1.47 (1.19–1.80), respectively.	Sleep restriction may be an independent risk factor for developing symptomatic T2D.	
The first National Health and Nutrition Examination Survey (NHANES I) [15]	Prospective (Cohort) study	Nine thousand men and women were followed over a period of 8 to 10 years.	Subjects with sleep durations of five or fewer hours (odds ratio = 1.47, 95% CI 1.03–2.09) and subjects with sleep durations of nine or more hours (odds ratio = 1.52, 95% CI 1.06–2.18) were significantly more likely to have T2D.	Short sleep duration could be a significant risk factor for T2D.	The association between long sleep duration and T2D incidence is more likely due to some unmeasured confounder such as poor sleep quality.
Kawakami et al. [16]	Prospective (Cohort) study	Two thousand six hundred forty-nine Japanese male employees with no medical history of T2D or other chronic illnesses at baseline followed for 8 years.	Thirty-eight cases of T2D. Those who experienced a high frequency of difficulty initiating sleep had a significantly higher age-adjusted hazard ratio (2.98, 95% CI 1.36–6.53) for T2D compared with those who experienced low-frequency difficulty initiating sleep.	Those who had sleep disturbances showed a two- to threefold higher risk of later onset T2D. The association was independent of known risk factors.	

(Continued)

TABLE 13.1 (*Continued*)
Table Summarizing Studies Showing Evidence of Relationship between Sleep Disturbance and Risk of Development of T2D

Study	Type of Study	Sleep Hygiene Factor	Associated Cardiometabolic Effect	Recommendations	Comments
Nilsson et al. [17]	Prospective (Cohort) study	Six thousand five hundred ninety-nine Swedish men without diabetes followed for an average of 15 years	Two hundred eighty-one (4.3%) of the men developed T2D. Results showed difficulties in falling asleep or regular use of hypnotics (odds ratio [OR] 1.52 [95% CI 1.05–2.20]) and resting heart rate (OR per 10 bpm 1.13 [0.99–1.30]) to be associated with development of T2D.	Sleep disturbances and elevated resting heart rate, in middle-aged men, are associated with an increased risk of T2D.	Higher resting heart rate could be interpreted as reflecting greater sympathetic nervous system activity, a mediator of the metabolic dysfunction associated with both short sleep duration and OSA. Sleep duration was self-reported in these studies and was not measured.
Cappuccio et al. [18]	Meta-analysis	Ten prospective studies, with 107,756 participants followed for a median of 9.5 years.	Relative risk for incidence of T2D was 28% higher with short sleep duration (defined as either ≤5 or <6 hours, 48% higher with long sleep duration (>8 hours), 57% higher with difficulty going to sleep, and 84% higher with difficulty staying asleep.		
Rawat et al. [55]	Cross-sectional study	Two hundred three adolescents. Sleep quality was measured by PSQI. Daytime sleepiness and chronotype were measured by Epworth Sleepiness Score and Morningness-Eveningness Questionnaire Self-Assessment version, respectively.	Evening chronotypes had higher mean value of BMI (23.06 kg/m² vs 22.50/21.89 kg/m², *p* 0.029), 2 hours blood glucose level following OGTT (131.84 vs 124.61/126.6; *p* < 0.001) and insulin resistance [(HOMA-IR) 2.97 vs 2.76/2.19; *p* 0.038] compared with morning and intermediate chronotypes.	Subjects with evening chronotype are more prone for development of MetS compared with subjects of intermediate and morning chronotypes if proper health policies are not adopted for adolescents.	

(Continued)

TABLE 13.1 (*Continued*)
Table Summarizing Studies Showing Evidence of Relationship between Sleep Disturbance and Risk of Development of T2D

Study	Type of Study	Sleep Hygiene Factor	Associated Cardiometabolic Effect	Recommendations	Comments
Ledda et al. [64]	Cross-sectional Study	One hundred thirty-seven HCSW and 135 HCNSW were enrolled, and fasting glucose, insulin, and HOMA-IR Index were evaluated.	Mean HOMA-IR Index levels in HCSW were above the cut-off (normal range: 2.5) and significantly higher (2.8 vs 1.5; p < 0.001) compared with HCNSW.	Shift work could be a risk factor in developing insulin resistance and MetS.	
Danilenko et al. [93]	Crossover, placebo-controlled randomized clinical trial	Thirty-four participants; 3-week in-home session of morning bright light treatment using a device of light-emitting diodes and a 3-week placebo session by means of a deactivated ion generator, separated by an off-protocol period.	With light, percentage fat, fat mass, and appetite were significantly lower (average fat reduction 0.35 kg) as compared to placebo.	Morning bright light treatment reduces body fat and appetite in overweight women and may be included in weight control programs.	
Dunai et al. [94]	Randomized controlled study	Twenty-five overweight and obese subjects were assigned to 6 weeks of moderate exercise with or without bright light treatment.	The addition of bright light significantly reduced body fat composition (p = 0.034)		The reduction in body fat mass was of particular importance, because visceral fat has been particularly implicated as a major factor in development of MetS.

(*Continued*)

TABLE 13.1 (*Continued*)
Table Summarizing Studies Showing Evidence of Relationship between Sleep Disturbance and Risk of Development of T2D

Study	Type of Study	Sleep Hygiene Factor	Associated Cardiometabolic Effect	Recommendations	Comments
Reid et al. [95]	Cross-sectional	Fifty-four participants. Light levels, sleep midpoint and duration were measured with wrist actigraphy (Actiwatch-L) for 7 days and compared with BMI.	MLiT500 was positively correlated with BMI ($r=0.51$, $p,0.001$), and midpoint of sleep ($r=0.47$, $p,0.01$)	Exposure to moderate levels of light at biologically appropriate times can influence weight, independent of sleep timing and duration.	
Cheung et al. [92]	Randomized controlled trial	Nineteen adults were randomized to 3 hours of blue-enriched light exposure on Day 3 starting either 0.5 hours after wake (morning group) or 10.5 hours after wake (evening group).	In both groups, insulin total area and HOMA-IR was increased, and subjective sleepiness was reduced with blue-enriched light compared to dim light.	The evening group had significantly higher glucose peak value during blue-enriched light exposure compared to dim light.	
The Child Heart and Health Study [99]	Cross-sectional survey	Four thousand four hundred ninety children aged 9–10 years; Fasting cardiometabolic risk markers, anthropometry measurements, and reported daily screen time were assessed.	Compared with children who had 1 hour or less of screen time daily, those who reported more than 3 hours had a 1.95 higher PI 4.5% higher skinfold thickness, 3.3% higher fat mass index, 9.2% higher leptin level, and 10.5% higher insulin resistance.	Strong graded associations between screen time, adiposity, and insulin resistance suggested that reducing screen time may facilitate early T2D prevention.	

(Continued)

TABLE 13.1 (Continued)
Table Summarizing Studies Showing Evidence of Relationship between Sleep Disturbance and Risk of Development of T2D

Study	Type of Study	Sleep Hygiene Factor	Associated Cardiometabolic Effect	Recommendations	Comments
Korean National Health and Nutrition Examination Surveys (KNHANES) [100]	Cross-sectional Survey	Screen time and incidence of MetS was assessed in 845 children and adolescents (10–18 years of age).	In comparison with the children and adolescents in the ST-Q1 ($\leq$16 hours for a week), the odds ratio for MetS of subjects in the ST-Q4 ($\geq$35 hours for a week) was 2.23 (95% CI, 1.02–4.86).	Physicians should be particularly cognizant of the likelihood of OSA in obese patients with T2D, especially among individuals with higher waist circumference and BMI.	
Sleep AHEAD study [109]	Cross-sectional study	Unattended polysomnography was performed in 306 participants.	84% of patients with T2D and obesity had OSA (with an AHI$\geq$5).		
Aronsohn et al. [110]	Cross-sectional study	Polysomnography studies and A1C in 60 patients with T2D.	A total of 77% of patients with T2D had OSA (AHI $\geq$5). Increasing OSA severity was associated with poorer glucose control	In patients with T2D, increasing severity of OSA is associated with poorer glucose control	

Abbreviations: AHI, apnea-hypopnea index; CI, confidence interval; HCNSW, health care non-shift workers; HCSW, health care shift workers; HOMA-IR, homeostasis model of assessment for insulin resistance; IGT, impaired glucose tolerance; MetS, metabolic syndrome; MLiT500, the mean light timing above 500 lux; OGTT, oral glucose tolerance test; PI, ponderal index (weight/height^3); PSQI, Pittsburgh sleep quality index; ST, screen time.

REFERENCES

1. Saeedi, P., et al., Global and regional diabetes prevalence estimates for 2019 and projections for 2030 and 2045: Results from the International Diabetes Federation Diabetes Atlas. *Diabetes Research and Clinical Practice*, 2019. **157**: p. 107843.
2. Touma, C. and S. Pannain, Does lack of sleep cause diabetes. *Cleveland Clinic Journal of Medicine*, 2011. **78**(8): pp. 549–558.
3. Centers for Disease Control and Prevention, Perceived insufficient rest or sleep among adults-United States, 2008. *MMWR. Morbidity and Mortality Weekly Report*, 2009. **58**(42): pp. 1175–1179.
4. Keith, S.W., et al., Putative contributors to the secular increase in obesity: exploring the roads less traveled. *International Journal of Obesity*, 2006. **30**(11): pp. 1585–1594.
5. Zoccoli, G., et al., The cerebral circulation during sleep: regulation mechanisms and functional implications. *Sleep Medicine Reviews*, 2002. **6**(6): pp. 443–455.
6. Pannain, S. and E. Van Cauter, Modulation of endocrine function by sleep-wake homeostasis and circadian rhythmicity. *Sleep Medicine Clinics*, 2007. **2**(2): pp. 147–159.
7. Somers, V.K., et al., Sympathetic-nerve activity during sleep in normal subjects. *New England Journal of Medicine*, 1993. **328**(5): pp. 303–307.
8. Zizi, F., et al., Sleep duration and the risk of diabetes mellitus: epidemiologic evidence and pathophysiologic insights. *Current Diabetes Reports*, 2010. **10**(1): pp. 43–47.
9. Gottlieb, D.J., et al., Association of sleep time with diabetes mellitus and impaired glucose tolerance. *Archives of Internal Medicine*, 2005. **165**(8): pp. 863–867.
10. Kuhn, E., et al., Metabolic reflection of sleep deprivation. *Activitas Nervosa Superior*, 1969. **11**: pp. 165–174.
11. Spiegel, K., R. Leproult, and E. Van Cauter, Impact of sleep debt on metabolic and endocrine function. *The Lancet*, 1999. **354**(9188): pp. 1435–1439.
12. Nedeltcheva, A.V., et al., Exposure to recurrent sleep restriction in the setting of high caloric intake and physical inactivity results in increased insulin resistance and reduced glucose tolerance. *The Journal of Clinical Endocrinology & Metabolism*, 2009. **94**(9): pp. 3242–3250.
13. Knutson, K.L., et al., Role of sleep duration and quality in the risk and severity of type 2 diabetes mellitus. *Archives of Internal Medicine*, 2006. **166**(16): pp. 1768–1774.
14. Ayas, N.T., et al., A prospective study of self-reported sleep duration and incident diabetes in women. *Diabetes Care*, 2003. **26**(2): pp. 380–384.
15. Gangwisch, J.E., et al., Sleep duration as a risk factor for diabetes incidence in a large US sample. *Sleep*, 2007. **30**(12): pp. 1667–1673.
16. Kawakami, N., N. Takatsuka, and H. Shimizu, Sleep disturbance and onset of type 2 diabetes. *Diabetes Care*, 2004. **27**(1): pp. 282–283.
17. Nilsson, P.M., et al., Incidence of diabetes in middle-aged men is related to sleep disturbances. *Diabetes Care*, 2004. **27**(10): pp. 2464–2469.
18. Cappuccio, F. and M.A. Miller, The epidemiology of sleep and cardiovascular risk and disease. *Sleep Epidemiology*, 2010: pp. 83–110.
19. Thomas, M., et al., Neural basis of alertness and cognitive performance impairments during sleepiness. I. Effects of 24 h of sleep deprivation on waking human regional brain activity. *Journal of Sleep Research*, 2000. **9**(4): pp. 335–352.
20. Spiegel, K., et al., Adaptation of the 24-h growth hormone profile to a state of sleep debt. *American Journal of Physiology-Regulatory, Integrative and Comparative Physiology*, 2000. **279**(3): pp. R874–R883.
21. Omisade, A., O.M. Buxton, and B. Rusak, Impact of acute sleep restriction on cortisol and leptin levels in young women. *Physiology & Behavior*, 2010. **99**(5): pp. 651–656.

22. Kumari, M., et al., Self-reported sleep duration and sleep disturbance are independently associated with cortisol secretion in the Whitehall II study. *The Journal of Clinical Endocrinology & Metabolism*, 2009. **94**(12): pp. 4801–4809.

23. Van Cauter, E., K.S. Polonsky, and A.J. Scheen, Roles of circadian rhythmicity and sleep in human glucose regulation. *Endocrine Reviews*, 1997. **18**(5): pp. 716–738.

24. Vgontzas, A.N., et al., Adverse effects of modest sleep restriction on sleepiness, performance, and inflammatory cytokines. *The Journal of Clinical Endocrinology & Metabolism*, 2004. **89**(5): pp. 2119–2126.

25. Simpson, N. and D.F. Dinges, sleep and inflammation. *Nutrition Reviews*, 2007. **65** (suppl_3): pp. S244–S252.

26. Vgontzas, A.N., et al., Circadian interleukin-6 secretion and quantity and depth of sleep. *The Journal of Clinical Endocrinology & Metabolism*, 1999. **84**(8): pp. 2603–2607.

27. Shearer, W.T., et al., Soluble TNF-α receptor 1 and IL-6 plasma levels in humans subjected to the sleep deprivation model of spaceflight. *Journal of Allergy and Clinical Immunology*, 2001. **107**(1): pp. 165–170.

28. Pradhan, A.D., et al., C-reactive protein is independently associated with fasting insulin in nondiabetic women. *Arteriosclerosis, Thrombosis, and Vascular Biology*, 2003. **23** (4): pp. 650–655.

29. Rifai, N. and P.M. Ridker, High-sensitivity C-reactive protein: a novel and promising marker of coronary heart disease. *Clinical Chemistry*, 2001. **47**(3): pp. 403–411.

30. Ridker, P.M., High-sensitivity C-reactive protein: potential adjunct for global risk assessment in the primary prevention of cardiovascular disease. *Circulation*, 2001. **103**(13): pp. 1813–1818.

31. Kritikou, I., et al., Sleep apnoea, sleepiness, inflammation and insulin resistance in middle-aged males and females. *European Respiratory Journal*, 2014. **43**(1): pp. 145–155.

32. Spiegel, K., et al., Leptin levels are dependent on sleep duration: relationships with sympathovagal balance, carbohydrate regulation, cortisol, and thyrotropin. *The Journal of Clinical Endocrinology & Metabolism*, 2004. **89**(11): pp. 5762–5771.

33. Esler, M., et al., Sympathetic nervous system and insulin resistance: from obesity to diabetes. *American Journal of Hypertension*, 2001. **14**(S7): pp. 304S–309S.

34. Sakurai, T., Roles of orexin/hypocretin in regulation of sleep/wakefulness and energy homeostasis. *Sleep Medicine Reviews*, 2005. **9**(4): pp. 231–241.

35. Wu, M.-F., et al., Hypocretin release in normal and narcoleptic dogs after food and sleep deprivation, eating, and movement. *American Journal of Physiology-Regulatory, Integrative and Comparative Physiology*, 2002. **283**(5): pp. R1079–R1086.

36. Rayner, D.V. and P. Trayhurn, Regulation of leptin production: sympathetic nervous system interactions. *Journal of Molecular Medicine*, 2001. **79**(1): pp. 8–20.

37. Van Der Lely, A.J., et al., Biological, physiological, pathophysiological, and pharmacological aspects of ghrelin. *Endocrine Reviews*, 2004. **25**(3): pp. 426–457.

38. Willie, J.T., et al., To eat or to sleep? Orexin in the regulation of feeding and wakefulness. *Annual Review of Neuroscience*, 2001. **24**(1): pp. 429–458.

39. Samson, W.K., M.M. Taylor, and A.V. Ferguson, Non-sleep effects of hypocretin/orexin. *Sleep Medicine Reviews*, 2005. **9**(4): pp. 243–252.

40. McHill, A. and K. Wright Jr, Role of sleep and circadian disruption on energy expenditure and in metabolic predisposition to human obesity and metabolic disease. *Obesity Reviews*, 2017. **18**: pp. 15–24.

41. Benedict, C., et al., Acute sleep deprivation reduces energy expenditure in healthy men. *The American Journal of Clinical Nutrition*, 2011. **93**(6): pp. 1229–1236.

42. Ip, M.S., et al., Obstructive sleep apnea is independently associated with insulin resistance. *American Journal of Respiratory and Critical Care Medicine*, 2002. **165**(5): pp. 670–676.

43. Punjabi, N.M., et al., Sleep-disordered breathing, glucose intolerance, and insulin resistance: the Sleep Heart Health Study. *American Journal of Epidemiology*, 2004. **160**(6): pp. 521–530.

44. Peschke, E., I. Bähr, and E. Mühlbauer, Melatonin and pancreatic islets: interrelationships between melatonin, insulin and glucagon. *International Journal of Molecular Sciences*, 2013. **14**(4): pp. 6981–7015.

45. Lee, Y.H., et al., Melatonin protects INS-1 pancreatic β-cells from apoptosis and senescence induced by glucotoxicity and glucolipotoxicity. *Islets*, 2020. **12**(4): pp. 87–98.

46. Cipolla-Neto, J., et al., Melatonin, energy metabolism, and obesity: a review. *Journal of Pineal Research*, 2014. **56**(4): pp. 371–381.

47. Beccuti, G. and S. Pannain, Sleep and obesity. *Current Opinion in Clinical Nutrition and Metabolic Care*, 2011. **14**(4): p. 402.

48. Calhoun, D.A. and S.M. Harding, Sleep and hypertension. *Chest*, 2010. **138**(2): pp. 434–443.

49. Nagai, M., S. Hoshide, and K. Kario, Sleep duration as a risk factor for cardiovascular disease-a review of the recent literature. *Current Cardiology Reviews*, 2010. **6**(1): pp. 54–61.

50. Dinges, D.F., et al., Cumulative sleepiness, mood disturbance, and psychomotor vigilance performance decrements during a week of sleep restricted to 4–5 hours per night. *Sleep*, 1997. **20**(4): pp. 267–277.

51. Panel, C.C., et al., Recommended amount of sleep for a healthy adult: a joint consensus statement of the American Academy of Sleep Medicine and Sleep Research Society. *Journal of Clinical Sleep Medicine*, 2015. **11**(6): pp. 591–592.

52. Carskadon, M., J. Mindell, and C. Drake, Contemporary sleep patterns of adolescents in the USA: results of the 2006 National Sleep Foundation Sleep in America poll. *Journal of Sleep Research*, 2006. **15**: p. 42.

53. Urbán, R., T. Magyaródi, and A. Rigó, Morningness-eveningness, chronotypes and health-impairing behaviors in adolescents. *Chronobiology International*, 2011. **28**(3): pp. 238–247.

54. Gangwar, A., et al., Circadian preference, sleep quality, and health-impairing lifestyles among undergraduates of medical university. *Cureus*, 2018. **10**(6): p. e2856.

55. Rawat, A., et al., Sleep quality and insulin resistance in adolescent subjects with different circadian preference: a cross-sectional study. *Journal of Family Medicine and Primary Care*, 2019. **8**(7): pp. 2502–2505.

56. Hasler, B.P., et al., Circadian rhythms, sleep, and substance abuse. *Sleep Medicine Reviews*, 2012. **16**(1): pp. 67–81.

57. Spruyt, K., D.L. Molfese, and D. Gozal, Sleep duration, sleep regularity, body weight, and metabolic homeostasis in school-aged children. *Pediatrics*, 2011. **127**(2): pp. e345–e352.

58. Sung, V., et al., Does sleep duration predict metabolic risk in obese adolescents attending tertiary services? A cross-sectional study. *Sleep*, 2011. **34**(7): pp. 891–898.

59. Koren, D., et al., Sleep architecture and glucose and insulin homeostasis in obese adolescents. *Diabetes Care*, 2011. **34**(11): pp. 2442–2447.

60. Skoufi, G.I., et al., Shift work and quality of personal, professional, and family life among health care workers in a rehabilitation center in Greece. *Indian Journal of Occupational and Environmental Medicine*, 2017. **21**(3): p. 115.

61. Knutsson, A., Health disorders of shift workers. *Occupational Medicine*, 2003. **53**(2): pp. 103–108.

62. Lowden, A., et al., Eating and shift work—effects on habits, metabolism, and performance. *Scandinavian Journal of Work, Environment & Health*, 2010. **36**: pp. 150–162.

63. Esquirol, Y., et al., Shift work and metabolic syndrome: respective impacts of job strain, physical activity, and dietary rhythms. *Chronobiology International*, 2009. **26**(3): pp. 544–559.

64. Ledda, C., et al., High HOMA-IR index in healthcare shift workers. *Medicina*, 2019. **55**(5): p. 186.

65. Zarrinpar, A., A. Chaix, and S. Panda, Daily eating patterns and their impact on health and disease. *Trends in Endocrinology & Metabolism*, 2016. **27**(2): pp. 69–83.

66. Asher, G. and U. Schibler, Crosstalk between components of circadian and metabolic cycles in mammals. *Cell Metabolism*, 2011. **13**(2): pp. 125–137.

67. Damiola, F., et al., Restricted feeding uncouples circadian oscillators in peripheral tissues from the central pacemaker in the suprachiasmatic nucleus. *Genes & Development*, 2000. **14**(23): pp. 2950–2961.

68. Reznick, J., et al., Altered feeding differentially regulates circadian rhythms and energy metabolism in liver and muscle of rats. *Biochimica et Biophysica Acta (BBA)-Molecular Basis of Disease*, 2013. **1832**(1): pp. 228–238.

69. Salgado-Delgado, R.C., et al., Shift work or food intake during the rest phase promotes metabolic disruption and desynchrony of liver genes in male rats. *PLoS One*, 2013. **8**(4): p. e60052.

70. Gupta, N.J., V. Kumar, and S. Panda, A camera-phone based study reveals erratic eating pattern and disrupted daily eating-fasting cycle among adults in India. *PLoS One*, 2017. **12**(3): p. e0172852.

71. Stenvers, D.J., et al., Circadian clocks and insulin resistance. *Nature Reviews Endocrinology*, 2019. **15**(2): pp. 75–89.

72. Fleur, L., A suprachiasmatic nucleus generated rhythm in basal glucose concentrations. *Journal of Neuroendocrinology*, 1999. **11**(8): pp. 643–652.

73. Van Cauter, E., et al., Modulation of glucose regulation and insulin secretion by circadian rhythmicity and sleep. *The Journal of Clinical Investigation*, 1991. **88**(3): pp. 934–942.

74. Reinke, H. and G. Asher, Crosstalk between metabolism and circadian clocks. *Nature Reviews Molecular Cell Biology*, 2019. **20**(4): pp. 227–241.

75. Saad, A., et al., Diurnal pattern to insulin secretion and insulin action in healthy individuals. *Diabetes*, 2012. **61**(11): pp. 2691–2700.

76. van Moorsel, D., et al., Demonstration of a day-night rhythm in human skeletal muscle oxidative capacity. *Molecular Metabolism*, 2016. **5**(8): pp. 635–645.

77. Scheer, F.A., et al., Adverse metabolic and cardiovascular consequences of circadian misalignment. *Proceedings of the National Academy of Sciences*, 2009. **106**(11): pp. 4453–4458.

78. Leproult, R., U. Holmbäck, and E. Van Cauter, Circadian misalignment augments markers of insulin resistance and inflammation, independently of sleep loss. *Diabetes*, 2014. **63**(6): pp. 1860–1869.

79. Wefers, J., et al., Circadian misalignment induces fatty acid metabolism gene profiles and compromises insulin sensitivity in human skeletal muscle. *Proceedings of the National Academy of Sciences*, 2018. **115**(30): pp. 7789–7794.

80. Oosterman, J.E., S. Wopereis, and A. Kalsbeek, The circadian clock, shift work, and tissue-specific insulin resistance. *Endocrinology*, 2020. **161**(12): p. bqaa180.

81. Sharma, A., et al., Glucose metabolism during rotational shift-work in healthcare workers. *Diabetologia*, 2017. **60**(8): pp. 1483–1490.

82. Morris, C.J., et al., Endogenous circadian system and circadian misalignment impact glucose tolerance via separate mechanisms in humans. *Proceedings of the National Academy of Sciences*, 2015. **112**(17): pp. E2225–E2234.

83. Wehrens, S.M., et al., Meal timing regulates the human circadian system. *Current Biology*, 2017. **27**(12): pp. 1768–1775.

84. Skene, D.J., et al., Separation of circadian-and behavior-driven metabolite rhythms in humans provides a window on peripheral oscillators and metabolism. *Proceedings of the National Academy of Sciences*, 2018. **115**(30): pp. 7825–7830.

85. Wright Jr, K.P., et al., Entrainment of the human circadian clock to the natural light-dark cycle. *Current Biology*, 2013. **23**(16): pp. 1554–1558.

86. De La Iglesia, H.O., et al., Access to electric light is associated with shorter sleep duration in a traditionally hunter-gatherer community. *Journal of Biological Rhythms*, 2015. **30**(4): pp. 342–350.

87. Stevens, R.G. and Y. Zhu, Electric light, particularly at night, disrupts human circadian rhythmicity: is that a problem? *Philosophical Transactions of the Royal Society B: Biological Sciences*, 2015. **370**(1667): p. 20140120.

88. Brainard, G.C., et al., Action spectrum for melatonin regulation in humans: evidence for a novel circadian photoreceptor. *Journal of Neuroscience*, 2001. **21**(16): pp. 6405–6412.

89. Berson, D.M., F.A. Dunn, and M. Takao, Phototransduction by retinal ganglion cells that set the circadian clock. *Science*, 2002. **295**(5557): pp. 1070–1073.

90. Lockley, S.W., G.C. Brainard, and C.A. Czeisler, High sensitivity of the human circadian melatonin rhythm to resetting by short wavelength light. *The Journal of Clinical Endocrinology & Metabolism*, 2003. **88**(9): pp. 4502–4505.

91. Thorne, H.C., et al., Daily and seasonal variation in the spectral composition of light exposure in humans. *Chronobiology International*, 2009. **26**(5): pp. 854–866.

92. Cheung, I.N., et al., Morning and evening blue-enriched light exposure alters metabolic function in normal weight adults. *PLoS One*, 2016. **11**(5): p. e0155601.

93. Danilenko, K.V., S.V. Mustafina, and E.A. Pechenkina, Bright light for weight loss: results of a controlled crossover trial. *Obesity Facts*, 2013. **6**(1): pp. 28–38.

94. Dunai, A., et al., Moderate exercise and bright light treatment in overweight and obese individuals. *Obesity*, 2007. **15**(7): pp. 1749–1757.

95. Reid, K.J., et al., Timing and intensity of light correlate with body weight in adults. *PLoS One*, 2014. **9**(4): p. e92251.

96. LeBlanc, A.G., et al., The ubiquity of the screen: an overview of the risks and benefits of screen time in our modern world. *Translational Journal of the American College of Sports Medicine*, 2017. **2**(17): pp. 104–113.

97. Hu, F.B., et al., Television watching and other sedentary behaviors in relation to risk of obesity and type 2 diabetes mellitus in women. *JAMA*, 2003. **289**(14): pp. 1785–1791.

98. Hu, F.B., et al., Physical activity and television watching in relation to risk for type 2 diabetes mellitus in men. *Archives of Internal Medicine*, 2001. **161**(12): pp. 1542–1548.

99. Nightingale, C.M., et al., Screen time is associated with adiposity and insulin resistance in children. *Archives of Disease in Childhood*, 2017. **102**(7): pp. 612–616.

100. Kang, H.-T., et al., Association between screen time and metabolic syndrome in children and adolescents in Korea: the 2005 Korean National Health and Nutrition Examination Survey. *Diabetes Research and Clinical Practice*, 2010. **89**(1): pp. 72–78.

101. Suchert, V., R. Hanewinkel, and B. Isensee, Sedentary behavior and indicators of mental health in school-aged children and adolescents: a systematic review. *Preventive Medicine*, 2015. **76**: pp. 48–57.

102. Costigan, S.A., et al., The health indicators associated with screen-based sedentary behavior among adolescent girls: a systematic review. *Journal of Adolescent Health*, 2013. **52**(4): pp. 382–392.

103. Chaput, J.P., et al., Modern sedentary activities promote overconsumption of food in our current obesogenic environment. *Obesity Reviews*, 2011. **12**(5): pp. e12–e20.

104. Fonken, L.K. and R.J. Nelson, The effects of light at night on circadian clocks and metabolism. *Endocrine Reviews*, 2014. **35**(4): pp. 648–670.

105. Wood, B., et al., Light level and duration of exposure determine the impact of self-luminous tablets on melatonin suppression. *Applied Ergonomics*, 2013. **44**(2): pp. 237–240.

106. Adams, S.K., J.F. Daly, and D.N. Williford, Article commentary: adolescent sleep and cellular phone use: recent trends and implications for research. *Health Services Insights*, 2013. **6**: p. HSI. S11083.

107. Caples, S.M., A.S. Gami, and V.K. Somers, Obstructive sleep apnea. *Annals of Internal Medicine*, 2005. **142**(3): pp. 187–97.
108. Punjabi, N.M. and V.Y. Polotsky, Disorders of glucose metabolism in sleep apnea. *Journal of Applied Physiology*, 2005. **99**(5): pp. 1998–2007.
109. Foster, G.D., et al., Obstructive sleep apnea among obese patients with type 2 diabetes. *Diabetes Care*, 2009. **32**(6): pp. 1017–1019.
110. Aronsohn, R.S., et al., Impact of untreated obstructive sleep apnea on glucose control in type 2 diabetes. *American Journal of Respiratory and Critical Care Medicine*, 2010. **181**(5): pp. 507–513.
111. Botros, N., et al., Obstructive sleep apnea as a risk factor for type 2 diabetes. *The American Journal of Medicine*, 2009. **122**(12): pp. 1122–1127.
112. Ioachimescu, O.C., et al., VAMONOS (Veterans Affairs' Metabolism, Obstructed and Non-Obstructed Sleep) study: effects of CPAP therapy on glucose metabolism in patients with obstructive sleep apnea. *Journal of Clinical Sleep Medicine*, 2017. **13**(3): pp. 455–466.
113. Labarca, G., et al., CPAP in patients with obstructive sleep apnea and type 2 diabetes mellitus: systematic review and meta-analysis. *The Clinical Respiratory Journal*, 2018. **12**(8): pp. 2361–2368.

14 Transculturalizing Lifestyle Medicine for Managing Cardiometabolic-Based Chronic Disease

Juan P. González-Rivas
St Anne's University Hospital (FNUSA) Brno
Harvard University TH Chan School of Public Health
Foundation for Clinic, Public Health, and Epidemiological
Research of Venezuela (FISPEVEN INC)

Ramfis Nieto-Martínez
Harvard University TH Chan School of Public Health
Foundation for Clinic, Public Health, and Epidemiological
Research of Venezuela (FISPEVEN INC)
LifeDoc Health

María M. Infante-García
St Anne's University Hospital (FNUSA) Brno
Foundation for Clinic, Public Health, and Epidemiological
Research of Venezuela (FISPEVEN INC)

Jeffrey I. Mechanick
Kravis Center for Cardiovascular Health at Mount Sinai Heart
Icahn School of Medicine at Mount Sinai

CONTENTS

DOI: 10.1201/9781003206637-14

299

ABBREVIATIONS

ABCD	Adiposity-Based Chronic Disease
BMI	Body Mass Index
CMBCD	Cardiometabolic–Based Chronic Disease.
CPA	Clinical Practice Algorithms
CPG	Clinical Practice Guidelines
CVD	Cardiovascular Disease
DBCD	Dysglycemia-Based Chronic Disease
HCP	Healthcare Professionals
MetS	Metabolic Syndrome
T2D	Type 2 Diabetes
SES	Socioeconomic Status
tDNA	transcultural Diabetes Nutrition Algorithm
WC	Waist Circumference

14.1 CULTURAL INFLUENCE OF LIFESTYLE ON CARDIOMETABOLIC DISEASE

Chronic cardiometabolic disease is a consequence of the complex interaction among risk factors that determine one's lifestyle, modeled by primary drivers (genetics, physical and non-physical environment, and behavior) and the biological response of the individual.[1] A deep focus on the non-physical environment draws close attention to aspects of culture, represented by belief systems, standards, practices, behaviors, language, social dictums, and political inclinations.[2] The terms culture, race, and ethnicity are based on different constructs and used in different contexts but remain nebulous due to overlapping popular connotations (Table 14.1). The American culture is no exception and lacks clarity. However, there are five main recognized ethnoracial populations in the U.S.: non-Hispanic Whites, African American (AA), Hispanic/Latino, Asian Americans, and American Indian/Alaska Native.[3] It is of

TABLE 14.1
Terminology and Definitions

Term	Definition
Acculturation	Adoption and assimilation of a different culture (usually a dominant culture) when cultures interact
Culture	Clustering of non-physical attributes common to a category of people, such as belief systems and values that influence customs, music, art, cooking, standards, practices, behaviors, social institutions and organizations, as well as psychological factors, language/linguistics, social practices, political ideology, interpretation of media, spirituality/religion, and structured disruption/deterioration (education, housing, poverty, crime, and discrimination); cultural classifications have significant overlap with ethnicity and are interpreted in terms of ethnocultural populations
Race	Clustering of physical/genetic attributes common to a category of people; these classifications are becoming less relevant and pragmatic in health care due to adverse perceptions (e.g., prejudice, bias, and structured racism) and therefore being re-interpreted in terms of ethnocultural populations
Ethnicity	Clustering of both non-physical and physical/genetic attributes common to a category of people, such as culture and race, genealogy, ancestry, geography, linguistics, and political ideology; ethnic classifications have significant overlap with culture and are interpreted in terms of ethnocultural populations
Transculturalization	Process of adapting evidence-based concepts and recommendations from one (source) ethnocultural population to a different (target) ethnocultural population
Transcultural medicine	Includes cultural elements in routine encounters between a healthcare professional and a patient, applicable to any ethnocultural population
Social Determinants of Health[4]	Conditions that influence health, in which people are born, grow, live, work, and age

Source: Adapted from Nieto-Martinez et al.[2]

utmost importance to realize that one's own ethnoracial background is based on self-report and not another person's determination. Within each ethnoracial population, there are specific demographic, biological, and cultural aspects that further characterize an individual and obviate the need to depend on historical biases associated with race. Thus, specific ethnocultural attributes apply for an individual and influence their own lifestyle, and by extension, their risk for cardiometabolic disease (Table 14.2). For example, a Hispanic man born in Miami, but descending from Argentine parents, is going to have a different set of beliefs, practices, behaviors, and social constructs than another Hispanic man born in California from Mexican parents. Each of these individuals may have acculturated to American life in different ways and from different starting points. To ensure and facilitate the adoption of recommendations from clinical practice guidelines (CPG) in such a way that promises the most precise and successful outcomes, healthcare professionals (HCPs) need to consider both biological determinants and social determinants (including ethnocultural factors) of health that influence individual responses.

TABLE 14.2

Selected Evidence on Biological and Social Determinants of Cardiometabolic Disease in U.S. Ethnocultural Populations

African American

Demographics/Ancestry	13.5% of U.S. population by 2017. Genomic analysis demonstrated a mixed ancestry: West African 73.2%–82.1%; European 16.7%–24.0%; and Native American 0.8%–1.2%.
Biology/Genetics	Project SuGAR identified a unique locus influencing body fat distribution, very-low-density-lipoprotein cholesterol low-density lipoprotein cholesterol, and particle size.[5]
	At comparable levels of abnormal adiposity and insulin resistance, AA adolescents with obesity showed higher levels of inflammation and lower concentrations of GLP-1 than Caucasians, which may synergistically lead to type 2 diabetes.[6]
	Genome-wide association studies (GWASs) of AA populations shows genetic relationships to elevated C-reactive protein, demonstrating a potential contributor for CVD.[7]
Behavior/Social determinants	Perceptions of the world: historical circumstances (e.g., being enslaved and experiencing poverty) and current experiences (e.g., racial minority and trust effects).
	Low socioeconomic status according to home ownership and income
	Significant socioeconomic status diversity and growing AA upper-middle class
Cultural Aspects	Hairstyles, fashion, dance, music, visual art, worldview, inner-city neighborhoods, and attendance at church
	Diet high in saturated fat, sodium, and starch
	Cooking leftovers into a mixture with consistency between stew and soup
	Sharing of food
	Cultivation and use of yams, peanuts, rice, okra, sorghum, grits, and incorporation of chicken, fish, macaroni and cheese, cornbread, black-eyed peas, and rice

Hispanic/Latino

Demographics/Ancestry	Predicted expansion from 17.6% (2015) to 24% (2065) of total U.S. population, with 63% Mexican, 9.2% Puerto Rican, 3.5% Cuban, and 24% from the rest of Latin America and Spain.
	Ancestry variation: Mexican American (31% Native American, 8% African, and 61% Spanish), Puerto Rican (19%, 37%, and 45%, respectively), and Cuban American (19%, 20%, and 62%, respectively).
Biology/Genetics	Abdominal obesity among Mexican Americans: highest in those born in the U.S. and Spanish speaking > those born in the U.S. and English speaking > those born in Mexico.
	The insulin sensitivity index is lowest for Latino/Hispanics, compared with Asian Americans, AA, and non-Latino whites
Behavior/Social Determinants	Language barriers: 21% not speaking English, and only 5% of physicians and 2% of nurses being Latino/Hispanic.
	More distrust of a healthcare professional of a different ethnicity or where there is a significant language barrier.
	Higher rates of living below the poverty level and being noncitizens.
	Education and household income rates are relatively low.

(Continued)

TABLE 14.2 (*Continued*)
Selected Evidence on Biological and Social Determinants of Cardiometabolic Disease in U.S. Ethnocultural Populations

Hispanic/Latino

Cultural Aspects   Food preferences: high-fat meats, fats and lards for cooking, fried foods, inadequate portion control, high-glycemic-index items, and some high-fiber items (e.g., corn and beans)

Physical inactivity is more prevalent among Latino/Hispanics (foreign-born > U.S.-born) than U.S. Caucasians

Hispanics present a high perceived discrimination, which is a form of social stress associated with mental and cardiovascular outcomes.[8]

Asian American

Demographics/Ancestry   Fastest growing racial group in the U.S. with 21 million people (2015) and is projected to be 34.4 million (8.2%) of the US population by 2060.

High population diversity: at least 23 countries, 19 languages, and four major religions represented, with varying incomes and education levels.

Acculturation to an "American way of life" has increased risks for chronic metabolic diseases

Biology/Genetics   Higher sarcopenic obesity due to decreased muscle mass and increased visceral adiposity, higher plasma no esterified fatty acid and triglycerides levels, hyperinsulinemia and insulin resistance, higher hs-CRP, lower adiponectin levels, and in some, reduced b-cell function.

South Asian population express 2–4 times higher level of Lipoprotein (a) [Lp(a)] than in whites.[9] High Lp(a) levels is a major determinant of cardiovascular events, especially at younger ages.

Behavior/Social determinants   Holidays (secular and religious) are frequent. Each holiday may have different dietary patterns (e.g., overeating or fasting patterns)

58.1% of Asian American adults have central obesity. U.S.-born Japanese American women have higher body fat amounts than their immigrant counterparts. Waist circumference is especially important in those of Asian ancestry.

Sedentary lifestyle is an important risk factor for cardiovascular disease in Asian Indians.

The Muslim custom requires fully covered attire (increases risk for vitamin D deficiency)

Sweating in public is an embarrassment

Cultural Aspects   Diet benefits: green tea, variety of vegetables and fruits, spices, low red meat consumption, beans and nuts, fish and seafood, fruit as desserts, whole grains, smaller portion sizes, and soy consumption.

Diet risks: white rice and other refined grains, use of animal fat and palm oil, unhealthy *trans* fats not labeled on packages, sweets, and snacks high in sugar, tea or coffee with too much added sugar, too much salt, excessive consumption of cured meats.

American Indian

Demographics/Ancestry   0.9% of the U.S. population identified as American Indian or Alaska Native alone and 1.7% in combination with another ethno racial population

(*Continued*)

TABLE 14.2 (Continued)

Selected Evidence on Biological and Social Determinants of Cardiometabolic Disease in U.S. Ethnocultural Populations

American Indian

Biology/Genetics	High overweight and obesity rates 71.7% (2005–2011)
Behavior/Social determinants	Value on extended family networks, emphasis on the collective, respect for authority figures (elders, in particular), and spirituality.
	The traditional diet of Native Americans is derived from a mixture of agriculture, hunting, and gathering wild foods.
	American Indians and Alaska Natives are disproportionally affected by exposure to environmental chemicals including toxic metals, contributing to the development of cardiovascular disease.[10]
Cultural Aspects	Forced displacement caused sedentarism.
	A less-healthy eating pattern emerged: disruption of family and tribal structure with residential schools and outlawing of religion and native languages.
	Tribal land was reduced and rights to fish, hunt, and collect wild foods were limited.

Source: Adapted from Mechanick et al.[11]

Abbreviations: AA, African American; GLP-1, Glucagon-Like Peptide 1.

14.2 PREVALENCE AND BURDEN OF CARDIOMETABOLIC DISEASE BY ETHNOCULTURAL POPULATIONS

The contrasting lifestyles, biology, and environment among ethnocultural groups are denoted in the different prevalence rates of cardiometabolic risk factors (Table 14.3). In 2015, the prevalence of tobacco use was 14% in the U.S., with higher prevalence rates in American Indians (21.9%) and AA men (20.9%), and the lowest prevalence rates in Asian females (2.6%).[12] In 2018, the prevalence of insufficient physical activity affected almost half of the population and was higher in AA and Asian females (59.5% and 56.8%, respectively), the group with the lowest prevalence rate was non-Hispanic White men (39.4%).[13] In 2013–2016, the prevalence of unhealthy nutrition affected about 80% of the U.S. population, but was lower in Asians (44.3%).[13] In 2015–2018, the prevalence of obesity affected about 43% of the U.S. population, higher in AA women (55.2%) and substantially lower in Asians (14.7%). In 2013–2016, the prevalence of diabetes was about 12% of the U.S. population, higher in AA (14.0%) and Hispanics (14.6%), and lower in non-Hispanic Whites (8.3%).[13] In 2015–2018, the prevalence of hypertension was about 49%, higher in AA (57.9%), and lower in non-Hispanic Whites and Hispanics (45.7% both groups).[13]

Cardiovascular disease (CVD) is the leading cause of death in the U.S., with approximately 957,000 deaths (291.9 per 100.000) in 2019,[14] disproportionally impacting each ethnocultural population. In 2018, compared with non-Hispanic Whites, AAs were 30% more likely to die from heart disease, AA men and women were 70% and 30% more likely to die from stroke, respectively, and 110% more

TABLE 14.3
Prevalence of Cardiovascular and Behaviors Risk Factor by Ethnocultural Population in the U.S.

Population Group	Smoking/Tobacco Used (2015)[12]	Physical Inactivity (2018)[13]	Unhealthy Nutrition (2013/2016)[13]	Cardiovascular and Behaviors Risk Factors					
				Obesity (2015/2018)[13]	Diabetes (2013/2016)[13]	Prediabetes (2013/2016)[13]	Hypertension (2015/2018)[13]	Hypercholesterolemia (2015/2018)[13]	Low-HDL (2015/2018)[13]
Non-Hispanic White									
Male	17.3	39.4	..	40.7	9.4	43.7	51.0	35.0	26.3
Female	16.0	45.3	..	38.7	7.3	32.2	40.5	41.8	7.4
Total	16.6	42.3	78.2	39.7	8.3	37.9	45.7	38.4	16.8
African American									
Male	20.9	46.7	..	38.2	14.7	31.9	58.3	31.0	17.0
Female	13.5	59.5	..	55.2	13.4	24.0	57.6	33.4	7.9
Total	16.8	53.1	81.9	46.7	14.0	27.9	57.9	32.4	12.4
Hispanic/Latino									
Male	13.1	48.3	..	44.0	15.1	48.1	50.6	37.7	32.0
Female	7.1	56.8	..	46.2	14.1	31.7	40.8	37.3	12.3
Total	10.1	52.5	83.7	45.1	14.6	39.9	45.7	37.5	22.1
Asian American				(2009)[16]	(2000/2006)[16]		(2004/2008)[16]	(2004/2008)[16]	
Male	12.0	..	..	13.5	12.8	47.1	51.0	38.6	26.4
Female	2.6	..	..	15.9	9.9	29.4	42.1	38.6	6.7
Total	7.0	..	44.3	14.7	11.3	38.2	46.5	38.6	16.5
American Indian/ Alaska Native									
Male	19.0	..	..	46.2	..	..	..	..	..
Female	24.0	..	..	45.5	..	..	..	..	..
Total	21.9	..	..	..	17.5	..	34.7%	40%	..

Source: Adapted from Virani SS et al.[13]

likely to die from diabetes;[15] American Indian/Alaska Natives had similar rates of heart disease and stroke than non-Hispanic Whites but were 130% more like to die from diabetes; Asians were 30% and 20% less likely to die from heart disease and stroke, respectively, with similar mortality rates of diabetes; Hispanics were 30% less likely to die from heart disease, had similar rates of stroke, and 30% times more likely to die from diabetes.[15]

14.3   RESPONSE TO THE STRESSOR ENVIRONMENT BY ETHNOCULTURAL GROUPS

Individuals from different environments are exposed to different levels and types of stressors. For example, individuals with lower socioeconomic status (SES) are exposed to higher levels of noise pollution, violence, discrimination, crowding, crime, etc.,[17] developing more physiological stress with higher basal levels of cortisol and catecholamine[18] and exhibiting more unhealthy behaviors, such as tobacco use, excessive alcohol use, physical inactivity, and poor nutrition than those with higher SES.[19] Allostatic load is a useful concept to describe this phenomenon by assessing the role of environmental characteristics and providing a mechanistic link to understand the biology underlying health disparities.[20–22] Allostatic load is a construct reflecting the nature, level, and accumulated hazard of physiological adaptations to stressors as part of the stress response.[23] This process involves many different physiological processes, interacting in complex, networked manners, with primary and secondary metabolic biomarkers that directly and indirectly predict CVD development and progression.[23]

The allostatic load score was evaluated in 5,765 adult women from the U.S. using ten biomarkers representing cardiovascular, inflammatory, and metabolic system functioning, from the National Health and Nutrition Examination Survey (NHANES) 1999–2004.[24] In this study, AA women manifested a higher allostatic load compared with other ethnocultural groups, as well as a higher allostatic load at younger ages, suggesting earlier health deterioration. Additionally, Mexican women not born in the U.S. had lower allostatic load scores than those born in the U.S.[24] This result was consistent with the evaluation of 1,410 adults assessed as part of the Texas City Stress and Health Study, 2004–2006, where AA men and women had higher allostatic load scores compared with other ethnical groups and that foreign-born Mexicans had lower allostatic load scores compared with U.S.-born Mexicans.[25] When the effect of acculturation was explored, the foreign-born Mexicans who had lived in the U.S. for 10 years or less were less likely to have a high allostatic load score than foreign-born Mexicans who had lived in the country for more than 10 years.[25] More-acculturated immigrants may adopt behaviors that harm their health, such as unhealthy diets, sedentary lifestyles, tobacco use, and alcohol consumption.[26]

14.4   TRANSCULTURAL LIFESTYLE MEDICINE

Cultural diversity and its effect on disease phenotype mandate attention to individual social determinants of health and understanding ethnocultural variables.

Transcultural medicine is a component of precision medicine aiming to include the cultural elements in the routine encounters between a HCP and patient to optimize outcomes.[2] Transcultural lifestyle medicine delivers pragmatic lifestyle recommendations, particularly focused on the adoption of healthy eating patterns, regular/sufficient physical activity, sleep hygiene, stress reduction, community engagement, and alcohol, tobacco, and substance cessation.[27] Successful implementation of lifestyle medicine in different ethnocultural populations requires transculturalization of clinical evidence. Transculturalization describes the process of adapting clinical recommendations from one culture to another, using source and target culture experts in an interactive setting, and a highly structured deliverable, such as an CPG or algorithm (CPA) (Table 14.1).[28] Optimally, this process is evidence-based and incorporates multiple validated components to significantly improve the prevention of a given chronic disease state, such as cardiometabolic disease. The transculturalization process addresses and narrows the gap between the HCP's and the patient's cultures, facilitating implementation of a more precise set of evidence-based recommendations (Figure 14.1).

14.5 TRANSCULTURAL ADAPTATION OF EVIDENCE

The transcultural Diabetes Nutrition Algorithm (tDNA) process is a validated methodology for transculturally adapting evidence-based recommendations to different ethnocultural groups and populations.[29] Initially, it was designed as a tool to facilitate the delivery of lifestyle modifications and nutrition therapy to people with

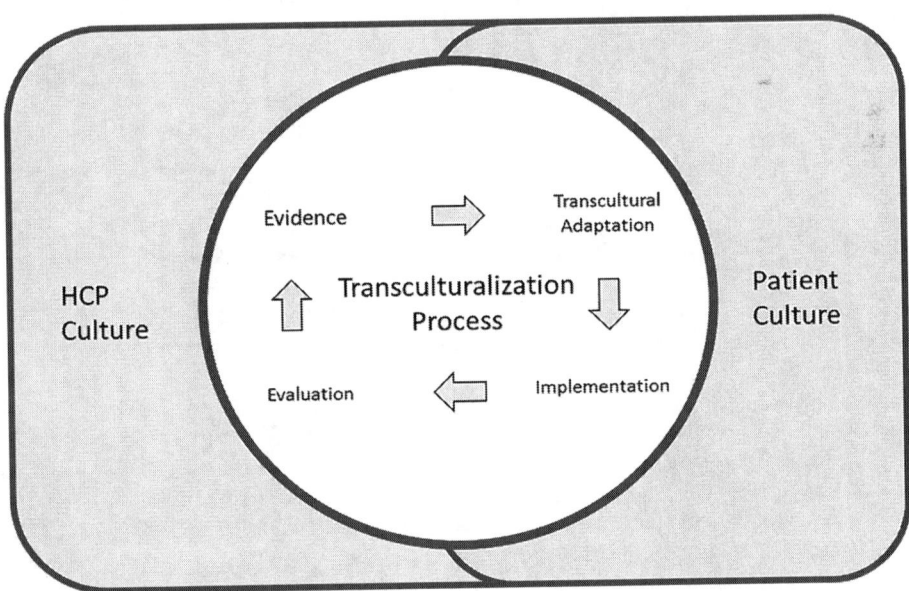

FIGURE 14.1 Transculturalization process to narrow the gap between the healthcare professional (HCP) and patient cultures.

prediabetes and T2D around the world, representing many different cultures, and resulting in the adaptation of existing CPG into new transculturalized CPA.[30] The tDNA has been adopted in many countries[31–37] and was validated in Malaysia.[38] The tDNA transcultural adaptation process is divided into five steps:

1. **Identification of the Target Population**: description of the population where the implementation is going to be delivered, with an emphasis on the ethnocultural and demographic characteristics, as well as cardiometabolic drivers.
2. **Identification of the Clinical Question**: description of the gap to address.
3. **Identification of the Appropriate Source Evidence Base**: analysis of the scientific evidence and derivative products/models (e.g., CPG and CPA) that address the problem.
4. **Identification of Experts in the Source and Target Populations**: experts in the scientific evidence from both the source and target population directly engage to address the cultural differences and adaptations using validated frameworks (e.g., the Ecological Validity Model[39]).
5. Synthesis of the transcultural recommendations and algorithm[30]
   a. **Creation of Nodes**: node-specific recommendations assist the process of transculturalization defining actions in the algorithm.
      i. **Diagnostic**: the nodes are organized according to *a priori* levels in the process (Figure 14.2). Each node ("N") has a numerical descriptor and represents different action levels; N1 – Screening or Aggressive Case Finding; N2 – Stratification; N3 – Diagnosis; N4 – Intervention; N5 – Metrics; N6 – Intervention; N7 – Follow-up. Additional levels can be included if necessary.

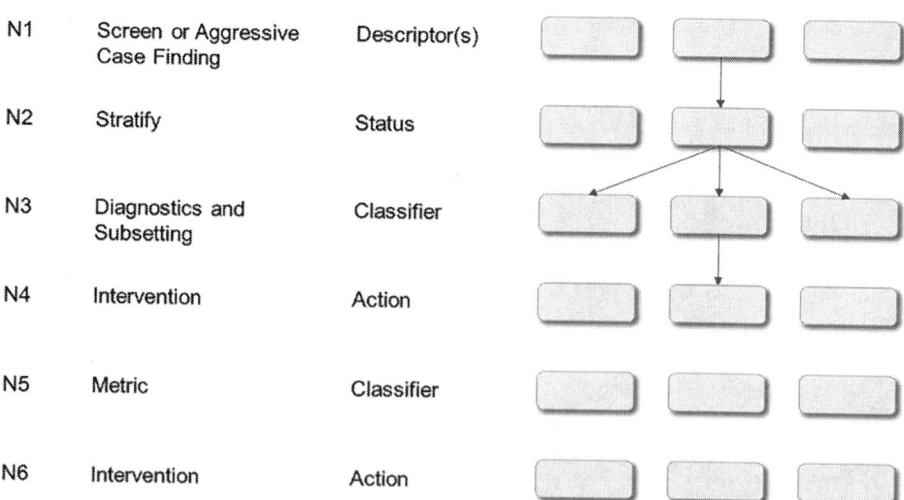

N1	Screen or Aggressive Case Finding	Descriptor(s)
N2	Stratify	Status
N3	Diagnostics and Subsetting	Classifier
N4	Intervention	Action
N5	Metric	Classifier
N6	Intervention	Action

FIGURE 14.2   Master clinical practice algorithm transculturalization template.[30]

ii. **Intervention**:
1. **Description**: ethnocultural characteristics of the target population are addressed in each node (e.g., prevalences, local anthropometrics, and cut-off values to define diagnosis) to fashion intervention strategies.
2. **Toolkit**: resources described/provided for tactical implementation of these strategies.
b. **Creation of Edges**: Each node offers a set of possible options (e.g., present, absent, ignored) and is connected to other nodes (within same or advanced levels) by edges (arrows from one node to another).
c. **Derivation of Specific Recommendations**: compilation of recommendations is distributed and published in a variety of formats (reviews, position papers, CPA/CPG, toolkits, etc.).
d. **Optimization of Topology**: the structure of the algorithm, in terms of node-edge relationships, is optimized over time based on feedback, performance, implementation metrics, and validation studies.

14.6 IMPLEMENTATION OF A TRANSCULTURALIZED CARDIOMETABOLIC MODEL USING LIFESTYLE MEDICINE

14.6.1 CONTEXTUALIZATION

Successful implementation of transculturalized lifestyle medicine approaches demands the evaluation and understanding of context (Table 14.4).[40] This includes elements that influence people's health and are part of the social determinants of health, which are commonly used to measure and understand health inequalities.[41–43] Adapting the recommendations to the context of an individual patient helps eliminate the potential barriers for successful adoption. For example, a qualitative survey of lifestyle coaches of the U.S. Diabetes Prevention Program reported that the general income and education level of the surrounding community shaped participants' interest in and reaction to the intervention.[44] In this case, out-of-pocket program fees, coupled with lower-incomes, were barriers to participation, whereas higher income is a facilitator.[44] However, in other cases, patients with more years of formal education paradoxically reacted negatively to the program because they perceived the content to be too basic.[44] The study highlighted that lifestyle coaching should have the flexibility to adapt the program to address challenges specific to their region and/or clinic, but the adaptations should be balanced with efforts to maintain program fidelity.[44] In another qualitative study that evaluated cancer survivors, Latinas reported among the barriers to adopting a healthy lifestyle, the negative impact of lack of knowledge of how to prepare healthy food relevant to their culture and the discrepancy between the food that they cook for their family members and the recommendations offered by their HCPs.[45]

14.6.2 COMPLICATION-BASED APPROACH

To mitigate the adverse effects of cardiometabolic risk factors, lifestyle medicine needs to be framed in a chronic care model focusing on modifiable primary (built

TABLE 14.4
Contextualization Factors

Category	Features
Physical	"Built" (human-made) environment
	Healthy/unhealthy food availability in restaurants, schools, workplace, and stores
	Food and water supply, food sourcing, food "deserts," pesticides, and endocrine disruptors
	Walking paths, public/private gyms, school fitness programs, green spaces, and parks
	Building design (elevators versus stairs), distances to walk, and handicapped access
	Security personnel, safe routes to schools, safe venues for exercise, city planning, community design, and energy supply
Non-physical	Culture, ethnicity, belief systems, and socio-political-economic factors
	Attitudes and customs toward food and eating, food policy and politics, and religious dictates
	Affordability of healthy foods (e.g., fresh fruits, fresh vegetables, and whole grains)
	Use of unhealthy, processed, and fast foods due to economics, availability, and affordability
	Attitudes and customs toward physical activity and exercise (e.g., not sweating in public)
	Screen time (e.g., television, games, and computer)
	Home and workplace stress including personal safety and crime (e.g., decreased sleep and increased use of comfort foods)
	Disparities in healthcare access (e.g., due to gender and socioeconomic class)
	Discrimination and stigmatization with obesity
	Confusion and ambiguity centered on the term "obesity"

Source: Adapted from Mechanick et al.[40]

[human-made] environment and behavioral) and secondary (metabolic) drivers, as well as relevant complications, rather than an array of surrogated markers to be interrogated, plugged into composite scoring systems, and associated with aggregated outcomes.[1] This traditional approach, exemplified by the metabolic syndrome (MetS) definition and the body mass index (BMI), was predicated on detection and interventions focused on specific biochemical markers. Unfortunately, this approach led to clinical inertia once markers were addressed leaving residual mechanisms intact. This approach also ignored specific actions prior to the appearance of abnormalities, essentially disregarding primordial and primary prevention strategies, stigma, and social determinants of health, as well as other ethnocultural, behavioral, and environmental components.[46,47]

In response to these shortcomings and based on the emerging recognition of "comprehensive care" and a "complications-centric" approach to cardiometabolic risk, various driver-based chronic disease models were conceived, formulated, and applied. These models are based on causal mechanisms, an eventual chronic disease state, and the need for early and sustainable preventive care. The Adiposity-Based Chronic Disease (ABCD) model paved the way for this initiative and described the impact of abnormal adiposity (function, distribution, and amount) interpreted in the physical and non-physical context of the individual.[47] The ABCD model targets the earliest possible prevention care to mitigate risk for weight-related complications, rather than simply targeting body weight or BMI. The ABCD model is divided into four stages that can be mapped to specific preventive care modalities. Stage 1 ("Risk") is created through the interactive of primary drivers (genetics, environment, and behavior) and amenable to population-based primordial preventive care. Stage 2 ("Predisease") results from an unhealthy lifestyle and produces mildly abnormal adiposity amount ("overweight" based on BMI cutoffs), distribution (based on waist circumference or body imaging [e.g., visceral fat or ectopic fat in the liver, kidney, pancreas, bone marrow, and epi/pericardium]), or function (based on biochemical testing [decreased adiponectin, increased high sensitivity C-reactive protein, increased interleukin-6, etc.]) and amenable to primary preventive care. Stage 3 ("Disease") results from a greater degree of abnormal adiposity ("obesity" is ABCD stage 3) and amenable to secondary prevention care. Stage 4 ("Complications") results from earlier pathophysiological mechanisms and produce a degree of symptom burden (mild, moderate, or severe), dependence on health care, increased healthcare expenditures, and mortality risk, best addressed with tertiary preventive care.[48,49] Transcultural factors with direct relevance to the ABCD model include genetic/biological differences among ethnocultural populations in adipose tissue, ethnicity adjusted anthropometrics (e.g., BMI and waist circumference [WC]), context (structural disruption and deterioration, social determinants of health, and other cultural factors), and disparities in access to quality health care, among others.[50]

A second driver-based chronic disease model was then developed for patients with or at risk for T2D and diabetes complications. The Dysglycemia-Based Chronic Disease (DBCD) model focuses on the spectrum from insulin resistance to prediabetes to T2D to CVD,[50] and encourages a proactive search for the earliest possible prevention action to mitigate complication risk; this is in contrast to a glucocentric approach, which simply targets blood glucose and hemoglobin A1c (A1C).[51] Similar to ABCD, DBCD is divided into the same four-stage schema. Stage 1 ("Risk") is an insulin resistance state with normoglycemia brought on by primary drivers and amenable to population-based primordial prevention. Insulin resistance also leads to macrovascular complications.[52] Stage 2 ("Predisease") is a prediabetes state resulting from an early β-cell defect and with mild hyperglycemia, amenable to primary prevention of T2D (e.g., the Diabetes Prevention Program[53]). About 10% of subjects with prediabetes already have hyperglycemia-related complications,[54] with about 70% progressing to T2D during their life.[55] Stage 3 ("T2D") results from a sustained β-cell defect and greater hyperglycemia that increases the development of complications, particularly microvascular, and is amenable to secondary preventive care. Stage 4 ("Complications") results from chronic insulin resistance and hyperglycemia and manifested by microvascular and/or macrovascular pathology; this stage is amenable to tertiary preventive care. Transcultural factors with direct relevance to the DBCD model include genetic/biological differences among ethnocultural populations in adipose tissue, inflammation, and β-cell function, potential ethnicity-related differences in diagnostic criteria, context (structural disruption and deterioration, social determinants of health, and other cultural factors), and disparities in access to quality health care (especially diabetes supplies, medications, and specialty care), among others.[56]

The ABCD and DBCD models are interconnected primarily by insulin resistance but also through convergence at dyslipidemia, hypertension, and inflammation levels, leading to CVD. Adipose tissue dysfunction is characterized by an imbalance of protective factors (e.g., adiponectin, nitric oxide, and protective prostaglandins) and increased activation of stress-related pathways leading to pathological adipokine release (e.g., resistin, visfatin, and leptin), low-grade inflammation, and immune cell infiltration.[57] Perivascular adipose tissue inflammation leads to vascular remodeling, superoxide production, and endothelial dysfunction with loss of nitric oxide bioavailability, contributing to vascular disease, atherosclerosis, and plaque instability.[57] Inappropriate adipose tissue distribution is associated with multiple cardiometabolic risks, contributing to hypertension, dyslipidemia, and other MetS traits.[58] This pathophysiological response can vary according to genetic/biological characteristics of the different ethnoracial groups. For example, AA shows blunted efficacy of some widely used antihypertensive drug classes (e.g., ACE inhibitors). Nevertheless, social, cultural, and other environment factors are still the critical determinants of poor hypertension control, especially in AA.[59] This is the basis for the next four-stage driver-based chronic disease model – cardiometabolic-based chronic disease (CMBCD) (Figure 14.3).[47] Stage 1 ("Risk") results from primary drivers and metabolic drivers (e.g., ABCD and DBCD, as well as other MetS traits

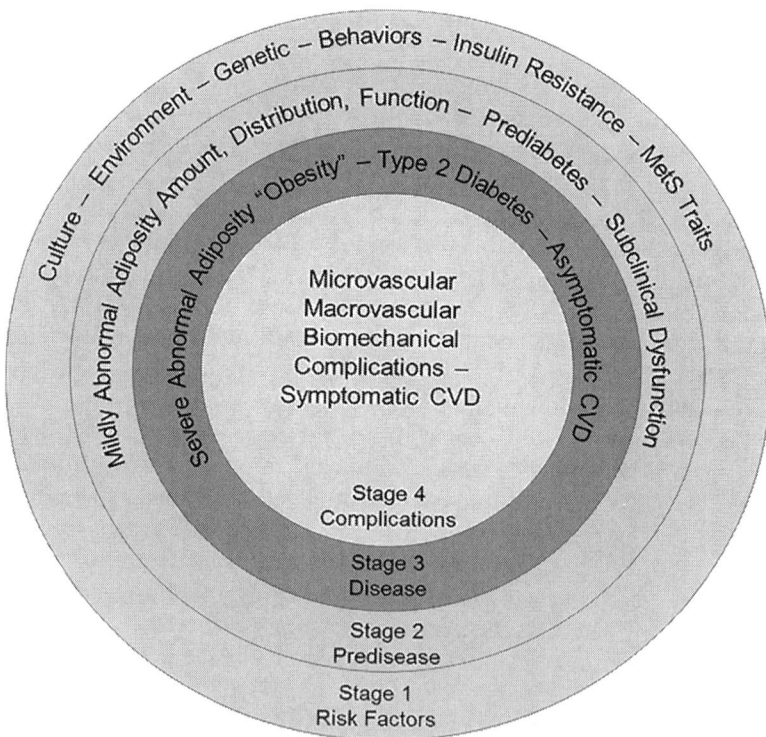

FIGURE 14.3   The cardiometabolic-based chronic disease model. Four stages of progression. Abbreviations: CVD, Cardiovascular Disease; MetS, Metabolic Syndrome.

[hypertension, dyslipidemia, and residual risk factors]) to initiate molecular alterations for CVD. CMBCD stage 1 is addressed with population-based primordial preventive care. Stage 2 ("Predisease") is characterized by cardiovascular alterations (atherosclerosis and structural cardiac abnormalities) that lead to CVD and amenable to primary preventive care. Stage 3 ("Disease") is characterized by early, asymptomatic coronary heart disease, atrial fibrillation, and heart failure and is amenable to secondary preventive care. Stage 4 ("Complications") is characterized by later, symptomatic coronary heart disease, atrial fibrillation, and heart failure and is amenable to tertiary preventive care. Transcultural factors with direct relevance to the CMBCD model include genetic/biological differences among ethnocultural populations in adipose tissue, inflammation, β-cell function, and the cardiovascular system, ethnicity-related differences in cardiovascular metrics, context (structural disruption and deterioration, social determinants of health, and other cultural factors), and disparities in access to quality health care (especially cardiovascular care), among others.[47,59]

14.6.3   Implementation: Case Study

14.6.3.1   Scenario

Vietnamese patient evaluated in California for Diabetes Risk Screening

14.6.3.2   Patient Presentation

A 36-year-old Vietnamese man is evaluated in a healthcare center in San Jose, California, U.S. He wants to know if he has T2D because, ever since arriving in the U.S., his dietary habits have worsened, resulting in weight gain and increased fasting blood sugar.

14.6.3.3   Cultural Factors

The Vietnamese population in the U.S. is estimated at 2.2 million,[3] the fourth-largest Asian American ethnic group. Approximately 32% of the total population in San Jose is Asian.

The attending U.S. physician interpreted the BMI of 23.5 kg/m² and the WC of 92 cm as normal based on criteria for the Caucasian population. The patient reported a previous fasting blood glucose of 115 mg/dL, but today's blood glucose was 90 mg/dL. The physician did not find any significant risk factors for T2D and recommended a new evaluation in 1 year and gave him a pamphlet with healthy recipes from American population guidelines. Because the patient's father developed T2D at age 28, the patient visited a second physician who recommended an oral glucose tolerance test, resulting in a blood glucose level at 2 hours post-challenge to be 234 mg/dL, diagnostic for T2D.

14.6.3.4   Analysis

What additional factors should the first physician have considered? This case illustrates the pitfalls of a purely glucocentric approach, without taking inventory of other risk factors (e.g., family history), other cardiometabolic risk factors (e.g., hypertension and dyslipidemia), and potential complications (e.g., foot and eye exams, renal function, and neurological exam). But more to the point, what transcultural components were not considered by the first physician? There are three main answers for Asians: dysglycemia pathophysiology, dietary patterns and food preferences, and other cultural and lifestyle behavioral trends.

At A1C levels below 7.1%, postprandial hyperglycemia in Asians contributes more to excess hyperglycemia than fasting glycaemia,[60] contributing to the development of T2D at younger ages and lower degrees of adiposity. Asians are considered to be overweight with a BMI ≥ 23 kg/m^2 and obesity with BMI ≥ 25 kg/m^2.[28] Also, specific WC cutoffs of 90 cm for men and 80 cm for women were recommended in the Asian population.[61] According to the ABCD and DBCD models,[48] Asians with a BMI ≥ 23 kg/m^2 need to be evaluated for dysglycemia and weight-related complications, and a checklist consulted for chronic care as provided by published CPG.[48] The initial approach should have been less focused on glucose alone, and more focused on the ramifications of dysglycemia – comprehensive care.

A transcultural adaptation of the interventions modeled by the Finnish Diabetes Prevention Study has been developed for South Asians, which could have also been used as a framework to implement lifestyle strategies with specific considerations according to the country where he is living and the effects of acculturation.[62] Medical nutritional therapy and a formal evaluation (i.e., screening, case finding, risk stratification, intervention, and follow-up) can be applied using the Asian version of the tDNA.[31] In this approach, nutritional recommendations incorporate cultural preferences. For example, considering the high consumption of dietary rice[21] and the high prevalence of postprandial hyperglycemia in Asians,[60] these transcultural dietary adaptations include the following:

- Reduce the intake of carbohydrates with a high glycemic index, such as "glutinous" short-grain rice and porridge and replace or mix them with grains and/or pulses (e.g., beans and lentils) with a lower glycemic index;[63]
- Increase the consumption of vegetables and fruits with a low glycemic index;
- Reduce the consumption of red meat;
- Increase the consumption of fish and shellfish and greater consumption of soy;
- Replace the use of animal fat and palm oil with healthier vegetable oils, such as canola, safflower, sunflower, walnut, and olive; and
- Reduce the consumption of foods rich in sodium, canned, and processed foods, encouraging the consumption of fresh foods.[11]

Healthy eating should be coupled with culturally adapted physical activity recommendations.[31] For example, some Asian cultures hold the beliefs that physical activity does not prevent complications and can be harmful: "the elderly should rest;" "it is unsafe for women to exercise outside the home;" and "sweating is embarrassing," limiting attendance to gyms. Based on this belief system, physical activity recommendations in Asians involving programs delivered through religious communities, such as mosques or temples, may be advised. There also are culturally appropriate forms of dance and other body movements that can be encouraged.[11]

14.7 CONCLUSION

Cardiometabolic disease creates symptom burdens that disproportionally affect different ethnocultural populations. Ethnicity and culture are constructs that include overlapping non-physical and physical attributes, which are better interpreted as ethnocultural populations, overcoming the adverse perceptions of race. Transcultural medicine incorporates the cultural elements that are relevant to routine encounters between HCP and patient, as well as guidelines, protocols, and policies that can optimize health care among different human populations. The gap between two distinct cultures can be narrowed using a transculturalization process of interpreting and translating scientific evidence. Multicultural populations are a particular challenge for HCPs globally. The U.S. is an example of a nation with an intermediate level of ethnocultural diversity. For context, a fractionalization analysis of ethnic, linguistic, and religious heterogeneity showed that the countries in Sub-Saharan Africa have the largest ethnical diversity, with Uganda leading with a fractionalization index of 0.93.[64] Asian countries are the most homogenous with the lowest index, such as Japan and South Korea, scoring 0.011 and 0.002, respectively. In this report, the U.S. score was 0.49.[64] Primary (genetics, environment, and behavior) and secondary/metabolic (ABCD, DBCD, hypertension, dyslipidemia, inflammation) drivers initiate and perpetuate the progression of CVD. Transcultural lifestyle medicine is the first step in the preventive care of CMBCD at any stage, addressing differences and the influence of cultural factors on various aspects of cardiometabolic risk including lifestyle, diagnosis cutoffs, response to interventions, and cardiometabolic phenotypes and outcome. In daily practice, HCPs could start from the understanding of the diverse ethnocultural groups under their care, incorporating relevant and adapted diagnostic measures, performance, and recommendations, that should be tracked, and then re-evaluated and integrated as part of the polices and protocols of their Centers, clinical service lines, or practices.

Disclosures:

Ramfis Nieto-Martínez received honoraria from Merck for lectures.
Jeffrey I. Mechanick received honoraria from Abbott Nutrition for lectures and serves on the Advisory Boards for Aveta.Life and Twin Health.

REFERENCES

1. Nieto-Martínez R, González-Rivas JP, Mechanick JI. Cardiometabolic risk: New chronic care models. *Journal of Parenteral and Enteral Nutrition.* 2021;45:85–92.
2. Nieto-Martinez R, Gonzalez-Rivas JP, Florez H, Mechanick JI. Transcultural endocrinology: Adapting type-2 diabetes guidelines on a global scale. *Endocrinology and Metabolism Clinics.* 2016;45:967–1009.
3. U.S. Census Bureau. Quickfacts: United States. Available online: https://www.census.gov/quickfacts/fact/table/us/pst045217. Accessed on April, 2019.
4. Center for Disease Control and Prevention (CDC). Social Determinants of Health. Available online: https://www.Cdc.Gov/nchhstp/socialdeterminants/faq.html. Accessed on August 01, 2021.

5. Divers J, Sale MM, Lu L, Chen WM, Lok KH, Spruill IJ, Fernandes JK, Langefeld CD, Garvey WT. The genetic architecture of lipoprotein subclasses in Gullah-speaking African American families enriched for type 2 diabetes: The Sea Islands genetic African American registry (Project SuGAR). *Journal of Lipid Research*. 2010;51:586–597.
6. Velasquez-Mieyer PA, Cowan PA, Perez-Faustinelli S, Nieto-Martinez R, Villegas-Barreto C, Tolley EA, Lustig RH, Alpert BS. Racial disparity in glucagon-like peptide 1 and inflammation markers among severely obese adolescents. *Diabetes Care*. 2008;31:770–775.
7. Carnethon MR, Pu J, Howard G, Albert MA, Anderson CAM, Bertoni AG, Mujahid MS, Palaniappan L, Taylor HA, Willis M, Yancy CW. Cardiovascular health in African Americans: A scientific statement from the American Heart Association. *Circulation*. 2017;136:e393–e423.
8. Balfour PC, Jr., Ruiz JM, Talavera GA, Allison MA, Rodriguez CJ. Cardiovascular disease in Hispanics/Latinos in the United States. *Journal of Latina/o Psychology*. 2016;4:98–113.
9. Palaniappan L, Garg A, Enas E, Lewis H, Bari S, Gulati M, Flores C, Mathur A, Molina C, Narula J, Rahman S, Leng J, Gany F. South Asian cardiovascular disease & cancer risk: Genetics & pathophysiology. *Journal of Community Health*. 2018;43:1100–1114.
10. Breathett K, Sims M, Gross M, Jackson EA, Jones EJ, Navas-Acien A, Taylor H, Thomas KL, Howard BV. Cardiovascular health in American Indians and Alaska natives: A scientific statement from the American Heart Association. *Circulation*. 2020;141:e948–e959.
11. Mechanick JI, Adams S, Davidson JA, Fergus IV, Galindo RJ, McKinney KH, Petak SM, Sadhu AR, Samson SL, Vedanthan R, Umpierrez GE. Transcultural diabetes care in the United States - a position statement by the American Association of Clinical Endocrinologists. *Endocrine Practice*. 2019;25:729–765.
12. American Lung Association. Tobacco Use in Racial and Ethnic Populations. American Lung Association; 2020. Available online: https://www.lung.org/stop-smoking/smoking-facts/tobacco-use-racial-and-ethnic.html. Accessed January 17, 2023.
13. Virani SS, Alonso A, Aparicio HJ, Benjamin EJ, Bittencourt MS, Callaway CW, Carson AP, Chamberlain AM, Cheng S, Delling FN, Elkind MSV, Evenson KR, Ferguson JF, Gupta DK, Khan SS, Kissela BM, Knutson KL, Lee CD, Lewis TT, Liu J, Loop MS, Lutsey PL, Ma J, Mackey J, Martin SS, Matchar DB, Mussolino ME, Navaneethan SD, Perak AM, Roth GA, Samad Z, Satou GM, Schroeder EB, Shah SH, Shay CM, Stokes A, VanWagner LB, Wang NY, Tsao CW. Heart disease and stroke statistics-2021 update: A report from the American Heart Association. *Circulation*. 2021;143:e254–e743.
14. Institute for Health Metrics and Evaluation (IHME). Global Burden Disease (GBD) Compare tool. University of Washington. Available online: http://vizhub.Healthdata.Org/gbd-compare. Accessed on January 17, 2023.
15. U.S Department of Health and Human Services Office of Minority Health. Minority Population Profiles 2018. Available online: https://minorityhealth.hhs.gov/omh/browse.aspx?lvl=2&lvlid=26. Accessed January 17, 2023.
16. Hutchinson RN, Shin S. Systematic review of health disparities for cardiovascular diseases and associated factors among American Indian and Alaska native populations. *PLoS One*. 2014;9:e80973.
17. Baum A, Garofalo JP, Yali AM. Socioeconomic status and chronic stress: Does stress account for SES effects on health? *Annals of the New York Academy of Sciences*. 1999;896:131–144.
18. Cohen S, Doyle WJ, Baum A. Socioeconomic status is associated with stress hormones. *Psychosomatic Medicine*. 2006;68:414–420.

19. Pampel FC, Krueger PM, Denney JT. Socioeconomic disparities in health behaviors. *Annual Review of Sociology.* 2010;36:349–370.
20. Szanton SL, Gill JM, Allen JK. Allostatic load: A mechanism of socioeconomic health disparities? *Biological Research for Nursing.* 2005;7:7–15.
21. Duru OK, Harawa NT, Kermah D, Norris KC. Allostatic load burden and racial disparities in mortality. *Journal of the National Medical Association.* 2012;104: 89–95.
22. Geronimus AT, Hicken M, Keene D, Bound J. "Weathering" and age patterns of allostatic load scores among blacks and whites in the United States. *American Journal of Public Health.* 2006;96:826–833.
23. McEwen BS, Nasveld P, Palmer M, Anderson RJ. Allostatic load a review of the literature. Published by the department of veterans' affairs, Canberra, 2012. P02297. Available online: https://www.Dva.Gov.Au/health-and-wellbeing/research-and-development/health-studies/allostatic-load-review-literature. Accessed on May 2018.
24. Chyu L, Upchurch DM. Racial and ethnic patterns of allostatic load among adult women in the United States: Findings from the national health and nutrition examination survey 1999–2004. *Journal of Women's Health.* 2011;20:575–583.
25. Peek MK, Cutchin MP, Salinas JJ, Sheffield KM, Eschbach K, Stowe RP, Goodwin JS. Allostatic load among non-Hispanic whites, non-Hispanic blacks, and people of Mexican origin: Effects of ethnicity, nativity, and acculturation. *American Journal of Public Health.* 2010;100:940–946.
26. Lara M, Gamboa C, Kahramanian MI, Morales LS, Bautista DEH. Acculturation and Latino health in the United States: A review of the literature and its sociopolitical context. *Annual Review of Public Health.* 2005;26:367–397.
27. Hamdy O, Mechanick JI. Transcultural applications to lifestyle medicine. In: Mechanick, J, Kushner, R, ed. *Lifestyle medicine. A manual for clinical practice.* Switzerland: Springer; 2016: 363.
28. Hegazi RA, Devitt AA, Mechanick JI. The transcultural diabetes nutrition algorithm: From concept to implementation. In: Watson RR, Dokken BB, eds. *Glucose intake and utilization in pre-diabetes and diabetes implications for cardiovascular disease.* Amsterdam: Elsevier Inc.; 2015:269–280.
29. Mechanick JI, Marchetti AE, Apovian C, Benchimol AK, Bisschop PH, Bolio-Galvis A, Hegazi RA, Jenkins D, Mendoza E, Sanz ML, Sheu WH, Tatti P, Tsang MW, Hamdy O. Diabetes-specific nutrition algorithm: A transcultural program to optimize diabetes and prediabetes care. *Current Diabetes Reports.* 2012;12:180–194.
30. Mechanick JI, Harrell RM, Allende-Vigo MZ, Alvayero C, Arita-Melzer O, Aschner P, Camacho PM, Castillo RZ, Cerdas S, Coutinho WF, Davidson JA, Garber JR, Garvey WT, Gonzalez FJ, Granados DO, Hamdy O, Handelsman Y, Jimenez-Navarrete MF, Lupo MA, Mendoza EJ, Jimenez-Montero JG, Zangeneh F, American Association of Clinical Endocrinologists, American College of Endocrinology. Transculturalization recommendations for developing Latin American clinical practice algorithms in endocrinology--proceedings of the 2015 Pan-American workshop by the American Association of Clinical Endocrinologists and American College of Endocrinology. *Endocrine Practice.* 2016;22:476–501.
31. Su HY, Tsang MW, Huang SY, Mechanick JI, Sheu WH, Marchetti A. Transculturalization of a diabetes-specific nutrition algorithm: Asian application. *Current Diabetes Reports.* 2012;12:213–219.
32. Joshi SR, Mohan V, Joshi SS, Mechanick JI, Marchetti A. Transcultural diabetes nutrition therapy algorithm: The Asian Indian application. *Current Diabetes Reports.* 2012;12:204–212.

33. Hussein Z, Hamdy O, Chin Chia Y, Lin Lim S, Kumari Natkunam S, Hussain H, Yeong Tan M, Sulaiman R, Nisak B, Chee WS, Marchetti A, Hegazi RA, Mechanick JI. Transcultural diabetes nutrition algorithm: A Malaysian application. *International Journal of Endocrinology*. 2013;2013:679396.

34. Gougeon R, Sievenpiper JL, Jenkins D, Yale JF, Bell R, Despres JP, Ransom TP, Camelon K, Dupre J, Kendall C, Hegazi RA, Marchetti A, Hamdy O, Mechanick JI. The transcultural diabetes nutrition algorithm: A Canadian perspective. *International Journal of Endocrinology*. 2014;2014:151068.

35. Galvis AB, Hamdy O, Pulido ME, Haje VAR, Molina HAL, Sánchez MEM, Bárcena DG, Huici T, Marchetti A, Hegazi R, Mechanick J. Transcultural diabetes nutrition algorithm: The Mexican application. *Journal of Diabetes & Metabolism*. 2014;5:1–10. Doi:10.4172/2155-6156.1000423

36. Moura F, Salles J, Hamdy O, Coutinho W, Baptista DR, Benchimol A, Marchetti A, Hegazi RA, Mechanick JI. Transcultural diabetes nutrition algorithm: Brazilian application. *Nutrients*. 2015;7:7358–7380.

37. Nieto-Martínez R, Hamdy O, Marante D, Marulanda M, Marchetti A, Hegazi R, Mechanick J. Transcultural diabetes nutrition algorithm (tDNA): Venezuelan application. *Nutrients*. 2014;6:1333–1363.

38. Chee WSS, Gilcharan Singh HK, Hamdy O, Mechanick JI, Lee VKM, Barua A, Mohd Ali SZ, Hussein Z. Structured lifestyle intervention based on a trans-cultural diabetes-specific nutrition algorithm (tDNA) in individuals with type 2 diabetes: A randomized controlled trial. *BMJ Open Diabetes Research & Care*. 2017;5:e000384.

39. Bernal G, Bonilla J, Bellido C. Ecological validity and cultural sensitivity for outcome research: Issues for the cultural adaptation and development of psychosocial treatments with hispanics. *Journal of Abnormal Child Psychology*. 1995;23:67–82.

40. Mechanick JI, Hurley DL, Garvey WT. Adiposity-based chronic disease as a new diagnostic term: The American Association of Clinical Endocrinologists and American College of Endocrinology position statement. *Endocrine Practice*. 2017;23:372–378.

41. de Villiers A, Steyn NP, Draper CE, Hill J, Dalais L, Fourie J, Lombard C, Barkhuizen G, Lambert EV. Implementation of the Healthkick intervention in primary schools in low-income settings in the Western Cape Province, South Africa: A process evaluation. *BMC Public Health*. 2015;15:818.

42. World Health Organization (WHO). Social Determinants of Health. Available online: https://www.who.int/social_determinants/sdh_definition/en/. Accessed on January 17, 2023.

43. Rubinstein A, Miranda JJ, Beratarrechea A, Diez-Canseco F, Kanter R, Gutierrez L, Bernabé-Ortiz A, Irazola V, Fernandez A, Letona P, Martínez H, Ramirez-Zea M. Effectiveness of an mHealth intervention to improve the cardiometabolic profile of people with prehypertension in low-resource urban settings in Latin America: A randomised controlled trial. *The Lancet Diabetes & Endocrinology*. 2016;4: 52–63.

44. Halley MC, Petersen J, Nasrallah C, Szwerinski N, Romanelli R, Azar KMJ. Barriers and facilitators to real-world implementation of the diabetes prevention program in large healthcare systems: Lifestyle coach perspectives. *The Lancet Diabetes & Endocrinology*. 2020;35:1684–1692.

45. Dolan HR, Alvarez AA, Freylersythe SJ, Penaloza I, Grijalva S, Taylor-Piliae R. Barriers and facilitators for adopting a healthy lifestyle among Latina cancer survivors: A qualitative descriptive study. *Supportive Care in Cancer*. 2022;30: 2649–2659.

46. Rubino F, Puhl RM, Cummings DE, Eckel RH, Ryan DH, Mechanick JI, Nadglowski J, Ramos Salas X, Schauer PR, Twenefour D, Apovian CM, Aronne LJ, Batterham RL, Berthoud HR, Boza C, Busetto L, Dicker D, De Groot M, Eisenberg D, Flint SW,

Huang TT, Kaplan LM, Kirwan JP, Korner J, Kyle TK, Laferrère B, le Roux CW. Joint international consensus statement for ending stigma of obesity. *Nature Medicine.* 2020;26:485–497.

47. Mechanick JI, Farkouh ME, Newman JD, Garvey WT. Cardiometabolic-based chronic disease, adiposity and dysglycemia drivers: JACC state-of-the-art review. *Journal of the American College of Cardiology.* 2020;75:525–538.

48. Garvey WT, Mechanick JI, Brett EM, Garber AJ, Hurley DL, Jastreboff AM, Nadolsky K, Pessah-Pollack R, Plodkowski R. American Association of Clinical Endocrinologists and American College of Endocrinology comprehensive clinical practice guidelines for medical care of patients with obesity. *Endocrine Practice.* 2016;22(Suppl 3):1–203.

49. Lauby-Secretan B, Scoccianti C, Loomis D, Grosse Y, Bianchini F, Straif K. Body fatness and cancer — viewpoint of the IARC Working Group. *New England Journal of Medicine.* 2016;375:794–798.

50. Joseph RP, Ainsworth BE, Keller C, Dodgson JE. Barriers to physical activity among African American women: An integrative review of the literature. *Women & Health.* 2015;55:679–699.

51. Mechanick JI, Garber AJ, Grunberger G, Handelsman Y, Garvey WT. Dysglycemia-based chronic disease: An American Association of Clinical Endocrinologists position statement. *Endocrine Practice.* 2018;24:995–1011.

52. Ormazabal V, Nair S, Elfeky O, Aguayo C, Salomon C, Zuñiga FA. Association between insulin resistance and the development of cardiovascular disease. *Cardiovascular Diabetology.* 2018;17:122

53. Ritchie ND, Baucom KJW, Sauder KA. Current perspectives on the impact of the national diabetes prevention program: Building on successes and overcoming challenges. *Diabetes, Metabolic Syndrome and Obesity: Targets and Therapy.* 2020;13:2949–2957.

54. Cade WT. Diabetes-related microvascular and macrovascular diseases in the physical therapy setting. *Physical Therapy.* 2008;88:1322–1335.

55. Nathan DM, Davidson MB, DeFronzo RA, Heine RJ, Henry RR, Pratley R, Zinman B. Impaired fasting glucose and impaired glucose tolerance: Implications for care. *Diabetes Care.* 2007;30:753–759.

56. Havranek EP, Mujahid MS, Barr DA, Blair IV, Cohen MS, Cruz-Flores S, Davey-Smith G, Dennison-Himmelfarb CR, Lauer MS, Lockwood DW, Rosal M, Yancy CW. Social determinants of risk and outcomes for cardiovascular disease. *Circulation.* 2015;132:873–898.

57. Guzik TJ, Skiba DS, Touyz RM, Harrison DG. The role of infiltrating immune cells in dysfunctional adipose tissue. *Cardiovascular Research.* 2017;113:1009–1023.

58. Lee JJ, Pedley A, Hoffmann U, Massaro JM, Levy D, Long MT. Visceral and intrahepatic fat are associated with cardiometabolic risk factors above other ectopic fat depots: The Framingham Heart Study. *The American Journal of Medicine.* 2018;131:684–692.

59. Mechanick JI, Farkouh ME, Newman JD, Garvey WT. Cardiometabolic-based chronic disease, addressing knowledge and clinical practice gaps: JACC state-of-the-art review. *Journal of the American College of Cardiology.* 2020;75:539–555.

60. Wang JS, Tu ST, Lee IT, Lin SD, Lin SY, Su SL, Lee WJ, Sheu WH. Contribution of postprandial glucose to excess hyperglycaemia in Asian type 2 diabetic patients using continuous glucose monitoring. *Diabetes/Metabolism Research and Reviews.* 2011;27:79–84.

61. WHO Expert Consultation. Appropriate body-mass index for Asian populations and its implications for policy and intervention strategies. *The Lancet.* 2004;363:157–163.

62. Wallia S, Bhopal RS, Douglas A, Bhopal R, Sharma A, Hutchison A, Murray G, Gill J, Sattar N, Lawton J, Tuomilehto J, McKnight J, Forbes J, Lean M, Sheikh A. Culturally adapting the prevention of diabetes and obesity in South Asians (PODOSA) trial. *Health Promotion International.* 2014;29:768–779.

63. Chan EM, Cheng WM, Tiu SC, Wong LL. Postprandial glucose response to Chinese foods in patients with type 2 diabetes. *Journal of the American Dietetic Association.* 2004;104:1854–1858.

64. Alesina; AF, Easterly; W, Devleeschauwer; A, Kurlat; S, Wacziarg. RT. *Fractionalization.* Harvard Institute of Economic Research (No. 1959). Discussion Paper; 2002.

15 Socioeconomics and Infrastructure

Jeffrey I. Mechanick
Kravis Center for Cardiovascular Health at Mount Sinai Heart
Icahn School of Medicine at Mount Sinai

Michael A. Via
Icahn School of Medicine at Mount Sinai

CONTENTS

15.1 INTRODUCTION

Lifestyle medicine is foundational, first-line, necessary, and indefinite in the management of all chronic diseases, with cardiometabolic-based chronic disease (CMBCD) being no exception (1,2). Unfortunately, the explosion of scientific studies for pharmacological and procedural interventions to manage chronic diseases, especially in later stages, continues to outpace scientific studies in lifestyle medicine, especially in early stages. Nevertheless, "research gaps" and "knowledge gaps" in lifestyle medicine are steadily narrowing. In this context, the challenge of implementing scientific information in lifestyle medicine has emerged, and from a pragmatic standpoint, become paramount in narrowing "practice gaps." In this chapter, the two most important and prevailing impediments to implementing lifestyle medicine for the management of CMBCD will be explored: socioeconomics and infrastructure. This is followed by a discussion of specific implementation science tools and an exemplar that can illustrate how these tactics address the socioeconomic and infrastructural challenges.

15.2   SOCIOECONOMIC CHALLENGES

15.2.1   SOCIAL DETERMINANTS OF CARDIOMETABOLIC HEALTH

In the 2-dimensional driver-based chronic disease (-BCD) models (1,2), there are primary (genetics, environment, and behavior) and metabolic (adiposity-[ABCD; (3)], dysglycemia-[DBCD; (4)], hypertension-[HBCD], and lipid-[LBCD] based chronic disease) drivers that progress along four discrete stages in a target clinical space (e.g., cardiovascular disease; CMBCD). A third dimension is introduced with each cell populated by social determinants of health (SDOH), which can vary across ethno-cultural populations (Table 15.1; Figure 15.1) (5–29). Though conventional emphasis in cardiometabolic care has been placed on the biological determinants of health and modifiable risks that are part of lifestyle, SDOH confer a greater element of

---

TABLE 15.1
Social Determinants of Health that Increase Cardiometabolic Risk[a]

Determinant	Description
Childhood development	Allostatic stress; abnormally increased adiposity (5–7)
Crime	Allostatic stress; decreases perceived safety (8,9)
Culture	Ethno-cultural factors (10,11)
Discrimination/oppression	Structural conflict (12,13)
Disparities in access to quality healthcare	Correlates with ethno-cultural and socioeconomic factors (14)
Education	Correlates with health literacy and access to care (12,15–17)
Employment	Correlates with socioeconomic factors (15)
Food insecurity	Unhealthy dietary pattern (18,19)
Housing/amenities	Structural deterioration (20)
Income/poverty	Correlates with access to care (9,12,15,16,21,22–24)
Religion/spirituality (R/S)	In certain cultures, decreased R/S associated with increased risk (25,26)
Work conditions	Unhealthy lifestyle in many workplaces (27,28)

[a] References in parentheses.

1D →

2D ↓ **3D = SDOH**

METABOLIC DRIVERS	STAGE 1 (RISK)	STAGE 2 (PREDISEASE)	STAGE 3 (DISEASE)	STAGE 4 (COMPLICATIONS)
ABCD	PRIMARY DRIVERS UNHEALTHY LIFESTYLE ABNORMAL ENERGETICS	OVERWEIGHT ABNORMAL ADIPOSITY	OBESITY ABNORMAL ADIPOSITY	Obesity related
DBCD	PRIMARY DRIVERS UNHEALTHY LIFESTYLE INSULIN RESISTANCE	PREDIABETES	TYPE 2 DIABETES	MICROVASCULAR MACROVASCULAR
HBCD	PRIMARY DRIVERS UNHEALTHY LIFESTYLE Δ ORGAN/HORMONAL	PREHYPERTENSION	HYPERTENSION	Hypertension related
LBCD	PRIMARY DRIVERS UNHEALTHY LIFESTYLE Δ ORGAN/HORMONAL	ABNORMAL LIPID	DYSLIPIDEMIA	Lipid related
CMBCD	METABOLIC SYNDROME TRAITS	SUBCLINICAL CARDIOVASCULAR DYSFUNCTION	ASYMPTOMATIC CVD	SYMPTOMATIC CVD

Vertical prevention bands (left to right): PRIMORDIAL PREVENTION | PRIMARY PREVENTION | SECONDARY PREVENTION | TERTIARY PREVENTION

← QUATERNARY PREVENTION →

FIGURE 15.1 Three-dimensional driver-based chronic disease model for cardiometabolic risk. *Cardiometabolic*-based Chronic Disease results from the complex interactions of *metabolic* drivers (abnormal adiposity [ABCD], dysglycemia [DBCD], hypertension [HBCD], lipids [LBCD], and other metabolic syndrome traits) that drive chronic *cardio*vascular disease (e.g., atherosclerosis, heart failure, and atrial fibrillation). The three-dimensions of this model are 1D = stages, 2D = drivers, and 3D = SDOH. The purpose of this model is to expose phenotypic targets for action, facilitate early and sustainable prevention (primordial, primary, secondary, tertiary, and quaternary), and reduce chronic disease burden at individual and population scales. Each cell represents a unique coordinate of (stage, driver, and SDOH) to optimize precision for preventive care. Horizontal arrows correspond to the natural history of each driver and CMBCD, and typically progress stepwise to the right, except for (1) insulin resistance, which can also leapfrog forward to macrovascular diabetes complications and (2) prediabetes, which can revert to normoglycemia or leapfrog forward to macro- and microvascular diabetes complications. Vertical arrows correspond to the aggregate natural history of all metabolic drivers to a metabolic syndrome trait and subsequent CVD risk. Abbreviations: 1D, first dimension; 2D, second dimension; 3D, third dimension; ABCD, adiposity-based chronic disease; CMBCD, cardiometabolic-based chronic disease; CVD, cardiovascular disease; DBCD, dysglycemia-based chronic disease; HBCD, hypertension-based chronic disease; LBCD, lipid-based chronic disease; SDOH, social determinants of health (adapted from Nieto-Martinez et al. (29)).

precision in driver-BCD models. More specifically, by detecting a precise phenotypic coordinate (stage, driver, and SDOH) as early as possible, there should be a greater likelihood for sustainable reduction in chronic disease burden. In a 2015 Scientific Statement from the American Heart Association, a critical role for SDOH was detailed in the context of cardiovascular disease (30).

The SDOH are nonbiological/medical factors that impact health and health outcomes (31). For CMBCD, Emeny et al. (32) postulated that a SDOH-exposome (personalized aggregate of environmental exposures) creates a redox rheostat that regulates reduction/oxidation stress circuitry (e.g., mediating effects of pollutants on cardiovascular disease). Andreacchi et al. (33) found that by incorporating various SDOH into a latent class analysis of data from the Canadian Longitudinal Study on Aging, novel obesity risk classifications emerged. Other demonstrable effects of various SDOH include:

- placental programming for cardiometabolic risk with maternal exposure to particulate matter (air pollution) (34);
- early life adversities and resilience on cardiometabolic risk (6,7);
- social capital/networks on physical activity (35); and
- low community socioeconomic position on preclinical atherosclerosis (associated with flat cortisol diurnal slope) (21).

Moreover, many SDOH exert effects through interactions with specific cardiometabolic risk factors:

- television viewing inversely correlates with physical activity, a modifiable cardiovascular risk factor, particularly in socioeconomically disadvantaged adolescents (36);
- diet quality inversely correlates with a continuous cardiometabolic risk score in Chinese children (37); and
- neighborhood characteristics (education, income, unemployment, and green space) correlate with lifestyle factors (tobacco, alcohol, physical activity, and weight gain) (15).

Food insecurity has negative effects on cardiometabolic risk in many studies of adults (and programs [e.g., 2009 Supplemental Nutrition Assistance Program] that decrease food insecurity can reduce these risks; 18), but this effect is less clear in children (19). Many SDOH affect cardiometabolic risk factors in complex ways, as observed during the humanitarian crisis in Venezuela (38), and likely involve determinants focused on psychosocial variables (e.g., social relationships, interpersonal violence, sexual orientation and gender identity) (39) and allostatic load (40). In contrast to various stressors promoting cardiometabolic risk, economic transition (i.e., expansion and development as in China) can lead to abnormally increased body mass index (41).

In a structural model of how various SDOH impact the metabolic syndrome, low socioeconomic position was the strongest causal factor, perhaps mediated through physical activity and stress-related eating (22). In a longitudinal latent class analysis using data from the 1970 British Cohort Study, early adulthood (ages 16–24 years) socioeconomic stress independently contributed to later life cardiovascular inequalities (23). This was confirmed by a study by Lee et al. (24) using data from the National Longitudinal Study of Adolescent to Adult Health. In another study that analyzed subsamples from the Midlife in the U.S. dataset, chronic macroeconomic stressors widened the educational gap in the population, adversely impacting biological and anthropometric risk factors in the metabolic syndrome (16). Mechanistically, the primary drivers are interpreted holistically as biology (genetics) and SDOH (environment) interacting at the epigenetic and physiological levels (42,43), to result in a personalized healthy or unhealthy behavior and lifestyle, to then impel metabolic drivers leading to cardiovascular disease (CVD).

Approaches to SDOH are implemented on two levels: patient (goal-oriented with focus on individual outcomes) and population (process-oriented with focus on broad-reaching policies). Efforts to address a pathological environment (e.g., obesogenic and/or diabetogenic) are very difficult, but can be accomplished through collaboration among healthcare professionals (HCPs; physicians, nurses, dietitians, advance practice providers, etc.) to create policies, beginning on a small scale (e.g., local/municipal) and then expanding to larger scales (e.g., state and federal). Robinson et al. (17) showed that a novel multi-level, multi-setting, multi-component intervention, based on behavioral change theory and cultural tailoring, was superior to a nutrition and health education control intervention to reduce body mass index in low socioeconomic class Latino/Hispanic children over 1 and 2 years. Among African American men, a high cardiometabolic risk population, the Black Barbershop Health Outreach Program was effective at hypertension and diabetes screening (44). The process of patient-centered care involves genuine interest in one's lifestyle with appropriate dialog about family, workplace, and recreational factors, as well as sources of structured conflict and deterioration, adversities due to the built environment, and lifestyle preferences. From this information, key SDOH can be identified for individual patients, leading to problem-solving discussions over multiple encounters. Drake et al. (45) demonstrated a correlation between social needs screening assessment data and cardiometabolic risk, affirming the need for validated predictive instruments for risk stratification, especially those that are sensitive to ethnocultural differences in SDOH.

15.2.2 Transcultural Factors

With an overarching premise to provide high-quality cardiometabolic lifestyle medicine care to all people, there must be a calculus to tailor interventions efficiently, without wasted resources or needless cost, based on objective assessments. This is the basic principle of quaternary prevention – to minimize overmedicalization. Nonbiological attributes of human beings cluster into meaningful categories defined by SDOH. In spite of a subtle distinction, transcultural factors are those SDOH that vary from one ethnicity to another. From a cardiometabolic standpoint, the major transcultural factors are dietary patterns, physical activity, behavior, sleep patterns, structured conflict and deterioration (i.e., poverty, crime, discrimination, housing, and education), religion and spirituality, and community engagement. The positive association of these transcultural factors with cardiometabolic risk has been demonstrated in Western (10) and Asian countries (11).

Transculturalization is the process of adapting transcultural factors in evidence-based clinical recommendations from a source population to a target population (46–48). A transculturalized CMBCD model has been validated by several reports concentrating on how the ABCD, DBCD, and CMBCD models differentially correlate transcultural cardiometabolic risk factors with specific cardiovascular endpoints in distinct populations (49–56). Most recently in the CARDIA study of young adults in four U.S. communities (12), the following transcultural factors differentially impacted "Black-White" CVD risk: discrimination, biological weathering, psychosocial stress, income status, education level, geocoding (a measure of segregation), diet quality, fast-food availability, and sedentary activity.

15.2.3 HEALTHCARE SYSTEM ECONOMICS

Cardiometabolic outcomes have improved of late but still fall short of expectations given recent advancements in basic and translational scientific research, clinical trials, technology (e.g., pharmaceuticals and procedures), and clinical practice guidelines. There are many explanations for this shortcoming, such as inadequate and inconsistent lifestyle change, poor attention to SDOH, inadequate implementation of preventive care, and most notably, the overarching impact of economics. In theory, economic considerations for clinical decision-making are predicated on the avoidance of unnecessary, expensive interventions, presuming that payments are made. However, in practice, evidence-based, guideline-directed prudent interventions, especially preventive lifestyle measures, are all too often poorly reimbursed, or not reimbursed at all. Standard fee-for-service payment models tend to reward high-cost care models, though alternative payment models (e.g., capitated per-member-per-month) may achieve similar levels of preventive care at lower cost (57). In effect, the management of CMBCD is hamstrung by inadequate reimbursement of necessary lifestyle medicine interventions, essentially forcing infrastructural changes and new implementation models.

The socioeconomic health gradient accounts for inequalities in cardiometabolic health. Among the many factors influencing this gradient, health behaviors (especially those pertaining to tobacco use) have proven to be the most important (58). Another dimension of socioeconomics in the cardiometabolic space relates to economic impact of different risk factors. Traditionally, adverse effects of cardiometabolic risks, alone or in combination, are considered linearly in terms of direct effects on healthcare expenses, lost wages, and decreased productivity (59). However, in a study on obesity and hospitalization by Gupta and Sheng (60), the adverse economic impact of abnormal adiposity was related more to the associated CMBCD and efforts to mitigate CMBCD stage progression than simply promoting weight loss and addressing ABCD alone. This observation is consistent with the driver-based chronic disease model paradigm.

One economic aspect of cardiometabolic care pertains to the timing and nature of *de-escalation*. This process is not only applied to the permissive decrease in a particular intervention and generally applies to pharmacotherapy, but it can also be applied to lifestyle interventions (e.g., decreased frequency of dietitian counseling sessions, liberalization of dietary recommendations, and less frequent/intense physical activity). The timing for de-escalation generally corresponds to an improved clinical/biochemical state, and though not always done nor guided by scientific evidence, it is justified by greater long-term adherence/sustainability, patient empowerment, and lower financial costs. The unwillingness for de-escalation on the part of the HCP is likely due to clinical training and a culture focused on escalation, as well as a dearth of scientific research on the topic. However, the willingness of de-escalation on the part of the patient is centered more on trust and inclusion in the decision-making process, rather than awareness of and attitudes about specific interventions (61).

15.3 INFRASTRUCTURAL CHALLENGES

Traditionally, cardiometabolic decision-making has been steeped in scientific evidence, which is predominantly pharmacologic, but well represented by lifestyle medicine.

Unfortunately, most lifestyle recommendations are not effectively implemented. This failing is in large part due to a lack of infrastructure that provides easily and promptly accessible counseling/instruction in nutrition, exercise, behavior, wearable technology use, etc. Infrastructure addresses the following domains of quality: patient experience, effectiveness, efficiency, timeliness, safety, equity, and sustainability (62). Three aspects of infrastructural change for cardiometabolic care are critical: the built environment, defragmentation, and creation of the lifestyle medicine center (LMC).

The built environment is human-made (super-size portions, running trails, elevators, unsafe commuting, etc.), in contrast to natural factors (climate, terrain, geography, etc.). There are various supporting elements to the built environment, including public services (urban infrastructure; (63)), public policy (especially on food prices, formulation, marketing, labeling, and assistance (64); e.g., National Menu Calorie Labeling Law (65), U.S. Food and Drug Administration Added Sugar Labeling Policy (66), and U.S. National Salt and Sugar Reduction Initiative (67)), equipment, information technology, accessibility, systems and processes, and human resources (62). As an example, the built environment can facilitate physical activity through better pedestrian/bicycle transportation systems, land use, and environmental design (68). Overall, the healthfulness of a built environment is inversely related to cardiometabolic risk (69). Beyond objective measures, even perceptions can make a difference. In a cross-sectional study in Australia by Baldock et al. (8), perceptions of increased walkable land, positive aesthetics, and less crime were associated with decreased metabolic syndrome occurrence. Moreover, according to a multi-level social-ecological framework, geospatial ("place-based") mismatches in the exposome will need to be addressed in order to reduce disparities in cardiometabolic risk (70).

Safety at home is a major concern when developing infrastructure. For instance, violence and discrimination, lack of sidewalks, and unleashed dogs are significant barriers to outdoor recreation, physical activity, and exercise in Black communities (13). Moreover, racial profiling and hypervigilance limit access to White communities (13). Both of these scenarios further disparities between Blacks and Whites in cardiometabolic health (13). Community intervention is often required to address food and pharmacy deserts that occur in areas typically more densely populated, with more renters than owners, more residents speaking English as a second language, less vehicle ownership, more people living under the federal poverty level, more Black and Latino/Hispanic residents, higher crime rates, and less available HCPs (9). These principles also apply to the workplace, where health promotion with more physical activity and higher diet quality impact cardiometabolic health (27). In a South African study on transforming the workplace to decrease cardiometabolic risk, four areas of change were identified: catering services, sports and physical activities, health and wellness services, and managerial support (28).

In the multi-morbidity chronic care model, there is typically more than one chronic condition afflicting a person and contributing to decreased quality of life and increased societal costs. The main challenge in addressing this complex healthcare problem begins with better characterization of chronic diseases, not only simply counting occurrences but also understanding interactions among different conditions and how they impact overall health (71). The problem is further challenged by implementing structured lifestyle interventions as part of comprehensive preventive care in various settings through life cycle, which is punctuated by acute events. To this end, community health workers can be better utilized to broaden the reach of and facilitate quality cardiometabolic care, especially in low-to-middle income areas (72).

Fragmentation of healthcare results from incomplete information and can compromise multi-morbid chronic care (73). Defragmentation primarily relates to a seamless model of clinical decision-making among different HCPs (e.g., integrating primary and specialty care into collaborative teams), settings (e.g., integrating outpatient and inpatient care to reduce rehospitalization), and administrative scenarios (e.g., integrating government, third-party payers, and different practice models to enhance efficiency, affordability, and access) (74–76). Defragmentation is facilitated by information technology that integrates and directs SDOH, medical/surgical management, and patient-generated data to a repository (electronic health record) for distribution as needed to patients, HCPs, and researchers (73). Defragmentation also applies to streamlining regulatory processes and relevant cost-benefit analyses, largely by minimizing or eliminating redundant policies and statutes (e.g., the Regulatory Flexibility and Paperwork Reduction Acts) (76). In effect, defragmentation of healthcare, especially the lifestyle medicine approach to cardiometabolic risk, which is still replete with incomplete knowledge, is necessitated though creative process (77).

The LMC is a real-world facility that addresses the above infrastructural challenges involving the built environment and fragmentation of healthcare delivery. Key aspects of a LMC strategy with core tactics have been detailed elsewhere (78) and are summarized below:

1. targeting primary and metabolic drivers in the multi-morbidity chronic care model with early and sustainable lifestyle change;
2. funding and identifying champions, teams, and needed resources for organizational preparedness;
3. materialization (conceptualization and operationalization) and optimization;
4. creation of clinical service lines, preventive care protocols and policies, and immersive physical and nonphysical environments; and
5. integration with community and attention to spirituality and culture.

15.4   IMPLEMENTATION SCIENCE

A major shortcoming in lifestyle medicine pertains to the translation of knowledge into action. Whereas strategy comprises a theoretical framework and set of long-term goals, tactics refer to near-term actions that allow realization of those goals. Implementation science is a formalism that focuses on factors along with outcomes, assists with tactical planning, and in the case of lifestyle medicine, is a major determinant of success. With respect to a strategic plan, the deliverables of implementation science are acceptability, adoption, appropriateness, feasibility, fidelity, cost, penetration, and sustainability (79). To achieve these deliverables, the following actions are recommended: engage a broad range of stakeholders to identify gaps and coproduce a knowledge base and strategic plan; build capacity to optimize delivery of interventions; and provide suitable training and resources (79). In addition, economic evaluation is a critical component of implementation science in healthcare and has been recently reviewed by Eisman et al. (80).

More implementation studies are needed to better align the rapid pace of clinical trial results with the sluggish adoption of these results into guideline-directed therapy (81). Implementation research is based on four models of causation (intervention theory [how plans/actions are built], framework [the structure of these plans/actions], middle-range theory [governing ideas between the routine and all-inclusive], and grand theory [explanations of social behavior, organization, and change]) and three methodological types (fidelity assessment [extent of intended implementation], process evaluation [factors affecting implementation], and complex evaluation [relating interventions and outcomes in different contexts]) (82).

Data-driven, value-based decision-making in cardiometabolic lifestyle medicine is needed to better prioritize coverage and care at multiple scales (81). Cross-domain (clinical medicine, research, social/behavioral science, marketing, economics, and public policy) collaboration will also be needed (83). As an example, this might take the form of community-based diabetes prevention programs that emphasize lifestyle medicine and not solely pharmacotherapy (84). Another example might be the study of "nudges" (predictably influencing behavior without restricting choice) on lifestyle to reduce cardiometabolic risk (85). These nudges can identify opportunities to improve care, measure various processes/outcomes, implement pragmatic actions, align stakeholders, compare effectiveness, and translate findings to scale (85).

15.4.1 GAPS

15.4.1.1 Research

Research gaps are "questions without answers." An example would include "What is the epidemiological association between abnormal adiposity, namely Stage 3 ABCD or Obesity, with COVID-19 severity?" Scientific substantiation of lifestyle interventions is oftentimes limited with these gaps typically filled by reported experience and opinion, but also potentially harmful unsubstantiated claims. The LMC can be a highly valued instrument in discovery science (i.e., epidemiological findings from mining registry data), prospective cohort studies, and randomized clinical trials, but a research agenda needs to be identified as these facilities are planned and developed. Research gaps can be exposed with scoping reviews and then followed up with systematic reviews, clinical practice guidelines, and a comprehensive knowledge translation platform that prioritizes pragmatism and relevance, over silo-thinking and self-interests, by stakeholders (86). This research platform can be part of routine LMC operations.

15.4.1.2 Knowledge

Knowledge gaps are "answers without awareness." An example would include the lack of recommendations for a healthier lifestyle and more aggressive obesity management in many areas of the world during the first wave of the COVID-19 pandemic, but after the initial associations of obesity with severe COVID-19 were published. In general, this applies to stakeholders involved with lifestyle medicine: HCPs, administrative staff, patients, third-party insurers, government decision-makers, community leaders, industry, etc. Knowledge gaps can also be exposed with scoping reviews, but they need to be addressed by formal educational and training programs. These programs can be incorporated into the planning and operations of a LMC as part of dedicated activities (face-to-face, web/cloud-based, or part of community engagement) and even construction of a lecture/conference room with audio/visual capabilities.

15.4.1.3 Practice

Practice gaps are "awareness without action." An example would include the paucity of fully operational LMCs specializing in healthy lifestyle, weight loss, obesity management, and preventive cardiology for all populations to prevent severe COVID and manage unhealthy behaviors from daily routine changes. This gap represents the crux of the LMC implementation problem: to translate strategy into tactics and successful, real-world outcomes on individual- and population-based scales. Practice gaps are exposed with systematic reviews and addressed with clinical practice guidelines, but having the human and physical resources at hand is what facilitates the implementation.

15.4.2   Logistics

In order to better understand and then implement measures that address research, knowledge, and practice gaps, it is necessary to apply structure, or an easily interpretable set of logistical steps, to the process.

15.4.2.1   Inception

After a deliberate, or even incidental, process of recognizing the gaps associated with lifestyle medicine (interpreted as a "need"), and then by consensus, recognizing there is a clear opportunity, healthcare leadership decides and commits to the creation of a *bona fide* LMC as part of an overarching strategy for preventive care for cardiometabolic health. After inception by leadership, funding and structure need to be discussed. Typically, funds are limited, but depending on institutional priorities, a funding level commensurate with the strategic plan begins the process. Ultimately, this culminates in a clinical service line in preventive cardiology or lifestyle medicine, with subordinated and dedicated programs mandated to a scale appropriate for the prespecified funding level, allowing for sustainability and growth over time. Integral to this inception process, and contemporaneously incorporated in the funding/structure steps above, is the creation of a mission statement, vision statement, strategic plan, and operational plan, followed by an organizational structure once human resources are delineated.

15.4.2.2   Champions

Perhaps the most important component of any successful initiative in healthcare delivery, particularly in the lesser-known field of lifestyle medicine, is identifying and empowering a champion – a person with leadership, managerial, and organization skills, as well as having an innovative and unique vision with ready access to necessary resources. Champions are already motivated and have likely formulated strategies and tactical approaches based on their own personal experiences and aspirations, but are simply lacking the necessary ingredients of timing, political support, teams, appropriate technologies, and most often, funding. Nevertheless, the first step after the inception of the LMC idea is an environmental scan for champions, a diligent selection/interview process, and then forging a firm commitment, anywhere from a handshake to a formal contract. One example of a champion in lifestyle medicine to diminish cardiometabolic risk is the diabetes care and education specialist, who provides leadership to a diabetes team, expertise with state-of-the-art diabetes technology (such as wearables), and the ability to defragment comprehensive diabetes and cardiometabolic care within the multi-morbid chronic care model (87,88). Another example of a champion is a peer who can lead exercise programs for older adults (89).

15.4.2.3 Teams

Once a champion in lifestyle medicine is identified to shepherd the LMC creation process, a leadership team must be assembled. Though leadership team members may be suggested by the institutional leadership during the inception process, it is critical that the champion have significant input. Leadership team members should be selected based on several desired (but not necessary) qualities:

- history of successful collaborations with the champion;
- skillset consistent with the problem at hand, namely creating and operating an LMC;
- potential for independent thinking and being a "force multiplier" (more effect for same effort);
- personality conducive to productive activities; and
- part of a diverse team, with respect to knowledge base, personality, experience, and capability as a constructive disruptor.

This diligent "prework" in assembling a highly qualified and functional team is a necessary step to assure correct decision-making and success of the LMC enterprise.

15.4.2.4 Resources

15.4.2.4.1 Physical

The physical resource component of the implementation process is identified according to three initial stages. In the first stage, knowledge, practice gaps, and how theses gaps can be closed with creation of a LMC are translated into action plans. The second stage is materialization, beginning with the first step – conceptualization – in terms of physical structure, design and architecture for an immersive (physical) environment, patient flow, and necessary supporting services and equipment (90). This is followed by the third stage or building out the conceived physical structure. Subsequent scale up (adding more services) and/or scale out (adding more locations) will require measured changes in this implementation process.

15.4.2.4.2 Human

Operationalization of the strategic plan is the second step of the materialization process, to be performed following conceptualization and building out, and ultimately takes the form of policies. These policies are spawned from beliefs vetted during the inception stage and manifested in the mission and vision statements. Once broad policies are agreed upon, then specific protocols can be devised and saved as enduring material, to be updated at regular intervals based on performance metrics or changes in strategic/operational goals.

The human resource component of this operationalization process extends from the above champion and leadership team, to include a compliment of faculty and staff that best match the mission, vision, strategy, and operational parameters of the enterprise. This fleshing out process, where detail takes the form of personnel with minimal gaps and acceptable redundancy, defines the organization structure and consists of a managerial template. There are three basic modalities for management that can be applied to a LMC for CMBCD care, ranging from a smaller scale single center to mid-level scale single center, to larger scale multi-center enterprise:

1. **Vertical**: a pyramidal top-down system where everyone has defined roles and accountability (higher levels control middle levels, who control lower levels), but decision-making and implementation can be slow with little autonomy and imagination, except where specific silos exist; this vertical format is typical and amenable to routine situations where a high level of structure is needed;

2. **Horizontal**: a more collaborative system that encourages shared decision-making, particularly at the lower levels, fostering autonomy and imagination but with more risk-taking and less guidance (there can be more conflict); this horizontal format may be more appropriate when there is a narrow time window for decision-making (e.g., a crisis) where efficiency and brainstorming are more valuable; and

3. **Diagonal**: a hybrid system with sharing of information and tasks among different levels, but care needs to be taken not to bypass critical persons; this diagonal format has a variable structure and can be tailored to a specific need at a specific time.

15.4.2.5   Community

The term community engagement is frequently used to describe not only an element of individual lifestyle change but also an element of how a LMC interacts and even guides urban infrastructure. In the first element, patients apply their life priorities to activities in the community setting (e.g., municipal center, school, house of worship, or charitable entity). In the second element, the LMC itself develops relationships with the neighboring built environment and public need.

15.4.2.6   Financial

Once operations begin, the financial status of the LMC requires dedicated and diligent monitoring by one or more members of the leadership team. The financial goal for the LMC has already been set (e.g., revenue neutrality for a mission that provides care to a large segment of patients in a lower socioeconomic class; or profit for a mission that provides care to population with sufficient out-of-pocket payments), and profit–loss statements need to be carefully monitored to ensure success and sustainability of the implementation efforts.

15.4.3 Technology

Leveraging technology is a critical component of implementation science. Technological advancements march to a much faster beat than behavioral trends and changes in clinical practice. These advancements must therefore be closely monitored, anticipated, and acted upon. Technology takes many forms, from cybersecurity and computing, to stand-alone devices and equipment, to wearables and cloud-based functions (91).

In a Scientific Statement from the American Heart Association in 2021 based on a systematic review of the literature (26 studies) (92), mobile health technologies were able to successively address implementation challenges in secondary CVD prevention, in the elderly, related to health behaviors and medication adherence. In Latin America, mobile technologies can address CMBCD by defragmenting care across an expanding mobile phone network involving the patient, HCP, and public, despite socioeconomic strains (93). Response rates are an important factor determining the cost-effectiveness and success of a preventive cardiology program. In a Dutch randomized controlled trial (94), the response rates of email invitations and digital reminders were comparable with those of standard face-to-face, written, telephonic, and mailed communications, but at lower cost and investment time, effectively improving implementation processes. Wearable physical activity trackers have provided valuable correlative information regarding cardiometabolic risk (95). In another Dutch study (96), technological nudges using a physical activity mobile app combined with supermarket-based healthy food choices and pricing strategies promoted healthy lifestyles in a low socioeconomic population.

Technology can also be leveraged across platforms to improve implementation. One example is a community-based registry (anthropometrics, cardiometabolic health assessment, and laboratory testing) and biorepository (serum, DNA, and RNA) to identify biocultural determinants of disparities affecting obesity and T2D care in the Latino community (97). On the contrary, technology oftentimes needs to be scaled down in order to reach implementation goals. As an example, in Esino Lario – a small mountain village in Northern Italy – a point-to-point telehealth infrastructure was devised and found to be feasible using off-the-shelf instruments, nonfasting lipid and metabolic biochemical markers, and nonmedical personnel (after brief training) (98).

An environmental scan should be performed during the conceptualization stage of physical resourcing to identify current available technologies based on services and operations, capabilities of available human resources, and cost factors guided by the business plan. An inventory of these items should be maintained and upgraded based on prevailing needs and perceived state-of-the-art to optimize CMBCD care in the LMC. Depending on the parameters identified during inception, a focus can then be better realized through an investment in innovative technology (i.e., significantly more advanced that what is typically used).

15.4.4 Sustainability

A key factor for success in any implementation effort is for the effect to last. This involves the following attributes: engagement of force multipliers (persons or technologies that increase effect from the same effort), nudges (e.g., electronic health record, wearable technologies, phone calls, electronic communications, regular face-to-face or virtual encounters, and cloud-based apps), adaptation (deliberate vertical escalation and de-escalation, coupled with horizontal thinking), and of course, success (theoretical/perceived, clinical outcomes, and economic viability).

At the HCP level, best practice alerts are nudges that can promote sustainability through guideline-directed care, deterrence of adverse events, and adaptation over time (e.g., using rapid-cycle randomized testing in a learning health system) (99). In addition, sustainability can occur through advanced training in preventive cardiology according to several models: endocrinology with specialization in cardiovascular disease; cardiology with specialization in prevention; or a dedicated cardiometabolic residency/fellowship program (100,101)

At an individual patient level, sustainability depends on a validated and consistently practiced behavioral medicine approach, consisting of motivational interviewing, positive messaging, and activation for change. Subsequent nudging is critical for durable benefits (91). An immersive nonphysical environment can nurture this process and is mediated by human resources and facilitated by policies and protocols (102). Immersive characteristics include friendly greetings, easy interfaces with technologies, in-person navigation with multiple "touches" (human caring through interaction) and warm hand-offs (e.g., direct/personal communications from navigator to medical assistant, medical assistant to clinician, clinician to advanced practice provider, advanced practice provider to nutritionist, nutritionist to exercise physiologist, and so forth), and efficient patient flow (102). Each of these activities requires ongoing training, evaluation, and optimization.

At a population level, critical features that can promote long-lasting success of a cardiometabolic LMC include community engagement and value to the urban infrastructure. This requires not only thought and planning, best applied during the inception stage, but also the scaled up and/or out LMC. Lessons about public program sustainability learned from the *Salud al Paso* initiative for chronic disease prevention in Ecuador include the following: incorporating a research program from the outset; monitoring adherence; reporting technical evidence to government overseers; fostering loyalty among human resources mainly through job security; improving screening processes especially in rural communities; and coordinating with other health institutions, ministries of public health, and various service networks (103). School-based lifestyle programs are critical for durable effects on cardiometabolic risk reduction. In a meta-analysis of 19 randomized controlled trials ($N = 11,988$ children aged 3–12 years), there was a significant initial improvement in waist circumference, diastolic blood pressure, and fasting insulin levels (104). Although feasible, long-term benefits remain to be demonstrated for this population.

15.4.4.1 Exemplars

The Center for Clinical Cardiovascular Health at Mount Sinai Heart is an example of a preventive cardiology clinical service line, integrating cardiac rehabilitation (with direct referrals from the cardiac catherization laboratory and inpatient cardiac surgery service), clinical cardiology and endocrinology, and lifestyle medicine programs within a large healthcare system in New York City (105). The principal mandate for the center was to create structure for early, successful, and sustainable change that prevented CMBCD progression, but with accessibility and affordability for all. From 2018 (year 1) to 2019 (year 2), there were significant increases in number of appointments, number of sessions, phase III cardiac rehabilitation volume, and medical fitness volume (105). Subsequently to 2022 (year 5), this program has continued to scale up with general medicine and infectious diseases clinical care, independent roles for advanced practice providers, diabetes technology (sensor and pump management), obesity care, wellness (primary prevention programs), specialty care (e.g., dedicated dysautonomia and peripheral arterial disease programs), and an expanded cloud-based educational webinar program. Clinical performance metrics after 5 years of operations will be analyzed and presented in 2022–2023. Other examples of LMCs providing effective cardiometabolic care that address socioeconomic and infrastructural challenges have been recently spotlighted: The Rippe Lifestyle Institute (106) and Northwestern Medicine Center for Lifestyle Medicine (107) in the United States, as well as many others globally (108).

15.5 CONCLUSIONS

The successful practice of lifestyle medicine is challenged by research, knowledge, and practice gaps, as well as implementation shortfalls unduly influenced by lack of standards of care, misinterpretation of markets, and a backdrop that fails to recognize the critical importance of preventive care. Management of CMBCD is not immune to these pressures, but it is possible to engineer successful and durable solutions. The key take-home points for creating a lifestyle medicine practice that focuses on cardiometabolic care, while also addressing socioeconomic and infrastructural challenges, are as follows:

1. begin with a robust, moderately ambitious, inception phase where the process is impelled by a clear, well-thought-out mission statement, vision statement, strategic plan, and business plan;
2. concurrently or subsequently, perform an environmental scan for local urban infrastructural, transcultural, and economic factors that impact patients' cardiometabolic profiles and preventive care needs;
3. then, implement tactics for translation, materialization (conceptualization and operationalization), organization, optimization, and potential scaling-up and scaling-out.

There are many research, knowledge, and practice gaps that need to be closed in cardiometabolic lifestyle medicine so that performance metrics can improve, clinical and economic burdens of CMBCD can decline, and overall population health can reach desired levels.

Disclosures:
Jeffrey I. Mechanick received honoraria from Abbott Nutrition for lectures and serves on the Advisory Boards for Aveta.Life and Twin Health.

REFERENCES

1. Mechanick JI, Farkouh ME, Newman JD, Garvey WT. Cardiometabolic-based chronic disease – adiposity and dysglycemia drivers. *J Am Coll Cardiol* 2020; 75: 525–538.
2. Mechanick JI, Farkouh ME, Newman JD, Garvey WT. Cardiometabolic-based chronic disease – addressing knowledge and clinical practice gaps in the preventive care plan. *J Am Coll Cardiol* 2020; 75: 539–555.
3. Mechanick JI, Hurley DL, Garvey WT. Adiposity-based chronic disease as a new diagnostic term: American Association of Clinical Endocrinologists and the American College of Endocrinology position statement. *Endocr Pract* 2017; 23: 372–378.
4. Mechanick JI, Garber AJ, Grunberger G, Handelsman Y, Garvey WT. Dysglycemia-based chronic disease: an American Association of Clinical Endocrinologists position statement. *Endocr Pract* 2018; 24: 995–1011.
5. Van Hulst A, Ybarra M, Mathieu M, et al. Determinants of new onset cardiometabolic risk among normal weight children. *Int J Obes* 2020; 44: 781–789.
6. Suglia SF, Appleton AA, Bleil ME, et al. Timing, duration, and differential susceptibility to early life adversities and cardiovascular disease risk across the lifespan: implications for future research. *Preventive Med* 2021; 153: 106736, doi:10.1016/j.ypmed.2021.106736.
7. Jimenez V, Sanchez N, Clark ELM, et al. Associations of adverse childhood experiences with stress physiology and insulin resistance in adolescents at risk for adult obesity. *Develop Psychobiol* 2021; 63: e22127.
8. Baldock K, Paquet C, Howard N, et al. Associations between resident perceptions of the local resident environment and metabolic syndrome. *J Environ Public Health* 2012; 2021: 589409, doi:10.1155/2012/589409.
9. Wisseh C, Hildreth K, Marshall J, et al. Social determinants of pharmacy deserts in Los Angeles county. *Racial Ethn Health Disparities* 2020, doi:10.1007/s40615-020-00904-6.
10. Johnson-Lawrence V, Zajacova A, Sneed R. Education, race/ethnicity, and multimorbidity among adults aged 30–64 in the National Health Interview Survey. *SSM Popul Health.* 2017; 3: 366–372.
11. Wang Y, Tan NC, Jafar TH. Ethnic variation, socioeconomic status, and factors associated with cardio-metabolic multi-morbidity among uncontrolled hypertension in multiethnic Singapore. *J Human Hypertension* 2021, doi:10.1038/s41371-020-00457-5.
12. Lloyd-Jones DM, Lewis CE, Schreiner PJ, et al. The Coronary artery risk development in young adults (CARDIA) study. *J Am Coll Cardiol* 2021; 78: 260–277.
13. Hornbuckle LM. Running while Black: a distinctive safety concern and barrier to exercise in White neighborhoods. *Prev Med Rep* 2021; 22: 101378.
14. Riley WJ. Health disparities: gaps in access, quality and affordability of medical care. *Trans Am Clin Climatol Assoc* 2012; 123: 167–174.
15. Kivimaki M, Batty GD, Pentti J, et al. Modifications to residential neighbourhood characteristics and risk of 79 common health conditions: a prospective cohort study. *Lancet Public Health* 2021; 6: e396–e407.
16. Jiang Y, Boylan JM, Zilioli S. Effects of the great recession on educational disparities in cardiometabolic health. *Ann Behav Med* 2021; 1–4, doi:10.1093/abm/kaab065.
17. Robinson TN, Matheson D, Wilson DM, et al. A community-based, multi-level, multi-setting, multi-component intervention to reduce weight gain among low socioeconomic status Latinx children with overweight or obesity: the Stanford GOALS randomized controlled trial. *Lancet Diabetes Endocrinol* 2021; 9: 336–349.
18. Samuel LJ, Szanton SL, Wolff JL, et al. Supplemental nutrition assistance program 2009 expansion and cardiometabolic markers among low-income adults. *Preventive Med* 2021; 150: 106678.

19. Te Vazquez J, Feng SN, Orr CJ, et al. Food insecurity and cardiometabolic conditions: a review of recent research. *Curr Nutrition Rep* 2021; doi:10.1007/s13668-021-00364-2.

20. Sims M, Kershaw KN, Breathett K, et al. Importance of housing and cardiovascular health and well-being: a scientific statement from the American Heart Association. *Circulation Cardiovasc Qual Outcomes* 2020; 13, doi:10.1161/HCQ.0000000000000089

21. Miller KG, Gianaros PJ, Kamarck TW, et al. Cortisol activity partially accounts for a relationship between community socioeconomic position and atherosclerosis. *Psychoneuroendocrinology* 2021; 131: 105292, doi:10.1016/j.psyneuen.2021.105292.

22. Smith KW, Krieger N, Kosheleva A, et al. A structural model of social determinants of the metabolic syndrome. *Ethnicity Dis* 2020; 30: 331–336.

23. Winpenny EM, Howe LD, van Sluijs EMF, et al. Early adulthood socioeconomic trajectories contribute to inequalities in adult cardiovascular health, independently of childhood and adulthood socioeconomic position. *J Epidemiol Community Health* 2021; 75: 1172–1180, doi:10.1136/jech-2021-216611.

24. Lee TK, Wickrama KAS, O'Neal CW. How early stressful life experiences combine with adolescents' conjoint health risk trajectories to influence cardiometabolic disease risk in young adulthood. *J Youth Adolescence* 2021; 50: 1234–1253.

25. Hemmati R, Bidel Z, Nazarzadeh M, et al. Religion, spirituality and risk of coronary heart disease: a matched case-control study and meta-analysis. *J Relig Health* 2019; 58: 1203–1216.

26. Kobayashi D, Shimbo T, Takahashi O, et al. The relationship between religiosity and cardiovascular risk factors in Japan: a large-scale cohort study. *J Am Soc Hypertens* 2015; 9: 553–562.

27. Amil S, Lemieux I, Poirier P, et al. Targeting diet quality at the workplace: influence on cardiometabolic risk. *Nutrients* 2021; 13: 2283.

28. Schouw D, Mash R, Kolbe-Alexander T. Transforming the workplace environment to prevent non-communicable chronic diseases: participatory action research in a South African power plant. *Global Health Action* 2018; 11: 1544336.

29. Nieto-Martinez R, Gonzalez-Rivas JP, Mechanick JI. Cardiometabolic risk – new chronic care models. *JPEN J Parenter Enteral Nutr* 2021; 45: S85–S92.

30. Havranek EP, Mujahid MS, Barr DA, et al. Social determinants of risk and outcomes for cardiovascular disease. *Circulation* 2015; 132: 873–898.

31. World Health Organization. Social determinants of health, 2021. https://www.who.int/health-topics/social-determinants-of-health#tab=tab_1.

32. Emeny RT, Carpenter DO, Lawrence DA. Health disparities: intracellular consequences of social determinants of health. *Toxicol Appl Pharmacol* 2021; 416: 115444, doi:10.1016/j.taap.2021.115444.

33. Andreacchi AT, Erbas Oz U, Bassim C, et al. Clustering of obesity-related characteristics: a latent class analysis from the Canadian Longitudinal Study on Aging. *Preventive Med* 2021; 153: 106739, doi:10.1016/j.ypmed.2021.106739.

34. Deyssenroth MA, Rosa MJ, Eliot MN, et al. Placental gene networks at the interface between maternal PM2.5 exposure early in gestation and reduced infant birthweight. *Environmental Res* 2021; 199: 111342, doi:10.1016/j.envres.2021.111342.

35. Cho SMJ, Lee H, Shim JS, et al. Association between social network structure and physical activity in middle-aged Korean adults. *Social Sci Med* 2021; 282: 114112, doi:10.1016/j.socscimed.2021.114112.

36. Gamble A, Beech BM, Blackshear C, et al. Changes in physical activity and television viewing from pre-pregnancy through postpartum among a socioeconomically disadvantaged perinatal adolescent population. *J Ped Adolescent Gynecol*, doi:10.1016/j.jpag.2021.06.009.

37. Liu M, Chen Q, Li Z, et al. Association between diet quality and cardiometabolic risk factor clustering stratified by socioeconomic status among Chinese children. *J Acad Nutr Dietet* 2021, doi:10.1016/j.jand.2021.03.009.

38. Gonzalez-Rivas JP, Mechanick JI, Ponte C, et al. Impact of the complex humanitarian crisis on the epidemiology of the cardiometabolic risk factors in Venezuela. *Clin Invest Arteriosclerosis* 2021, doi:10.1016/j.arteri.2021.04.002.

39. Trudel-Fitzgerald C, Chen Y, Singh A, et al. Psychiatric, psychological, and social determinants of health in the Nurse' Health Study Cohorts. *Am J Public Health* 2016; 106: 1644–1649.

40. Nobel L, Roblin DW, Becker ER, et al. Index of cardiometabolic health: a new method of measuring allostatic load using electronic health records. *Biomarkers* 2017; 22: 394–402.

41. Bu T, Popovic S, Huang H, et al. Relationship between national economic development and body mass index in Chinese children and adolescents aged 5–19 from 1986 to 2019. *Front Pediatr* 2021; 9: 671504.

42. Clausing ES, Non AL. Epigenetics as a mechanism of developmental embodiment of stress, resilience, and cardiometabolic risk across generations of Latinx immigrant families. *Front Psychiat* 2021; 12: 69827.

43. Jhun M, Mendelson M, Wilson R, et al. A multi-ethnic epigenome-wide association study of leukocyte DNA methylation and blood lipids. *Nat Commun* 2021; 12: 3987.

44. Releford BJ, Frencher SK, Yancey AK, et al. Cardiovascular disease control through barbershops: design of a nationwide outreach program. *J Natl Med Assoc* 2010; 102.

45. Drake C, Lian T, Trogdon JG, et al. Evaluating the association of social needs assessment data with cardiometabolic health status in a federally qualified community health center patient population. *BMC Cardiovasc Disord* 2021; 21: 342.

46. Mechanick JI, Marchetti AE, Apovian C, et al. Diabetes-specific nutrition algorithm: a transcultural program to optimize diabetes and prediabetes care. *Curr Diab Rep* 2021; 12: 180–194.

47. Mechanick JI, Harrell R, Allende-Vigo MZ, et al. Transculturalization recommendations for developing Latin American clinical practice algorithms in endocrinology – proceedings of the 2015 Pan-American Workshop by the American Association of Clinical Endocrinologists and American College of Endocrinology. *Endocr Pract* 2016; 22: 476–501.

48. Mechanick JI, Adams S, Davidson JA, et al. Transcultural diabetes care in the United States – a position statement by the American Association of Clinical Endocrinologists. *Endocr Pract* 2019; 25: 729–765.

49. Gonzalez-Rivas JP, Mechanick JI, Pantaleon Hernandez J, Infante-Garcia MM, Pavlovska L, Medina-Inojosa JR, Kunzova S, Nieto-Martinez R, Broz J, Busetto L, Maranhao Neto GA, Lopez-Jimenez F, Urbanova J, Stokin GB. Prevalence of adiposity-based chronic disease in middle-aged adults from Czech Republic. The Kardiovize Study. *Obes Sci Pract* 2021, doi:10.1002/osp4.496.

50. Gonzalez-Rivas JP, Mechanick JI, Infante-Garcia MM, Medina-Inojosa JR, Pavlovska L, Hinomaz O, Zak P, Kunzova S, Nieto-Martinez R, Skladana M, Broz J, Pantaleon Hernandez J, Lopez-Jimenez F, Stokin GB. Prevalence of dysglycemia-based chronic disease (DBCD) in European population: a new paradigm to address diabetes burden. The Kardiovize Study. *Endocr Pract* 2021, doi:10.1016/j.eprac.2020.10.003.

51. Maranhao Neto GA, Pavlovska I, Polcrova A, Mechanick JI, Infante-Garcia MM, Pantaleon J, Araujo MA, Nieto-Martinez R, Gonzalez-Rivas JP. Prediction of cardiorespiratory fitness in Czech adults: normative values and association with cardiometabolic health. *Int J Environ Res Public Health* 2021, 18, 10251, doi:10.3390/ijerph181910251.

52. Polcrova A, Pavlovska I, Marahao GA, Kunzova S, Infante-Garcia MM, Medina-Inojosa JR, Lopez-Jiminez F, Mechanick JI, Nieto-Martinez R, Stokin GB, Pikhart H, Gonzalez-Rivas JP. Visceral fat area and cardiometabolic risk: the Kardiovize Study. *Obes Res Clin Pract Mar* doi: 10.1016/j.orcp.2021.03.005.

53. Pavlovska I; Mechanick JI; Maranhao Neto GA; Infante-Garcia MM; Nieto-Martinez R; Kunzova S; Polcrova A; Vysoky R; Medina-Inojosa JR; Lopez-Jimenez F; Stokin GB; González-Rivas JP. Arterial stiffness and cardiometabolic-based chronic disease: the Kardiovize Study. *Endocr Pract* 2021:S1530–891X(21)00085-9, doi: 10.1016/j.eprac.2021.03.004.

54. González-Rivas JP, Mechanick JI, Iglesias-Fortes R, De-Oliveira-Gomes D, Silva J, Valencia J, Figueroa E, Duran M, Ugel E, Infante-Garcia MM, Marulanda MI, Nieto-Martinez R. Optimal waist circumference cutoff values to predict cardiometabolic alterations in a Venezuelan national representative sample. The EVESCAM study. *Arch Cardiol Mex* 2021; 91: 272–280.

55. Nieto-Martinez R, Gonzalez-Rivas JP, Ugel E, Duran M, Davila E, Constantino R, Garcia A, Mechanick JI, Ines Marulanda M. Cardiometabolic risk factors in Venezuela. The EVESCAM study: a national cross-sectional survey in adults. *Primary Care Diabetes* 2020, doi: 10.1016/j.pcd.2020.07.006.

56. Rabizadeh S, Rajab A, Mechanick JI, Moosaie F, Rahimi Y, Nakhjavani M, Esteghamati A. LDL/Apo B ratio predict coronary heart disease in Type 2 diabetes independent of aSCVD risk score: a case-cohort study. *Nutr Metab Cardiovasc Dis* 2021, doi:10.1016/j.numecd.2021.01.013.

57. Ukhanova M, Marino M, Angier H, et al. The impact of capitated payment on preventive care utilization in community health clinics. *Preventive Med* 2021; 145: 106405.

58. Petrovic D, de Mestral C, Bochud M, et al. The contribution of health behaviors to socioeconomic inequalities in health: a systematic review. *Preventive Med* 2018; 113: 15–31.

59. McQueen RB, Ghushchyan V, Olufade T, et al. Incremental increases in economic burden parallels cardiometabolic risk factors in the US. *Diabetes Metab Syndr Obes Targets Ther* 2016; 9: 233–241.

60. Gupta N, Sheng Z. Beyond weight: examining the association of obesity with cardiometabolic related inpatient costs among Canadian adults using linked population based survey and hospital administrative data. *BMC Health Serv Res* 2021; 21: 54.

61. Crutzen S, Baas G, Abou J, et al. Barriers and enablers of older patients to deprescribing of cardiometabolic medication: a focus group study. *Front Pharmacol* 2020; 11: 1268.

62. Luxon L. Infrastructure – the key to healthcare improvement. *Future Hosp J* 2015; 2: 4–7.

63. Padron NA. The role of physical infrastructure on health and well-being. In Mechanick JI, Kushner RF. *Creating a Lifestyle Medicine Center*, Springer, New York, 2020, pp. 47–56.

64. Huang Y, Pomeranz J, Wilde P, et al. Adoption and design of emerging dietary policies to improve cardiometabolic health in the US. *Curr Atheroscl Rep* 2018; 20: 25.

65. Liu J, Mozaffarian D, Sy S, et al. Health and economic impacts of the national menu calorie labeling law in the United States. *Circ Cardiovasc Qual Outcomes* 2020; 13: e006313.

66. Huang Y, Kypridemos C, Lee Y, et al. Cost-effectiveness of the US Food and Drug Administration added sugar labeling policy for improving diet and health. *Circulation* 2019; 139: 2613–2624.

67. Shangguan S, Mozaffarian D, Sy S, et al. Health impact and cost-effectiveness of achieving the national salt and sugar reduction initiative voluntary sugar reduction targets in the United States: a micro-simulation study. *Circulation*, doi:10.1161/CIRCULATIONAHA.121.053678.

68. Omura JD, Carlson SA, Brown DR, et al. Built environment approaches to increase physical activity. *Circulation* 2020; 142: e160–e166.

69. Le Gal C, Dale MJ, Cargo M, et al. Built environments and cardiometabolic morbidity and mortality in remote indigenous communities in the Northern Territory, Australia. *Int J Environ Res Public Health* 2020; 17: 769, doi:10.3390/ijerph17030769.

70. Tamura K, Curlin K, Neally SJ, et al. Geospatial analysis of neighborhood environmental stress in relation to biological markers of cardiovascular health and health behaviors in women: protocol for a pilot study. *JMIR Res Protoc* 2021; 10: e29191.

71. Coste J, Valderas JM, Carcaillon-Bentata, L. Estimating and characterizing the burden of multimorbidity in the community: a comprehensive multistep analysis of two large nationwide representative surveys in France. *PLoS Med* 2021; 18: e1003584.

72. Babagoli MA, Nieto-Martinez R, Gonzalez-Rivas JP, et al. Roles for community health workers in diabetes prevention and management in low- and middle-income countries. *Cad Saude Publica* 2021; 37: e00287120.

73. Byrd TF, Ahman FS, Liebovitz DM, et al. Defragmentating heart failure care – medical records integration. *Heart Failure Clin* 2020; 16: 467–477.

74. Perish E, Meltzer D, McDonald E. Models for caring for patients with complex lifestyle, medical, and social needs. In Mechanick JI, Kushner RF. *Creating a Lifestyle Medicine Center*, Springer, New York, 2020, pp. 37–46.

75. Jencks SF. Defragmenting care. *Ann Intern Med* 2010; 153: 757–758.

76. Shapiro S. Degragmenting the regulatory process. *Risk Analysis* 2011; 31: 893–901.

77. Mechanick JI. Methods of creative cognition in medical diagnosis. *Mt Sinai J Med* 1987; 54: 348–354.

78. Mechanick JI, Kushner RF. *Creating a Lifestyle Medicine Center*, Springer, New York, 2020.

79. Adsul P, Perez LG, Oh A, Chambers DA. Implementation science across lifestyle medicine interventions. In Mechanick JI, Kushner RF. *Creating a Lifestyle Medicine Center*, Springer, New York, 2020, pp. 29–36.

80. Eisman AB, Kilbourne AM, Dopp AR, et al. Economic evaluation in implementation science: making the business case for implementation strategies. *Psychiatric Res* 2020; 283: 112433.

81. Bhatt AS, Vaduganathan M, Butler J. Growing mismatch between evidence generation and implementation in heart failure. *Am J Med* 2020; 133: 525–527.

82. Ridde V, Perez D, Robert E. Using implementation science theories and frameworks in global health. *BMJ Global Health* 2020; 5: e002269.

83. Bhatt AS, Solomon SD, Vaduganathan M. Prioritizing dissemination and implementation science in cardiometabolic medicine. *JAMA* 2021; 326: 311–313.

84. Weber MB, Hassan S, Quarells R, et al. Prevention of type 2 diabetes. *Endocrinol Metab Clin N Am* 2021; 50: 387–400.

85. Patel MS, Volpp KG, Asch DA. Nudge units to improve the delivery of health care. *N Engl J Med* 2018; 378: 214–216.

86. Wensing M, Grol R. Knowledge translation in health: how implementation science could contribute more. *BMC Med* 2019; 17: 88.

87. Greenwood DA, Howell F, Scher L, et al. A framework for optimizing technology-enabled diabetes and cardiometabolic care and education. *Diab Educ* 2020; 46: 315–322.

88. Isaacs D, Cox C, Schwab K, et al. Technology integration: the role of the diabetes care and education specialist in practice. *Diabetes Educ* 2020; 46: 323–334.

89. Bouchard DR, Olthuis JV, Bouffard-Levasseur V, et al. Peer-led exercise program for ageing adults to improve physical functions – a randomized trial. *Eur Rev Aging Phys Act* 2021; 18: 2, doi:10.1186/s11556-021-00257-x.

90. Engineer A. Immersive physical environment: office interiors and preparedness. In Mechanick JI, Kushner RF. *Creating a Lifestyle Medicine Center*, Springer, New York, 2020, pp. 95–110.

91. Mechanick JI, Zhao S. Wearable technologies in lifestyle medicine. In Mechanick JI, Kushner RF. *Creating a Lifestyle Medicine Center*, Springer, New York, 2020, pp. 133–144.

92. Schorr EN, Gepner AD, Dolansky MA, et al. Harnessing mobile health technology for secondary cardiovascular disease prevention in older adults. *Circ Cardiovasc Qual Outcomes* 2021; 14: e000103.

93. Beratarrechea A, Diez-Canseco F, Irazola V, et al. Use of m-health technology for preventive interventions to tackle cardiometabolic conditions and other non-communicable diseases in Latin America – challenges and opportunities. *Prog Cardiovasc Dise* 2016; 58: 661–673.

94. Badenbroek IF, Mielen MM, Hollander M, et al. Feasibility and success rates of response enhancing strategies in a stepwise prevention program for cardiometabolic diseases in primary care. *BMC Family Pract* 2020; 21: 228.

95. Rykov Y, Thach T, Dunleavy G, et al. Activity tracker-based metrics as digital markers of cardiometabolic health in working adults: cross-sectional study. *JMIR Mhealth Uhealth* 2020; 8: e16409.

96. Stuber JM, Mackenbach JD, de Boer FE, et al. Reducing cardiometabolic risk in adults with a low socioeconomic position: protocol of the Supreme Nudge parallel cluster-randomised controlled supermarket trial. *Nutrition J* 2020; 19: 46.

97. Shaibi GQ, Coletta DK, Vital V, et al. The design and conduct of a community-based registry and biorepository: a focus on cardiometabolic health in Latinos. *Clin Trans Sci* 2013; 6: 429–434.

98. Malacarne M, Gobbi G, Pizzinelli P, et al. A point-to-point simple telehealth application for cardiovascular prevention: the ESINO LARIO experience. Cardiovascular prevention at point of care. *Telemed e-Health* 2009; 15: 80–86.

99. Horowitz LI, Kuznetsova M, Jones SA. Creating a learning health system through rapid-cycle, randomized testing. *N Engl J Med* 2019; 381: 1175–1179.

100. Saeed A, Dabhadkar K, Virani SS, et al. Cardiovascular disease prevention: training opportunities, the challenges, and future directions. *Curr Atheroscl Rep* 2018; 20: 35.

101. De Oliveira Correia E, Mechanick JI. Medical residency in Brazil in the era of chronic diseases: the need for cardiometabolic medicine residency. *Arq Bras Cardiol* 2022; 118: 655–658.

102. Johnson JH. Immersive non-physical environment: high-touch and human resources. In Mechanick JI, Kushner RF. *Creating a Lifestyle Medicine Center*, Springer, New York, 2020, pp. 111–118.

103. Sacoto F, Torres I, Lopez-Cevallos DF. Sustainability in chronic disease prevention: lessons from the Salud al Paso program in Ecuador. *Rev Panam Salud Publica* 2021; 45: 1–7.

104. Pozuelo-Carrascosa DP, Cavero-Redondo I, Herraiz-Adillo A, et al. School-based exercise programs and cardiometabolic risk factors: a meta-analysis. *Pediatrics* 2018; 142: e20181033.

105. Johnson JH, Al-Kazaz M, Mechanick JI. The Marie-Josée and Henry R. Kravis Center for Clinical Cardiovascular Health at Mount Sinai Heart. In Mechanick JI, Kushner RF. *Creating a Lifestyle Medicine Center*, Springer, New York, 2020, pp. 309–326.

106. Rippe JM. Rippe Lifestyle Institute: establishing the academic basis for lifestyle medicine. In Mechanick JI, Kushner RF. *Creating a Lifestyle Medicine Center*, Springer, New York, 2020, pp. 283–288.

107. Kushner RF, Herrington HR. Northwestern medicine center for lifestyle medicine. In Mechanick JI, Kushner RF. *Creating a Lifestyle Medicine Center*, Springer, New York, 2020, pp. 289–298.

108. Nieto-Martinez R, Gonzalez-Rivas JP, Mechanick JI. Survey of international centers that incorporate lifestyle medicine. In Mechanick JI, Kushner RF. *Creating a Lifestyle Medicine Center*, Springer, New York, 2020, pp. 345–254.

16 Synthesis and Core Recommendations for Using Lifestyle Medicine to Reduce Dysglycemia and Cardiometabolic Risk

Michael A. Via
Icahn School of Medicine at Mount Sinai

Jeffrey I. Mechanick
Kravis Center for Cardiovascular Health at Mount Sinai Heart
Icahn School of Medicine at Mount Sinai

CONTENTS

DOI: 10.1201/9781003206637-16

16.1 PART 1: PROBLEM – WHY IS STRUCTURED LIFESTYLE MEDICINE NEEDED IN THE DYSGLYCEMIA AND CARDIOMETABOLIC SPACES?

16.1.1 ASPECT 1: EPIDEMIOLOGY – LINKING DYSGLYCEMIA AND OTHER DETERMINANTS WITH CARDIOMETABOLIC RISK

The considerable burden of noncommunicable cardiometabolic disease in modern societies is among the greatest health challenges of our time. Insulin resistance, pre-diabetes, type 2 diabetes (T2D), and atherosclerotic cardiovascular disease (ASCVD; CVD) are highly prevalent. Both the development and progression of these cardiometabolic conditions depend significantly on lifestyle and societal factors. Prior to 1960, T2D, obesity, and other signs of insulin resistance were rare, with a prevalence of T2D of less than 1%, compared with a current T2D prevalence of 10.6% only 60 years later.[1] Additionally, the prevalence of metabolic syndrome (MetS) is currently 30%–35% in the U.S. population, depending on definition, and the prevalence of insulin resistance is 75%.[1] Among patients with T2D, 32% demonstrate clinically apparent ASCVD, while at least 75% have subclinical atherosclerosis, demonstrable through imaging studies.[2,3]

Behaviors and lifestyle choices are responsible for the vast majority of risk factors for dysglycemia- and transculturalized cardiometabolic-based chronic diseases (DBCD; tCMBCD).[4] While some risk factors are not modifiable, such as age, sex, and genetics, a comprehensive lifestyle intervention can significantly alter the course of insulin resistance and its pathophysiological consequences through effects on modifiable factors, such as abnormal adiposity, dysglycemia, hypertension, dyslipidemia, tobacco use, physical inactivity, and unhealthy eating, as well as other MetS traits (e.g., inflammation and thrombosis) and behaviors (alcohol consumption, poor sleep hygiene, and various social determinants of health).[4] In short, the information gleaned from a slew of statistical-based classifiers associating biological and social determinants with DBCD/tCMBCD risk supports the clinical emphasis on lifestyle medicine to optimize cardiometabolic health.

16.1.2 ASPECT 2: MECHANISMS – MAPPING LIFESTYLE INTERVENTIONS TO CARDIOMETABOLIC RISK REDUCTION

Examination of the daily practices employed by our distant ancestors provides insights as to what may constitute a healthy lifestyle for present-day humans. The hunter–gatherer lifestyle has been utilized by humans during most of the time since the emergence of *Homo sapiens*. Ancient members of our species carry mostly identical genomes, but very different gastrointestinal microflora and epigenomes, and they have substantially reduced cardiometabolic risk.[5,6] The many published examples of hunter–gatherer peoples that were suddenly exposed to westernized culture and then rapidly accrued a high prevalence of T2D[7–9] should amplify this important message: *daily lifestyle choices and exposures drastically affect insulin resistance and cardiometabolic health.*

In the modern world, an understanding of the arc of metabolic regulation and risks that occur at all life stages for an individual patient, including epigenetic phenomena affecting primordial processes, metabolic control during growth and development, energy homeostasis during adulthood, and the dysregulation that leads to prediabetes, T2D, and cardiometabolic disease can guide clinical practice in lifestyle medicine.

One of the most significant barriers to successful lifestyle change is the long time-frame required for implementation, monitoring, and adaptation. Messaging is also an issue as most patients will focus on immediate changes in certain surrogate markers (weight, body mass index [BMI], hemoglobin A1c [A1C], low-density lipoprotein cholesterol, blood pressure, etc.) rather than being "healthy." With respect to abnormal adiposity, which includes pathological ectopic fat, most clinical approaches exclusively focus on body weight, but sustained weight loss for most patients is extremely difficult. In the Swedish Obesity Study, enrolled patients opted for bariatric surgery or served as a control group that were essentially included in a long-term-monitored lifestyle intervention.[10] Though not directly measured in the study, patients who volunteered for trial inclusion were likely to be well-motivated and health-conscious by virtue of wanting to participate. However, in this control group, initial modest weight loss was followed by weight regain to baseline with continued weight gain over the ensuing 20 years.[10] However, the studies reviewed in this book portray a different angle: Weight loss is noted, but also reduction in associated morbidities, such as reduced rates of T2D, microvascular diabetic complications, and ASCVD, as well as other significant improvements in health consequences and even quality of life.[11–13]

Due to the modest weight loss that is commonly seen with lifestyle change, many professional medical organizations recommend setting achievable weight loss goals, recognizing real-world limitations and patient/physician frustrations that may develop.[14–17] In some individuals, significant weight loss is achieved, but the majority of patients show a modest improvement.

The multiple benefits of a lifestyle intervention cover many aspects of health beyond weight loss. Significant improvement in markers of well-being and depression was seen among patients with T2D that underwent a lifestyle intervention.[12] Cardiovascular risk was reduced among patients who successfully lost weight.[18] Additionally, increased physical fitness, quality of life, as well as reduced urinary incontinence, reduced sleep apnea, and even remission of T2D were noted in the lifestyle group.[18] Similar findings were even more pronounced within trials at earlier stages, such as the Diabetes Prevention Project, that showed a great reduction in T2D incidence among patients with prediabetes who followed a lifestyle intervention.[11]

One common thread among these large trials is the main interventional focus on diet and exercise. Undoubtedly, the aspects of dietary pattern and physical activity are important variables central to a healthy lifestyle. However, addressing other targets, such as sleep, environmental lighting, screen time, the chronobiology of food consumption, tobacco cessation and alcohol moderation, and stress management, can further improve outcomes. Still other potential targets include the avoidance of endocrine-disrupting chemicals (EDC), which is extremely challenging in the modern world. The ubiquity and diversity of EDCs makes some exposure unavoidable, but attempts to reduce exposures should be incorporated in a healthy lifestyle.

To sum up, the relationships among manifold risk factors conferred by primary drivers (genetics, environment, and behavior) of lifestyle with healthy versus unhealthy cardiometabolic phenotypes can be understood in terms of drivers, mechanisms, and networking effects.[19] Thus, in contrast to statistical-based classifiers informed by epidemiological studies, network-based classifiers informed by evolutionary studies, basic research, and clinical trials can be very useful for designing lifestyle medicine interventions to mitigate DBCD/tCMBCD development and progression.

16.1.3   Aspect 3: Wanting Preventative Care versus Doing Preventive Care

Current models of medical care often focus on disease management. By detecting patients earlier with predisease (or even pre-predisease as in DBCD/tCMBCD stage 1 "risk"), economic and clinical burdens can be remarkably lower.[14,20,21] Moreover, clinical inertia by healthcare professionals may be less when practice standards embrace early intervention, well before any disease metrics become evident.[14,20,21] A series of attainable lifestyle targets can generate a great impact on the lives of individual patients by delaying and preventing disease progression.[17] Unfortunately, the virtues of preventive care, as obvious as they may seem, and as clear as the supporting evidence may be, is not enough to close research gaps (questions without answers), knowledge gaps (answers without awareness), and practice gaps (awareness without action) in cardiometabolic lifestyle medicine. Pragmatically, the next steps to close these gaps, respectively, are as follows: (1) conduct relevant, well-designed studies; (2) facilitate engaging educational and training programs in lifestyle medicine with a focus on preventive care; and (3) create succinct, regularly updated evidence-based clinical practice guidelines and algorithms and leverage implementation science to bring excellence and uniformity to clinical practice, such as the creation of lifestyle medicine centers and clinical service lines that can scale up and out over time and engage with communities.

What are the specific hurdles to the implementation of lifestyle medicine in the dysglycemia/cardiometabolic space? One is a general poor understanding of the problem on the part of the patients, and oftentimes the healthcare professional. For instance, although obesity and diabetes are easily diagnosed, a scientific explanation with companion educational activities for complex connections to cardiovascular risk is generally elusive and supplanted with more simplified, linear rationales: Stress causes overeating causes obesity causes heart disease; or genetics causes insulin resistance causes diabetes causes atherosclerosis. These simplified lines of reasoning fail to account for recalcitrance to therapies and rising rates of obesity, T2D, and other cardiometabolic conditions.[22] In fact, it is the complexity of interactions between biological and social determinants of health in the framework of driver-based chronic disease models (e.g., DBCD/tCMBCD) that expose multiple lifestyle medicine targets.[22] Again, this shortcoming can be addressed by closing research, knowledge, and practice gaps.

Another hurdle pertains to difficulties with lifestyle medicine research, especially at early stages of disease. Clinical trials would require a large base of enrollees, and long-term follow-up, presenting a formidable challenge.[23] Pragmatic solutions (e.g., measurements with low cost and high benefit; Bayesian designs) can move the science and practice of lifestyle medicine forward.[23]

16.2   PART 2: PREMISE – CORRECT MODELING OF CHRONIC DISEASE LEADS TO TACTICAL ADVANTAGES

16.2.1   Aspect 1: The 3-Dimensional Cardiometabolic-Based Chronic Disease Model

The process of developing the three-dimensional tCMBCD model as an umbrella device to guide early and sustainable preventive care is given below:[14,20,24–26]

- development of new framework for obesity management as a complications-centric (not BMI-centric) adiposity-based chronic disease (ABCD) incorporating not only abnormally high adiposity amount, but also abnormal adiposity distribution (especially with ectopic fat) and function (i.e., the adipocyte secretome);
- development of new framework for T2D management, which considers prediabetes not in isolation but rather as part of a spectrum from insulin resistance to prediabetes, to T2D, to vascular complications;
- interpretation of a two-dimensional CMBCD model consisting of staged progression over time (risk to predisease to disease to complications) and multiple metabolic drivers (ABCD, DBCD, and other MetS traits) with CVD phenotypes (focusing on atherosclerosis, heart failure, and atrial fibrillation);
- incorporation of a third dimension for each 2×2 (stage $\times$ driver) cell consistent of individual social determinants of health and transcultural factors; and
- further development of hypertension- and dyslipidemia based chronic disease as additional metabolic drivers for tCMBCD.

The tCMBCD model offers several key advantages: (1) unique configuration of how biological/metabolic and social determinants of health interact in generating CVD; (2) exposing early stages as statistically and mechanistically relevant opportunities for intervention that can mitigate development or progression of this chronic disease; and (3) codifying this preventive paradigm in terms of primordial (prevention of stage 1 "risk" and stages 1–2 "predisease"), primary (prevention of stages 2–3 "disease"), secondary (prevention of stages 3–4 "complications), and tertiary (prevention of suffering and mortality in stage 4).[5,6] In early stages (1 and 2), an intensive lifestyle alone may be sufficient. In later stages (3 and 4), changes in lifestyle add significant benefit to optimal pharmacological and procedural therapies.[17] Despite the management of specific metabolic drivers, patients with DBCD/tCMBCD may still exhibit increased risk for CVD.[27] This "residual risk" supports the role of lifestyle change, which has broad, robust networking effects.[25,26] Central to this model are healthcare professionals who are prepared for leadership, care coordination, follow-up reevaluation, education, and clinical testing.[14,17,28] Application of the tCMBCD model encourages the design of innovative education systems, new health policies and legislation, health-conscious built environments, reformed reimbursement systems, better messaging and health literacy, and enhanced community engagement.[14,17,29]

16.2.2 Aspect 2: The Patient as an Agent of Change

Central to chronic care models, strategic goals, and the initial tactical step is patient activation for change. All of the potential interventions suggested by the tCMBCD model involve patient actions.[29] At initial and follow-up encounters, each patient should be assessed for readiness to change and for their conviction. Action plans should be individualized to the patient, with patient autonomy prioritized in any suggested change. Early achievements that are more easily reached can serve as a foundation with confidence to reach more substantial change. In this manner, stepwise implementation and refinement can lead to significant transformation over time. Any actions taken should be praised, and if possible, obstacles should be anticipated. For the success of a lifestyle intervention, maintenance over the long term is paramount.[17] Setbacks to progression commonly occur. For example, orthopedic injuries, or conditions such as osteoarthritis can curtail

physical activity. Holidays or vacations can trigger dietary regression. Continued reinforcement can be helpful with re-evaluation and revision at each subsequent visit.[29]

16.2.3   Aspect 3: The Specialized Field of Lifestyle Medicine

Lifestyle medicine is revealed as a necessary intervention by the tCMBCD model,
the various inferred preventive modalities, and the critical role for motivational interviewing and behavioral change. The term "Lifestyle Medicine" was first coined by the
1999 premier textbook in the field, edited by Dr. James Rippe,[30] with the American
College of Lifestyle Medicine serving as a strong voice advocating for recognition and
implementation of this burgeoning field. Other professional medical organizations,
such as the National Academy of Medicine,[31] the World Health Organization,[32] the
American College of Physicians,[33] The American Academy of Pediatrics,[34] American
Association of Clinical Endocrinologists,[24] the Endocrine Society,[35] the European
Society of Endocrinology,[36] the American College of Cardiology,[16] the American
Heart Association,[16] and the American Diabetes Association,[37] recognize the paramount role for lifestyle modification in the management of chronic diseases, especially those in the dysglycemic and cardiometabolic spaces. In 2013, the American
Medical Association defined obesity as a disease,[38] highlighting the importance of
clinicians, as well as various socioeconomic and health policy platforms to advance
care for patient with this dominant cardiometabolic driver. *The Exercise is Medicine*
program developed by the American College of Sports Medicine places exercise as
a crucial daily activity for clinicians, with a recommendation that daily time spent in
physical activity be included as a vital sign for each patient encounter.[39] Additionally,
clinicians are encouraged to explicitly write for exercise as a prescription.

Despite these initiatives and the subsequent evidence-based guidelines that
emerged, the amount of time dedicated to actually addressing aspects of lifestyle
medicine within medical education and training is vanishingly small. A survey of
physicians showed 22% of respondents reported no formal education in nutrition
during medical school.[40] In cases where education is provided, time dedicated is
minimal, perhaps a single lecture or even only part of a single lecture, with almost no
time dedicated to physical activity or other lifestyle targets.[40] In post-graduate training, 70% of medical residents report receiving minimal to no nutritional training.

Specific nutrition fellowship training programs exist in the United States and elsewhere; however, these are small in number and outside the oversight of the American
College of Graduate Medical Education (ACGME). Moreover, board certification
in nutrition or lifestyle medicine is not available through the American Board of
Medical Specialties (ABMS). Current certification programs such as those offered
through the American College of Lifestyle Medicine, the Obesity Society, or the
National Board of Physician Nutrition Specialists hold much less weight in comparison with certifications provided through the ABMS.[41,42] As with residency, specialty
training programs in related fields such as in cardiology, endocrinology, and sleep
medicine often have minimal exposure and little formalized teaching of lifestyle
medicine or nutrition.[28] In a national survey of endocrine fellowship program direc-
tors, approximately half of the responding programs offer no education in nutrition.[28]
This is despite nutrition training being an ACGME requirement for an endocrine
fellowship. Additionally, about one-third of endocrine programs that do report
their educational curricula had 5 hours or less of nutritional education over a 2-year

fellowship.[28] It comes as no surprise that in a poll of patients, only 26% report they receive adequate nutritional guidance after visits to their physician.[40] Furthermore, other aspects of lifestyle medicine (behavioral medicine, exercise physiology, sleep hygiene, etc.) also commonly fall by the wayside.[17]

The lack of lifestyle medicine education is symptomatic of a systems failure in healthcare that also gives lifestyle medicine practice and research short shrift. Increased time in direct patient care that emphasizes lifestyle medicine, as well as formal educational sessions in lifestyle medicine during medical training, can diminish knowledge and practice gaps.[28] Systemic improvements, including reimbursement models that promote disease prevention, policies that support a healthy built environment, and empowered and motivated patients that lead to better outcomes, all work together to drive the practice of lifestyle medicine.

16.3 PART 3: EVIDENCE – LIFESTYLE MEDICINE AS AN EVOLVING SCIENCE

Lifestyle medicine practice and education are informed by evidence, and this process needs to be fluid with a trajectory impelled by high-quality research. This results in a growing body of knowledge that leads to novel approaches to healthy lifestyle change. For example, a recent review suggests clear benefit of coffee consumption to reduce cardiometabolic risk.[43] This is based on many observational and cohort studies, and on a limited trial that used mendelian randomization. However, considering this level of evidence, should one advise a patient who currently does not drink coffee to commence this practice? At least we can be reassured that coffee consumption does not appear harmful, and the consistent epidemiological findings are highly suggestive of benefit. But unfortunately, the standard needed for recommendation, that is, multiple randomized controlled trials (RCT), do not exist for coffee consumption.

Scientific study in the field of lifestyle medicine is difficult. For many aspects of lifestyle, conducting an RCT to gauge the effects of behavior change over a lifetime may be impractical or outright impossible due to time or blinding limitations (for example, a patient cannot be blinded to coffee consumption, tobacco use, or exercise).[23] Outside of RCTs, observational trials with strong methodology, diverse strategies, and consistent findings may serve as suitable surrogates, especially in cases in which mechanisms of action are well understood.[23] Continued accumulation of observational data, combined with RCT studies where possible, provide the basis for further development in lifestyle medicine.

16.4 SYNTHESIS AND CORE RECOMMENDATIONS

To put all this information together, three broad steps are conducted. In step 1, the process of translating content in this book into core recommendations as take-home messages begins with a synoptic account of key points and recommendations for each chapter (Table 16.1). In step 2, commonalities, affirmed concepts, and emergent concepts are then discerned (Table 16.2). Finally, in step 3, a core set of recommendations is formulated with a specific action plan to facilitate tactical implementation that can be adapted to specific healthcare scenarios (Table 16.3). It is hoped that readers of this book will be further inspired to use this array of action plans as a starting point for their own customized initiative to launch a successful lifestyle medicine practice in the dysglycemia and cardiometabolic spaces.

TABLE 16.1
Summary of Chapter Key Points and Preliminary Recommendations

Chapter 1: Epidemiology and Public Health Challenges of Cardiometabolic-Based Chronic Disease	• Noncommunicable disease affecting insulin resistance and adiposity, especially ectopic fat, is highly common. The approximate prevalence of insulin resistance is 75% and metabolic syndrome is 35%.[1,44] • Predisease imposes considerable risk and is underappreciated in the current healthcare system. Diabetic retinopathy, nephropathy, and neuropathy are each present in 4%–5% of patients with prediabetes. A 20% increase in risk for cardiovascular disease and a 10-fold increase in heart failure are observed in patients with prediabetes.[45,46] • Pragmatic and effective approaches to patients at early chronic disease stages is centered on lifestyle medicine, while patients with complications at later stages still benefit from adjustments to lifestyle choices.[14,17,20]
Recommendation 1	Hypervigilance should be exercised in case finding for dysglycemic and cardiometabolic drivers of chronic disease. Suspicion should be raised among patients with conditions that are associated with insulin resistance, or in patients with family history of T2D or cardiometabolic disease. Sufficient encounter time and structure dedicated to lifestyle evaluation and treatment is necessary.
Chapter 2: Evolutionary Biology of Cardiometabolic-Based Chronic Disease	• *Homo sapiens* first appeared approximately 200,000 years ago with metabolic physiology are adapted to a hunter–gatherer lifestyle. However, evidence from the fossil record suggests that CVD existed among humans even in these pristine conditions.[47] • Studies of present-day hunter–gatherer tribes show essentially no dysglycemia, but similar metabolic rates and calorie consumption to people who follow modern lifestyles.[48] • Among the primary drivers, inherited genetic variability may explain only a small fraction of cardiometabolic disease in current populations, whereas epigenetic phenomena exert a significant influence, and behavioral/environmental factors exert the greatest influence on cardiometabolic risk.[4] • The prevalence of T2D in the United States has increased approximately 10-fold since the 1960s, when the diagnosis of this condition was first possible.[49]
Recommendation 2	Opportunities should be intensively sought out for effective prevention of dysglycemia and CVD since seemingly "normal" modern lifestyles are actually novel for our species and may be maladaptive for human physiology.
Chapter 3: Mechanisms of Cardiometabolic-Based Chronic Disease	• Cardiac metabolism is affected by systemic inflammation, insulin resistance, and local dysfunctional/ectopic adipose tissue, including peri-/epi-cardial fat and intracardiomyocyte lipid accumulation.[20,21,25] • Cardiac energy sources change under conditions, such as insulin resistance, favoring lipid oxidation, and reduced efficiency, associated with cardiometabolic risk.[50] • Lipotoxicity and glucotoxicity impair cardiomyocyte function.[51] • High risk for HF is observed in patients with insulin resistance.[52]

(Continued)

TABLE 16.1 (*Continued*)
Summary of Chapter Key Points and Preliminary Recommendations

Recommendation 3	Preventive strategies should be based on the diverse mechanisms that drive cardiac dysfunction/disease in patients with DBCD and tCMBCD.
Chapter 4: Endocrine Disruptors	• Over 1,000 industrial chemicals interfere with biological homeostasis in humans; many are associated with increased cardiometabolic risk.[53]
	• Knowledge in this field relies on animal models and epidemiological studies.
	• Minimizing exposure to EDC may be beneficial; however, full avoidance of EDC is unrealistic given the ubiquity of these substances.[53]
	• Government policies and societal directives are among the strongest platforms to reduce EDC risk.[54]
Recommendation 4	For patients, identifying EDC exposures must be part of the routine history. For populations, minimizing EDC exposure must be a societal priority.
Chapter 5: Primordial Prevention of Cardiometabolic-Based Chronic Disease	• Primordial prevention is mitigating the development of risk and predisease.
	• Cardiometabolic disease risk begins *in utero* and accumulates in childhood.[55]
	• Learned health behaviors during childhood can influence subsequent lifestyle choices and eventually chronic disease risks in adulthood.[55]
	• Education, reinforcement, structured activities, and community engagement at early ages can mitigate cardiometabolic risk factors.[56]
Recommendation 5	Formal health education and active encouragement of healthy lifestyle choices should be applied in women who are pregnant, infants, children, and adolescents; this is an emerging requirement for population health, especially for CVD.
Chapter 6: Primary Prevention of Type 2 Diabetes in the Context of Cardiometabolic Risk	• Primary prevention is mitigating the progression of predisease to disease. Patients with prediabetes are identified by impaired glucose tolerance, impaired fasting glucose, and/or A1C levels of 5.7%–6.4% and exhibit high risk for T2D development as well as cardiometabolic disease.[11] Patients with one or more cardiometabolic drivers are at increased risk for CVD.
	• Long-term randomized trials that implement a lifestyle intervention of regular physical activity and dietary modification show reduction and delay of T2D development, as well as reduced risk for CVD.[11]
Recommendation 6	Once dysglycemic/cardiometabolic risk factors or predisease are detected, evidence-based primary prevention strategies and tactics should be implemented to prevent T2D/CVD.
Chapter 7: Secondary Prevention Example: Using Lifestyle Medicine in Patients with Type 2 Diabetes	• Secondary prevention is mitigating the progression of early, asymptomatic disease to later, symptomatic disease, often with complications.
	• A successful lifestyle intervention among patients who developed T2D demonstrates reduced cardiometabolic risk, renal impairments, diabetic neuropathy, erectile dysfunction, depression, obstructive sleep apnea, hepatosteatosis, and urinary incontinence, as well as improvements in hypertension and the lipid profile.[57]

(Continued)

TABLE 16.1 (*Continued*)
Summary of Chapter Key Points and Preliminary Recommendations

Recommendation 7	Once a patient has T2D/CVD, evidence-based secondary prevention strategies and tactics should be implemented to prevent disease progression with/without complications (e.g., adopting a healthy dietary patterns such as a Mediterranean diet; moderate-to-intense physical activity such as 30–45 minutes daily for 5 days per week; cardiac rehabilitation; dedicated sufficient time for sleep; and stress-reduction protocols).
Chapter 8: Tertiary Prevention using Lifestyle Medicine for Cardiometabolic-Based Chronic Disease	• Tertiary prevention is mitigating the adverse effects of complications; this primarily involves medications and procedures but should also include healthy lifestyle changes. • Specifically, after the development of complications including atherosclerosis, heart failure, atrial fibrillation, end-stage renal disease, neuropathy, and retinopathy, lifestyle modifications still provide benefits to patients by improvement in daily function, disease burden, and quality of life.[58–60]
Recommendation 8	Even with T2D/CVD complications, healthy lifestyle changes must be implemented since they can improve clinical outcomes (e.g., healthy dietary patterns, physical activity as tolerated, behavioral therapy, and improved sleep hygiene).
Chapter 9: The Mediterranean Diet	• Cultures and available foods from the Mediterranean region determine dietary patterns that are high in fruits, vegetables, legumes/pulses, whole grains, nuts, olives and olive oil, poultry and fish, and in some cases, wine.[61] • Significant reduction in the incidence of T2D/CVD and their complications is demonstrated in observational studies and large randomized clinical trials involving patients at all stages of DBCD and tCMBCD.[13]
Recommendation 9	A Mediterranean diet should be discussed with patients with DBCD/tCMBCD and implemented if possible to mitigate DBCD/CMBCD risks, development, and progression.
Chapter 10: The Vegan Diet	• Ingestion of animal proteins and fats is associated with development of T2D, while lower rates of T2D are observed among patients following vegetarian and vegan lifestyles.[62] • Patients with T2D adherent to a plant-based diet require less glucose lowering medication and demonstrate improvement in glycemia.[62] • Hypertension and hyperlipidemia are also improved with a plant-based diet.[62]
Recommendation 10	Plant-based diets should be discussed with patients with DBCD/tCMBCD and implemented if possible to improve dysglycemia and cardiometabolic health.
Chapter 11: Physical Activity	• Physical activity is beneficial for glucose and lipid metabolism, cardiac, adipose, and endothelial function, hypothalamic regulation of energy metabolism, systemic inflammation, and sleep quality.[63] • Staying physically active mitigates DBCD and tCMBCD development and progression through multiple mechanisms.[63,64]

(Continued)

TABLE 16.1 (*Continued*)
Summary of Chapter Key Points and Preliminary Recommendations

Recommendation 11	All patients should be physically active as tolerated, with a reasonable target of 30–45 minutes of moderate- to high-intensity physical activity for 5 days per week.
Chapter 12: Behavioral Modification	• Psychological stress and the resulting allostatic load can exacerbate insulin resistance, abnormal adiposity, and other cardiometabolic risks through increased cortisol secretion, increased catecholamine release, autonomic dysfunction/sympathetic activation, and systemic inflammation.[65] • Patients with high levels of stress demonstrate an odds ratio of 5.7 for abdominal obesity, 6.2 for hypertension, 7.9 for T2D, and 4.3 for atherosclerotic cardiometabolic disease.[66]
Recommendation 12	Behavioral therapies, often with pharmacotherapy, should be initiated in patients with DBCD/tCMBCD in conjunction with multidisciplinary, comprehensive lifestyle change when there is significant psychological stress or refractoriness to preventive care.
Chapter 13: Sleep Hygiene	• Sleep quality and quantity can affect insulin resistance and cardiometabolic risk through several mechanisms, including influence on circadian rhythms, systemic inflammation, hormonal regulation of metabolism, and pancreatic β-cell function.[67] • Other factors affecting circadian rhythms contribute to insulin resistance and cardiometabolic risk, including timing of dietary intake, day and night light exposures, shift work, and timing of sleep.[68] • Obstructive sleep apnea is highly prevalent among patients with prediabetes, T2D, and CVD.[69]
Recommendation 13	At least 7 hours of sleep should be targeted each night, along with diminished nocturnal light intensity, minimized nocturnal screen exposure, bright light exposure in daytime hours, minimal to no late night snacking or meals, and case finding and treatment for obstructive sleep apnea.
Chapter 14: Transculturalizing Lifestyle Medicine for Managing Cardiometabolic-Based Chronic Disease	• Ethnocultural factors greatly influence patient risks for DBCD/tCMBCD development and progression, affecting beliefs, practices, and behaviors.[70] • All lifestyle recommendations must take into account ethnocultural factors to optimize care and clinical outcomes.[70]
Recommendation 14	Cultural sensitivity and understanding should be addressed in all patients when implementing lifestyle medicine recommendations.
Chapter 15: Socioeconomics and Infrastructure	• Social determinants of health are nonbiological factors that impact a patient's health. In the modern world, these factors contribute significantly to abnormal adiposity, insulin resistance, and cardiometabolic risk.[71] • Social determinants of health, such as highest level of education, housing, income level, employment status, available green space, and food insecurity correlate with lifestyle choices such as tobacco use, alcohol moderation, physical activity, and healthy dietary patterns.[72] • Lifestyle medicine centers and clinical service lines can optimize DBCD/tCMBCD preventive care plan infrastructure.

(*Continued*)

TABLE 16.1 (*Continued*)
Summary of Chapter Key Points and Preliminary Recommendations

Recommendation 15	An inventory of social determinants of health should be conducted as part of the history in all patients. Preventive care plans should incorporate relevant social determinants of health. Optimal infrastructure for lifestyle medicine should be engineered to reduce population-based DMBCD/tCMBCD risks.

Abbreviations: A1C, hemoglobin A1c; tCMBCD, transculturalized cardiometabolic-based chronic disease; CVD, cardiovascular disease; DBCD, dysglycemia-based chronic disease; EDC, endocrine disrupting compounds; HF, heart failure; T2D, type 2 diabetes.

TABLE 16.2
Commonalities, Affirmed Concepts, and Emergent Concepts in Lifestyle Medicine to Reduce Dysglycemia and Cardiometabolic Risk[a]

Commonalities	Affirmed Concepts	Emergent Concepts
Chronic disease mechanisms	Multi-morbid chronic care models are useful	DBCD/tCMBCD as driver-based chronic disease models
Central role for insulin resistance	Mechanistic relationships with MetS traits	ABCD, DBCD, tCMBCD intersect at insulin resistance
Evidence-based preventive care	Epidemiological and clinical trial data support lifestyle medicine and preventive care in DBCD/tCMBCD management	Validation studies needed for DBCD/tCMBCD models
Case finding for intervention	Prevalence rates are growing and associated with increased burden (QALY, DALY, etc.)	Prevalence rates are higher than expected for ABCD/DBCD/CMBCD based on obesity, T2D, and CVD studies
Lifestyle medicine implementation	Components of healthy lifestyles are necessary parts of DBCD/tCMBCD preventive care	DBCD/tCMBCD modeling exposes specific opportunities for lifestyle change based on networked biological, social, and transcultural factors
Population-based action	Cardiometabolic health can be optimized at population level through policy and infrastructural change	The creation of lifestyle medicine centers and clinical service lines can optimize implementation of DBCD/tCMBCD preventive care

Abbreviations: ABCD, adiposity-based chronic disease; DALY, disability-adjusted life year; DBCD, dysglycemia-based chronic disease; tCMBCD, transculturalized cardiometabolic-based chronic disease; CVD, cardiovascular disease; MetS, metabolic syndrome; QALY, quality-adjusted life year.

[a] Commonalities are recurrent discussion points among chapters, representing areas of emphasis by different authors. Affirmed concepts are statements in one or more chapters that are based on commonalities and consistent with current beliefs and practice standards. Emergent concepts are statements in one or more chapters that are based on commonalities but are novel, need to be validated, and can potentially be used to enhance and improve current practice standards.

TABLE 16.3
Four Core Recommendations and Action Plans for Lifestyle Medicine to Reduce Dysglycemia and Cardiometabolic Risks[a]

Core Recommendation	Action Plan
1. To implement aggressive case finding for insulin resistance in any patient at risk for DBCD/tCMBCD	Until validated commercially available classifiers are available for routine insulin resistance testing, patients should be evaluated for primary drivers: (1) genetics (i.e., family history; markers when available), (2) environment (unhealthy built environments; high prevalence rates of cardiometabolic risk factors), and (3) behavior (unhealthy; high stress)
2. To conduct well-designed epidemiological and clinical trial studies on the effects of various lifestyle interventions on DBCD/tCMBCD stage progression	Identify research gaps, develop a research platform, and incorporate the following in a lifestyle medicine infrastructure: (1) funding strategy; (2) integrated clinical registry; and (3) dedicated research team with a data scientist
3. To routinely discuss healthy lifestyles in all patients with DBCD/tCMBCD and then initialize a lifestyle medicine preventive care plan	Develop policies and protocols for lifestyle medicine and incorporate in the routine operations of lifestyle medicine centers and clinical service lines
4. To reduce dysglycemia and cardiometabolic risk at a population level	Create policy through interactions with government, beginning on a small scale (e.g., municipalities) and then once successful, to increase scale (e.g., state then national). To create lifestyle medicine centers and clinical service lines with strong community engagement.

Abbreviations: DBCD, dysglycemia-based chronic disease; tCMBCD, transculturalized cardiometabolic-based chronic disease.

[a] Core recommendations represent a distillation of relevant affirmed and emergent concepts that are also actionable.

Disclosures:
Jeffrey I. Mechanick received honoraria from Abbott Nutrition for lectures and serves on the Advisory Boards for Aveta.Life and Twin Health.

REFERENCES

1. Tamayo T, Schipf S, Meisinger C, et al. Regional differences of undiagnosed type 2 diabetes and prediabetes prevalence are not explained by known risk factors. *PLoS One* 2014; **9**(11): e113154.
2. Gast KB, Tjeerdema N, Stijnen T, Smit JW, Dekkers OM. Insulin resistance and risk of incident cardiovascular events in adults without diabetes: meta-analysis. *PLoS One* 2012; **7**(12): e52036.
3. Lei MH, Wu YL, Chung SL, Chen CC, Chen WC, Hsu YC. Coronary artery calcium score predicts long-term cardiovascular outcomes in asymptomatic patients with type 2 diabetes. *J Atheroscler Thromb* 2021; **28**(10): 1052–62.

4. Locke AE, Kahali B, Berndt SI, et al. Genetic studies of body mass index yield new insights for obesity biology. *Nature* 2015; **518**(7538): 197–206.

5. Adler CJ, Dobney K, Weyrich LS, et al. Sequencing ancient calcified dental plaque shows changes in oral microbiota with dietary shifts of the neolithic and industrial revolutions. *Nat Genet* 2013; **45**(4): 450–5.

6. Crujeiras AB, Diaz-Lagares A, Moreno-Navarrete JM, et al. Genome-wide DNA methylation pattern in visceral adipose tissue differentiates insulin-resistant from insulin-sensitive obese subjects. *Transl Res* 2016; **178**: 13–24.

7. Bennett PH, Burch TA, Miller M. Diabetes mellitus in American (Pima) Indians. *Lancet* 1971; **2**(7716): 125–8.

8. O'Dea K. Marked improvement in carbohydrate and lipid metabolism in diabetic Australian aborigines after temporary reversion to traditional lifestyle. *Diabetes* 1984; **33**(6): 596–603.

9. Zimmet P, Taft P, Guinea A, Guthrie W, Thoma K. The high prevalence of diabetes mellitus on a Central Pacific Island. *Diabetologia* 1977; **13**(2): 111–5.

10. Carlsson LMS, Sjoholm K, Jacobson P, et al. Life expectancy after bariatric surgery in the Swedish obese subjects study. *n engl j med* 2020; **383**(16): 1535–43.

11. Diabetes Prevention Program (DPP) Research Group. The diabetes prevention program (DPP): description of lifestyle intervention. *Diabetes Care* 2002; **25**(12): 2165–71.

12. Rubin RR, Wadden TA, Bahnson JL, et al. Impact of intensive lifestyle intervention on depression and health-related quality of life in type 2 diabetes: the Look AHEAD Trial. *Diabetes Care* 2014; **37**(6): 1544–53.

13. Estruch R, Ros E, Salas-Salvado J, et al. Primary prevention of cardiovascular disease with a mediterranean diet supplemented with extra-virgin olive oil or nuts. *N Engl J Med* 2018; **378**(25): e34.

14. Mechanick JI, Garber AJ, Grunberger G, Handelsman Y, Garvey WT. Dysglycemia-based chronic disease: an American Association of Clinical Endocrinologists Position Statement. *Endocr Pract* 2018; **24**(11): 995–1011.

15. Apovian CM, Aronne LJ, Bessesen DH, et al. Pharmacological management of obesity: an endocrine society clinical practice guideline. *J Clin Endocrinol Metab* 2015; **100**(2): 342–62.

16. Jensen MD, Ryan DH, Apovian CM, et al. 2013 AHA/ACC/TOS guideline for the management of overweight and obesity in adults: a report of the American College of Cardiology/American Heart Association task force on practice guidelines and the obesity society. *Circulation* 2014; **129**(25 Suppl 2): S102–38.

17. Rippe JM. Lifestyle medicine: the health promoting power of daily habits and practices. *Am J Lifestyle Med* 2018; **12**(6): 499–512.

18. Steinberg H, Jacovino C, Kitabchi AE. Look inside Look AHEAD: why the glass is more than half-full. *Curr Diab Rep* 2014; **14**(7): 500.

19. Mechanick JI, Zhao S, Garvey WT. The Adipokine-Cardiovascular-Lifestyle Network: translation to clinical practice. *J Am Coll Cardiol* 2016; **68**(16): 1785–803.

20. Mechanick JI, Farkouh ME, Newman JD, Garvey WT. Cardiometabolic-based chronic disease, adiposity and dysglycemia drivers: JACC state-of-the-art review. *J Am Coll Cardiol* 2020; **75**(5): 525–38.

21. Mechanick JI, Hurley DL, Garvey WT. Adiposity-based chronic disease as a new diagnostic term: the American Association of Clinical Endocrinologists and American College of Endocrinology position statement. *Endocr Pract* 2017; **23**(3): 372–8.

22. Mozaffarian D. Perspective: Obesity-an unexplained epidemic. *Am J Clin Nutr* 2022; **115**(6): 1445–50.

23. Katz DL, Karlsen MC, Chung M, et al. Hierarchies of evidence applied to lifestyle Medicine (HEALM): introduction of a strength-of-evidence approach based on a methodological systematic review. *BMC Med Res Methodol* 2019; **19**(1): 178.

24. Garvey WT, Mechanick JI, Brett EM, et al. American Association of Clinical Endocrinologists and American College of Endocrinology comprehensive clinical practice guidelines for medical care of patients with obesity. *Endocr Pract* 2016; **22**(7): 1–203. Available at https://www.aace.com/publications/guidelines.
25. Mechanick JI, Farkouh ME, Newman JD, Garvey WT. Cardiometabolic-based chronic disease, addressing knowledge and clinical practice gaps: JACC state-of-the-art review. *J Am Coll Cardiol* 2020; **75**(5): 539–55.
26. de Oliveira Correia ET, Mechanick JI, Dos Santos Barbetta LM, Jorge AJL, Mesquita ET. Cardiometabolic-based chronic disease: adiposity and dysglycemia drivers of heart failure. *Heart Fail Rev* 2022.
27. Gimeno Orna JA, Ortez Toro JJ, Peteiro Miranda CM. Evaluation and management of residual cardiovascular risk in patients with diabetes. *Endocrinol Diabetes Nutr* 2020; **67**(4): 279–88.
28. Bassin SR, Kohm K, Fitzgerald N, Cohen DA. An assessment of nutrition education in endocrinology fellowship programs in the United States. *Endocr Pract* 2021; **28**(3): 310–14.
29. Koenigsberg MR, Corliss J. Diabetes Self-management: facilitating lifestyle change. *Am Fam Physician* 2017; **96**(6): 362–70.
30. Rippe JM. *Lifestyle Medicine*. London, England: Blackwell Science; 1999.
31. Kumanyika S. *Getting to Equity in Obesity Prevention: A New Framework. NAM Perspectives.* Discussion Paper. National Academy of Medicine; 2017.
32. Chaput JP, Willumsen J, Bull F, et al. 2020 WHO guidelines on physical activity and sedentary behaviour for children and adolescents aged 5–17 years: summary of the evidence. *Int J Behav Nutr Phys Act* 2020; **17**(1): 141.
33. Snow V, Barry P, Fitterman N, Qaseem A, Weiss K, Clinical Efficacy Assessment Subcommittee of the American College of P. Pharmacologic and surgical management of obesity in primary care: a clinical practice guideline from the American College of Physicians. *Ann Intern Med* 2005; **142**(7): 525–31.
34. Daniels SR, Hassink SG, Committee on Nutrition. The role of the pediatrician in primary prevention of obesity. *Pediatrics* 2015; **136**(1): e275–92.
35. Bray GA, Heisel WE, Afshin A, et al. The science of obesity management: an endocrine society scientific statement. *Endocr Rev* 2018; **39**(2): 79–132.
36. Pasquali R, Casanueva F, Haluzik M, et al. European Society of Endocrinology clinical practice guideline: endocrine work-up in obesity. *Eur J Endocrinol* 2020; **182**(1): G1–G32.
37. Davies MJ, D'Alessio DA, Fradkin J, et al. Management of hyperglycemia in type 2 diabetes, 2018. A consensus report by the American Diabetes Association (ADA) and the European Association for the Study of Diabetes (EASD). *Diabetes Care* 2018; **41**(12): 2669–701.
38. Kyle TK, Dhurandhar EJ, Allison DB. Regarding obesity as a disease: evolving policies and their implications. *Endocrinol Metab Clin North Am* 2016; **45**(3): 511–20.
39. Garber CE, Blissmer B, Deschenes MR, et al. American College of Sports Medicine position stand. Quantity and quality of exercise for developing and maintaining cardiorespiratory, musculoskeletal, and neuromotor fitness in apparently healthy adults: guidance for prescribing exercise. *Med Sci Sports Exerc* 2011; **43**(7): 1334–59.
40. Aggarwal M, Devries S, Freeman AM, et al. The deficit of nutrition education of physicians. *Am J Med* 2018; **131**(4): 339–45.
41. Lipner RS, Hess BJ, Phillips RL, Jr. Specialty board certification in the United States: issues and evidence. *J Contin Educ Health Prof* 2013; **33**(Suppl 1): S20–35.
42. Apovian CM, Shah MS, Ruth MR, et al. Board certification and credentialing in nutrition. *JPEN J Parenter Enteral Nutr* 2010; **34**(6 Suppl): 78S–85S.

43. van Dam RM, Hu FB, Willett WC. Coffee, caffeine, and health. *N Engl J Med* 2020; **383**(4): 369–78.

44. Fowler JR, Tucker LA, Bailey BW, LeCheminant JD. Physical activity and insulin resistance in 6,500 NHANES adults: the role of abdominal obesity. *J Obes* 2020; **2020**: 3848256.

45. Beulens J, Rutters F, Ryden L, et al. Risk and management of pre-diabetes. *Eur J Prev Cardiol* 2019; **26**(2_suppl): 47–54.

46. Pandey A, Vaduganathan M, Patel KV, et al. Biomarker-based risk prediction of incident heart failure in pre-diabetes and diabetes. *JACC Heart Fail* 2021; **9**(3): 215–23.

47. Andrews P, Johnson RJ. Evolutionary basis for the human diet: consequences for human health. *J Intern Med* 2020; **287**(3): 226–37.

48. Pontzer H, Raichlen DA, Wood BM, et al. Energy expenditure and activity among Hadza hunter-gatherers. *Am J Hum Biol* 2015; **27**(5): 628–37.

49. Diabetes Data and Statistics. CDC. http://www.cdc.gov/diabetes/statistics/. Accessed January 17, 2023.

50. Wall SR, Lopaschuk GD. Glucose oxidation rates in fatty acid-perfused isolated working hearts from diabetic rats. *Biochim Biophys Acta* 1989; **1006**(1): 97–103.

51. Peterson LR, Herrero P, Schechtman KB, et al. Effect of obesity and insulin resistance on myocardial substrate metabolism and efficiency in young women. *Circulation* 2004; **109**(18): 2191–6.

52. Lai L, Leone TC, Keller MP, et al. Energy metabolic reprogramming in the hypertrophied and early stage failing heart: a multisystems approach. *Circ Heart Fail* 2014; **7**(6): 1022–31.

53. Guo W, Pan B, Sakkiah S, et al. Persistent organic pollutants in food: contamination sources, health effects and detection methods. *Int J Environ Res Public Health* 2019; **16**(22): 4361.

54. Takagi K. Study on the biodegradation of persistent organic pollutants (POPs). *J Pestic Sci* 2020; **45**(2): 119–23.

55. Virani SS, Alonso A, Aparicio HJ, et al. Heart disease and stroke statistics-2021 update: a report from the American Heart Association. *Circulation* 2021; **143**(8): e254–e743.

56. Santos-Beneit G, Fernandez-Jimenez R, de Cos-Gandoy A, et al. Lessons learned from 10 years of preschool intervention for health promotion: JACC state-of-the-art review. *J Am Coll Cardiol* 2022; **79**(3): 283–98.

57. Garvey WT. Long-term health benefits of intensive lifestyle intervention in the Look AHEAD study. *Obesity (Silver Spring)* 2021; **29**(8): 1242–3.

58. Arnett DK, Blumenthal RS, Albert MA, et al. 2019 ACC/AHA guideline on the primary prevention of cardiovascular disease: a report of the American College of Cardiology/American Heart Association task force on clinical practice guidelines. *Circulation* 2019; **140**(11): e596–e646.

59. Morseth B, Lochen ML, Ariansen I, Myrstad M, Thelle DS. The ambiguity of physical activity, exercise and atrial fibrillation. *Eur J Prev Cardiol* 2018; **25**(6): 624–36.

60. Zilliox LA, Russell JW. Physical activity and dietary interventions in diabetic neuropathy: a systematic review. *Clin Auton Res* 2019; **29**(4): 443–55.

61. Davis C, Bryan J, Hodgson J, Murphy K. Definition of the Mediterranean diet; a literature review. *Nutrients* 2015; **7**(11): 9139–53.

62. Barnard RJ, Jung T, Inkeles SB. Diet and exercise in the treatment of NIDDM. The need for early emphasis. *Diabetes Care* 1994; **17**(12): 1469–72.

63. Stanford KI, Goodyear LJ. Exercise and type 2 diabetes: molecular mechanisms regulating glucose uptake in skeletal muscle. *Adv Physiol Educ* 2014; **38**(4): 308–14.

64. Schuttler D, Clauss S, Weckbach LT, Brunner S. Molecular mechanisms of cardiac remodeling and regeneration in physical exercise. *Cells* 2019; **8**(10): 1128.

65. Hackett RA, Steptoe A. Type 2 diabetes mellitus and psychological stress - a modifiable risk factor. *Nat Rev Endocrinol* 2017; **13**(9): 547–60.

66. Carlsson AC, Nixon Andreasson A, Wandell PE. Poor self-rated health is not associated with a high total allostatic load in type 2 diabetic patients--but high blood pressure is. *Diabetes Metab* 2011; **37**(5): 446–51.

67. Touma C, Pannain S. Does lack of sleep cause diabetes? *Cleve Clin J Med* 2011; **78**(8): 549–58.

68. Wright KP, Jr., McHill AW, Birks BR, Griffin BR, Rusterholz T, Chinoy ED. Entrainment of the human circadian clock to the natural light-dark cycle. *Curr Biol* 2013; **23**(16): 1554–8.

69. Foster GD, Sanders MH, Millman R, et al. Obstructive sleep apnea among obese patients with type 2 diabetes. *Diabetes Care* 2009; **32**(6): 1017–9.

70. Mechanick JI, Marchetti AE, Apovian C, et al. Diabetes-specific nutrition algorithm: a transcultural program to optimize diabetes and prediabetes care. *Curr Diab Rep* 2012; **12**(2): 180–94.

71. Havranek EP, Mujahid MS, Barr DA, et al. Social determinants of risk and outcomes for cardiovascular disease: a scientific statement from the American Heart Association. *Circulation* 2015; **132**(9): 873–98.

72. Kivimaki M, Batty GD, Pentti J, et al. Modifications to residential neighbourhood characteristics and risk of 79 common health conditions: a prospective cohort study. *Lancet Public Health* 2021; **6**(6): e396–e407.

Index

Note: **Bold** page numbers refer to tables and *italic* page numbers refer to figures.

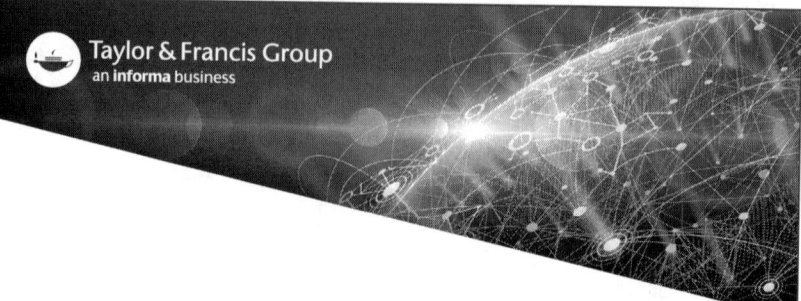
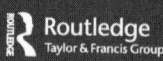
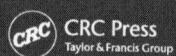